Maternal and Child Health in India

This book examines the process of information diffusion and the challenges of spreading awareness about maternal and child health (MCH) outcomes in India, with a special focus on Bihar – a state in eastern India.

Investing in the health of women and children results in significant and long-lasting economic and social benefits to society. Analysing the National Family Health Survey data, the volume explores the role that access to information has on the adoption of MCH practices. It also explores regional variations – between Empowered Action Group (EAG) states and non-EAG states and also across EAG states – in the impact of information networks. Using appropriate econometric methods, the authors study the role of peer effects and grass-roots health workers in bringing about a change in attitude within communities. The book looks at the process of information dissemination between the grass-roots health workers and the target women and brings to the forefront the intricacies of patriarchal family dynamics that hinder women from accessing basic maternal and child healthcare needs. Based on grass-roots experiences, the book provides sharp insights from the field for the benefit of researchers, policymakers, and activists.

Rich in empirical data, this book will be of interest to academics and researchers of development economics, public health policy and practice, community health, healthcare administration and management, primary healthcare and family practice, and health and social care.

Mousumi Dutta is Professor in the Economics Department at Presidency University, Kolkata, West Bengal, India.

Saswata Ghosh is Associate Professor at the Institute of Development Studies Kolkata, Kolkata, West Bengal, India.

Zakir Husain teaches in the Economics Department at Presidency University, Kolkata, West Bengal, India.

Maternal and Child Health in India

Networks and Information Diffusion

Mousumi Dutta, Saswata Ghosh and
Zakir Husain

Routledge
Taylor & Francis Group
LONDON AND NEW YORK

First published 2025
by Routledge
4 Park Square, Milton Park, Abingdon, Oxon OX14 4RN

and by Routledge
605 Third Avenue, New York, NY 10158

Routledge is an imprint of the Taylor & Francis Group, an informa business

British Library Cataloguing-in-Publication Data
A catalogue record for this book is available from the British Library

Library of Congress Cataloging-in-Publication Data
Names: Dutta, Mousumi, author. | Ghosh, Saswata, author. |
Husain, Zakir, author.
Title: Maternal and child health in India: networks and information diffusion / Mousumi Dutta, Saswata Ghosh, and Zakir Husain.
Description: Abingdon, Oxon; New York, NY: Routledge, 2024. |
Includes bibliographical references and index.
Identifiers: LCCN 2024006882 (print) | LCCN 2024006883 (ebook) |
ISBN 9781032514741 (hardback) | ISBN 9781032813264 (paperback) |
ISBN 9781003499251 (ebook)
Subjects: MESH: Maternal Health | Child Health | Maternal-Child Health Services | Health Services Accessibility | Information Dissemination | Community Networks | India
Classification: LCC RG965.I4 (print) | LCC RG965.I4 (ebook) |
NLM WQ 105 | DDC 362.198200954–dc23/eng/20240405
LC record available at https://lccn.loc.gov/2024006882
LC ebook record available at https://lccn.loc.gov/2024006883

ISBN: 978-1-032-51474-1 (hbk)
ISBN: 978-1-032-81326-4 (pbk)
ISBN: 978-1-003-49925-1 (ebk)

DOI: 10.4324/9781003499251

Typeset in Sabon
by Deanta Global Publishing Services, Chennai, India

Contents

Figures

Tables

Acknowledgements

The study was funded by a research grant (Grant No. 18013) from the International Growth Center, UK. We are grateful to the staff at both the UK office and their Indian counterparts. The COVID-19 pandemic posed considerable problems to the study, calling for great flexibility. The IGC staff cheerfully accommodated all our requests, enabling its smooth completion. In particular, we would like to express our gratitude to Mr. Kumar Das and Ms. Ani Bhagtiani for their support and encouragement during the execution of the project.

Among others, we would like to thank Prof. Anjan Mukherji, Professor Emeritus at Jawaharlal Nehru University, and a member of the Departmental Research Advisory Committee of the Economics Department, Presidency University. His encouragement motivated us to apply to IGC for funding. Dr. Diganta Mukherjee, Sampling and Official Statistics Unit, Indian Statistical Institute, Kolkata commented on our methodology; his suggestions have improved our report significantly.

The survey was facilitated by JEEViKA. We are grateful to the Chief Executive Officer cum State Mission Director, Sri Balamurugan D, IAS, for granting us permission to undertake the survey. The advice and suggestions received from Mr. Apollonerius Purty, State Program Manager – Health & Nutrition Strategy, and Dr. Ritesh Kumar, Program Manager (IB) were invaluable.

We would not have been able to complete the study without the assistance provided by the Research Assistants – Ms. Debamita Guha and Ms. Jhinuk Banerjee. They worked hard and sincerely throughout their tenure and steadily supplied us with inputs that we had demanded at short notice. The survey was undertaken by Ms. Madhulika Mitra, Mr. Prabir Ghosh, the late Mr. Pankaj Kumar, Mr. Asit Kumar, Ms. Archita Dey, Mr. Megnath Mondol, Mr. Pranab Mazumdar, and Mr. Madhusudan Das. We thank them for their hard work and sincere efforts. In particular, we would like to single out the support and assistance extended by Mr. Pankaj Kumar. Whenever we required any information about the survey or districts studied, he always responded to our queries. The study would not have been completed without him. He was responsible for the excellent quality of data collected. We deeply regret his untimely passing away during the COVID-19 pandemic. We are also grateful to respondents who shared their personal information and experience with us.

We would like to acknowledge the comments and suggestions received from the two anonymous reviewers of the study and from the participants of the IGC and IUSSP conferences where we presented our findings.

Finally, we are grateful to the Hon'ble Vice Chancellor, Prof. Anuradha Lohia, for her encouragement. Prof. Sankar Basu and Prof. Joydeep Mukhopadhyay, the then Deans of Mathematics and Natural Sciences, helped us in various ways. The administration – particularly, Dr. Debajyoti Konar (Registrar), Ms. Pritha Ghosh (Assistant Registrar) – facilitated the survey and enabled its smooth execution. We would also like to thank our Departmental colleagues and staff – particularly Prof. Indrajit Ray (Cardiff University), the then Infosys Chair Professor of Economics at Presidency University – for their support and encouragement.

Mousumi Dutta
Zakir Husain
Saswata Ghosh
January 28, 2021

Chapter 1

Maternal and child health outcomes in India

Where do we stand?

1.1 Introduction

The notion of health as a driver of economic growth was first emphasised by Mushkin (1962) and Grossman (1972). This idea was taken up by the neo-classical growth theorists (Barro, 1998; Fogel, 2004; Mankiw et al., 1992) who extended the Solow model by adding health as a form of human capital. Simultaneously, empirical studies by Strauss and Thomas (1998), Schultz (1999), Bloom et al. (2004), and others provided evidence on the impact of health on growth.

Health and nutrition have a close synergy with other sectors of the economy as well. For example, investing in basic nutrition during pregnancy and infancy has a substantially positive effect on early childhood development, which, in turn, significantly contributes to educational attainment (D. Bloom et al., 2003; Jamison, 2006). Countries experiencing a demographic transition also enjoy a demographic dividend (Bloom et al., 2003), with a bulge in the labour force relative to overall population size. This means less dependency, more savings, and faster economic growth (Jamison, 2006; The World Bank, 2006). Foreign companies often avoid investment in countries with a high burden of disease because of concerns about their own workers' health, the possibility of high turnover and absenteeism, and the potential loss of workers with "institutional knowledge" of the firm (Haacker, 2004). Once such fears are allayed through sustained progress in health and nutrition policy, there will be a considerable improvement in the investment climate and inflow of foreign direct investment. There is substantial empirical evidence in support of investing in women, children, and adolescents (Every Woman Every Child, 2016, p. 16). Such investment facilitates desirable adult outcomes like height, schooling, income or assets, offspring birthweight, body mass index, glucose concentrations, and blood pressure (Victora et al., 2008).

DOI: 10.4324/9781003499251-1

1.2 Progress towards sustainable development goals: A global picture

Although the post-1970 decades had witnessed a substantial improvement in the status of health and nutrition, persistent challenges had remained – particularly concerning the status of maternal and child health. For instance, almost 11 million children die every year (Every Woman Every Child, 2016), mainly from preventable causes such as diarrhoea and malaria (Mathers et al., 2006). Globally, one child or young adolescent died every five seconds in 2018 (UN Inter-agency Group for Child Mortality Estimation, 2019). Most of the deaths occurred in the first year of birth – mortality rates were 18 per 1000 live births for children below one month, and 11 for children between 1 and 12 months (UN Inter-agency Group for Child Mortality Estimation, 2019). About 28% of such deaths occurred in Central and South Asia, making this region – along with sub-Saharan Africa – a hotspot (UN Inter-agency Group for Child Mortality Estimation, 2019). Studies reveal that malnutrition is the major cause of high childhood mortality (Horton, 2008). A study using data from 2005 reports that 20% of children are underweight and 32% are stunted (Black et al., 2008). In India, undernutrition accounts for 68% of the total under-5 deaths, and it is the leading risk factor for health loss for all ages; it is responsible for 17% of the total disability-adjusted life years (India State-Level Disease Burden Initiative Malnutrition Collaborators & Collaborators, 2019).

The situation was equally concerning with respect to maternal health. In South and Central Asian countries, more than 10% of women aged 15–49 years were shorter than 145 cm; about one out of every five women suffered from undernutrition,[1] while this proportion was about 40% in India (Black et al., 2008). Undernutrition during pregnancy had adverse consequences on pregnancy outcomes, increasing chances of complicated pregnancies, restricted intrauterine growth, and maternal mortality (Black et al., 2008). The latter has unfavourable consequences bearing on child health. Statistics revealed that more than 0.30 million women died during pregnancy and childbirth in 2017, of which 12% occurred in India (WHO, 2017).

Thus, "Maternal and child undernutrition remain pervasive and damaging conditions in low-income and middle-income countries" (Black et al., 2008, p. 5). Consequently, both the millennium development goals (MDGs) and sustainable development goals (SDGs) emphasises the importance of improving maternal and child health (MCH) outcomes – both for their intrinsic worth, and also their long-run socio-economic benefits. While the fifth MDG was to "Improve maternal health" (UNDP, 2015), the third SDG was to "Ensure healthy lives and promote well-being for all at all ages" (UNDP, 2015).

The adoption of the sustainable development goals in 2016, in particular, introduced a new era for the global health and development community (McArthur et al., 2018). The preceding millennium development goals (MDGs) had set targets to reduce the mortality rate for children under 5 years by two-thirds and the maternal mortality ratio by three-quarters between 1990 and 2015, with special focus on the poorest countries. A study estimates that child mortality and maternal mortality ratio were reduced by an estimated 55% and 44%, respectively, while countries classified as "least developed" by the United Nations experienced a 60% decline in child mortality and 52% decline in maternal mortality (UN Inter-agency Group for Child Mortality Estimation, 2017). It saved 10.1 million and as many as 19.4 million additional children's and mothers' lives compared with pre-MDG trajectories (McArthur et al., 2018), with substantial improvements occurring in sub-Saharan Africa (McArthur et al., 2018).

In the last decade substantial progress has been made with regard to the improvement of MCH and attainment of SDG targets (Gordillo-Tobar et al., 2017; Raina et al., 2023). A World Bank study reports that maternal mortality decreased by 44% over the past 25 years with an annual rate of reduction of 2.4%; however, to reach the SDG target 3.1, maternal mortality rate (MMR) must decrease by 7.5% annually (Gordillo-Tobar et al., 2017). The study also observes that, despite significant progress in reducing the under-five mortality rate (U5MR), neonatal mortality rate (NMR) reduction has been slow. Consequently, while the gains made so far needs to be substantiated,

> further actions are required by the region and the countries to address the challenges of widespread inequities, suboptimal quality of care in maternal, newborn and child health, emerging priorities like still births, birth defects, early childhood development, and preparedness against emergencies like the current pandemic and climate change.
>
> (Raina et al., 2023, p. 11)

A recent study, analysing the composite coverage index (CCI) estimated for 70 low and middle-income countries (LMICs) using Bayesian hierarchical models, also reports that there has been considerable progress globally with respect to the improvement of maternal and child health (Rahman et al., 2023). However, the study also observes that further efforts are needed in LMICs. Only 18 such countries are projected to reach the 80% CCI target by 2030. The CCI is projected to increase in Asian countries (in southern Asia from 51.8% in 2000 to 89.2% in 2030; in southeastern Asia from 58.8% to 84.4%; in central Asia from 70.3% to 87.0%; in eastern Asia from 76.8% to 82.1%; and in western Asia from 56.5% to 72.1%), Africa (in sub-Saharan Africa from 46.3% in 2000 to 72.2% in 2030 and in northern Africa from 55.0% to 81.7%), and Latin America and the Caribbean (from 67.0% in 2000 to 83.4% in 2030). Across LMICs, considerable horizontal inequities in coverage are observed. For instance, CCIs are relatively higher in urban areas, among affluent groups and among more educated women (Rahman et al., 2023).

1.3 From MDG to SDG: Performance of India and Bihar

The global performance in attaining MDGs with respect to MCH outcomes had, however, been poor. India belonged to the group of 88 countries that were seriously off-target with respect to meeting MDGs. According to United Nations Development Programme (UNDP), India had attained the targets for reducing poverty by half, accomplished gender parity in primary school enrolment, and made barely successful progress in providing clean drinking water. However, India fell short of achieving the targets for reducing hunger, primary school completion, and access to sanitation facilities (Ministry of Statistics & Programme Implementation, 2006). The progress with respect to improving MCH outcomes has been poor to moderate:

> The fourth Millennium Development Goal aims to reduce mortality among children under five by two-thirds. India's Under Five Mortality (U5MR) declined from 125 per 1,000 live births in 1990 to 49 per 1,000 live births in 2013. The MDG target is 42 per 1000, which suggests that India is moderately on track, largely due to the sharp decline in recent years. ... From a Maternal Mortality Rate (MMR) of 556 per 100,000 live births in 1990–91, India is required to reduce MMR to 139 per 100,000 live births by 2015. Between 1990 and 2006, there has been some improvement in the Maternal Mortality Rate (MMR), which has declined to 167 per 100,000 live births in 2009. However, despite this, India's progress on this goal has been slow and off track.
>
> (Government of India, 2005)

On the whole, one could argue that India had more or less accomplished the targets in the field of basic universal education, gender equality in education, and global economic growth, but failed to make any significant progress in the improvement of health indicators related to mortality, morbidity, and various environmental factors, which contributed to the poor health status of the population (Nath, 2011).

After the failure to attain all MDGs, significant shifts in health strategies were adopted in recent times. Emphasis was given on water and sanitation through the *Swachh Bharat* Mission to reduce the spread of communicable diseases; a National Food Security Act was enacted and a well-targeted National Nutrition Mission (or *Poshan Abhiyan*) was introduced to combat the menace of undernutrition; eVIN (electronic vaccine intelligence network) was introduced to track and improve immunization coverage; ANMOL (Auxiliary Nurse Midwives or ANM online) was implemented to extend better maternal and newborn care services. Despite these efforts, inequities in availability, accessibility, and utilisation of MCH services persisted across states and among vulnerable sections of the society (Awasthi et al., 2016; Balarajan et al., 2011; Gandhi et al., 2022; Panda & Mohanty, 2019). According to the State Health Index Report of 2019, India had to go a long way in improving the affordability and cost of healthcare, lack of health awareness, and reducing the gap between better-performing and poor-performing states (Niti Ayog, The World Bank, and Ministry of Health & Family Welfare, 2019).[2] Considerable regional variations in attaining MCH-related targets were reported, with states like Bihar, Uttar Pradesh, Assam, and others lagging behind. Bihar was a prime example of states lagging behind with respect to other states (Ali & Chauhan, 2020; Dasgupta et al., 2021; Hiwale & Chandra Das, 2022).

The state of Bihar – located in the eastern part of India and a resource-constrained state – has a long history related to poor health indicators, including utilisation of MCH services. At the onset of the National Rural Health Mission (NRHM; subsequently expanded to cover urban areas and renamed as National Health Mission) in 2005, Bihar was listed as one of the High Focus states, and special attention was paid to improving health indicators. Although early breastfeeding practices, institutional delivery, and utilisation of ICDS services have increased substantially during the last two decades, malnutrition continued to be the largest risk factor instigating an increased number of deaths and disability (Indian Council of Medical Research et al., 2017). The study also reports that iron-deficiency anaemia caused the most years lived with disability for both sexes during 2016. The latest round of the National Family Health Survey (International Institute of Population Studies, 2017) also reports that 11.0% of women aged 15–19 years were pregnant and had given birth to a child at the time of the survey (India: 6.8%); moreover, 63.1% of pregnant women were suffering from anaemia (India: 52.2%). The percentage of women receiving antenatal care (ANC) was very poor – only 25.2% (India: 58.1%) of pregnant women received at least four check-ups. Institutional delivery took place for 76.2% cases (India: 88.6%). Even among the urban educated and affluent section, maternal health indicators are substantially lower than that of similar socio-economic groups in other states.

A World Bank study reported that, in Bihar, nutritional outcomes were a major challenge before policymakers:

> 48.3% of children aged under 5 years in the state are stunted (low height-for-age), 43.9% are underweight (low weight-for-age) and 20.8% are wasted (low weight-for-height). Poor infant and young child feeding practices, among other determinants, are key contributors to these poor nutritional outcomes. Only 53.5% children under 6 months of age are exclusively breastfed, 30.7% children aged 6–8 months receive solid or semi-solid food and breastmilk and a negligible 7.3% children aged 6–23 months receive a minimum acceptable diet, which includes breastmilk, minimum meal frequency and diet diversity.
>
> (The World Bank, 2016, p. 1)

It has also been observed that neonatal mortality was relatively high in Bihar, and the utilisation of maternal care was very low and inequitable (Kumar et al., 2014). Another study, based on population-based data, reported a significant burden of stillbirths in Bihar, suggesting that addressing these must become an important part of maternal and child health initiatives (Kochar et al., 2014). The study also reported high induced abortion in the more developed districts and an inverse relationship between induced abortion and neonatal mortality rates. These findings have programmatic implications. A major reason underlying the poor state of maternal and child health in Bihar was the inadequate quality of ANC services (Dandona et al., 2022). Improving maternal health outcomes in accordance with the SDG is, therefore, a major challenge before policymakers in Bihar.

1.4 Improving MCH outcomes

1.4.1 National Rural Health Mission

The NRHM was launched on 12th April 2005 throughout India to carry out the necessary architectural corrections in the basic healthcare delivery system. While NRHM covers the entire country, it focuses on states with weak public health indicators and/or weak health infrastructure. Bihar is one such state. The mission seeks to provide effective healthcare to the rural population, and has the following objectives:

- Reduction in child and maternal mortality.
- Universal access to public healthcare services for food and nutrition, sanitation, and hygiene with emphasis on services addressing women's and children's health and universal immunization.
- Prevention and control of communicable and non-communicable diseases, including locally endemic diseases.
- Access to integrated comprehensive primary health care.
- Population stabilisation, gender, and demographic balance.
- Revitalise local health traditions and mainstream AYUSH.
- Promotion of healthy lifestyles.

In 2015, the NRHM was extended to include urban areas under its purview, and renamed as National Health Mission (NHM).

To attain the above objectives, the NRHM emphasised on grass-roots level interventions like creating the capacity of Panchayati Raj Institutions to own, control, and manage public health services; promoting access to improved healthcare at the household level through female Accredited Social Health Activists (ASHA),[3] private–public partnerships, etc.

In Bihar, the State Programme Implementation Plans (PIP) prepared to implement the NRHM focused on reducing maternal, infant, and neonatal mortality, and controlling fertility rates (State Health Society, 2011). This was to be attained through a significant upscaling of availability, accessibility, and utilisation of MCH services. Simultaneously, special schemes such as

Muskaan, MAMTA – addressing child health, providing incentives to health staff – were introduced.

1.4.2 Impact of NRHM in Bihar

Such attempts have had limited success. A recent study on Bihar has reported a significant improvement in the MCH indicators after the inception of the NRHM in 2005 (Ghosh & Husain, 2019).

However, as may be seen from Figures 1.1 and 1.2, Bihar still lags behind the all-India average, particularly if we consider the proportion of women availing any ANC services (). The continuum of maternal care[4] is also poor (Husain et al., 2022):

> The State has achieved some progress in terms of output indicators, however the maternal mortality, child mortality and population growth continue to be a cause of serious concern to the state's development efforts. In terms of key health indicators, Bihar is among the low performing states. Though the state fares reasonably well in terms of its Infant Mortality Rate (56) as against the national average (53) and NMR (42.1) as against national average of 45, it continues to be among the poorer performing states in terms of TFR and MMR.
>
> (State Health Society, 2011, p. 34)

Overall, the situation in Bihar, vis-à-vis the all-India picture, may be seen in Table 1.1.

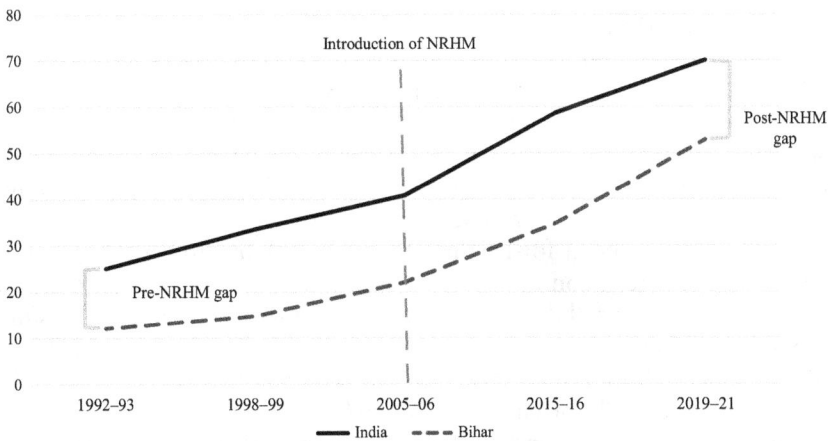

Figure 1.1 Institutional delivery in India and Bihar: A snapshot.
Source: Fact sheets of NFHS.

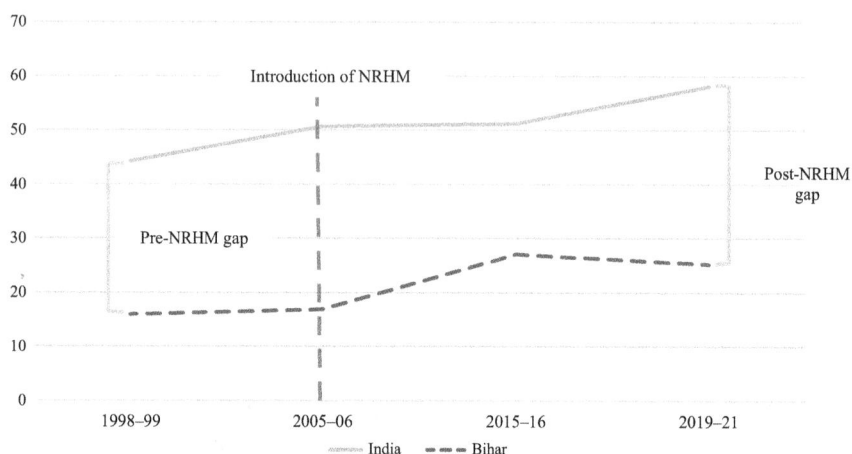

Figure 1.2 Percentage of pregnant women availing any ANC service in India and Bihar: A comparative picture.

Source: Fact sheets of NFHS.

The utilisation of maternal healthcare services is restricted to specific socio-economic groups. For instance, women belonging to rural, non-literate, poor, SC/ST, and non-Hindu households are less likely to opt for institutional delivery; older women, and those belonging to minority communities and socially marginalised sections, are also less likely to deliver in private facilities (Ghosh & Husain, 2019). Therefore, ensuring horizontal equity and a continuum of care, particularly in rural areas, remain major challenges before the policymakers.

Child health outcomes are also not satisfactory in Bihar (Ghosh & Husain, 2019; International Institute of Population Sciences, 2015). The state has the highest rates of undernutrition in the country (International Institute for Population Sciences and ICF & International Institute for Population Sciences, 2021). About 48% of children aged under five years are stunted (low height-for-age), 44% are underweight (low weight-for-age), and 21% are wasted (low weight-for-height) (International Institute of Population Sciences, 2015). Key contributors to these poor nutritional outcomes are poor infant and young child feeding practices (Ghosh & Husain, 2019). Only 53.5% of children under age 6 months are exclusively breastfed, 30.7% of children aged 6–8 months receive solid or semi-solid food and breastmilk, and a negligible 7.3% of children aged 6–23 months receive an adequate diet (minimum meal frequency and four or more food groups) (International Institute of Population Sciences, 2015).

Table 1.1 Demographic and health scenario in Bihar vis-à-vis all-India

Demographic and health indicators	Bihar 1992–93	Bihar 2015–16	Bihar 2019–21	All-India 1992–93	All-India 2015–16	All-India 2019–21
Sex ratio (females/1000 male)	956	1062	1090	944	991	1020
Child sex ratio (0–6 years)	944	934	908	946[2]	919	929
Percentage of 6+ population that is Literate	**44.6**	**66.9**	**NA**	**56.3**	**75.7**	**NA**
Percentage of 6+ female population that is literate	28.6	49.6	NA	43.3	68.4	71.5
Infant mortality rate	89.2	48	46.8	78.5	40.7	35.2
Child mortality rate	127.5	58.0	56.4	109.3	49.7	41.9
Total fertility rate	4.0	3.4	3.0	3.4	2.2	2.0
Percentage of mothers with at least three ANC check-ups	30.7	27.0	25.2[5]	43.8[3]	51.2	58.1[5]
Percent of deliveries attended by skilled attendants	19.0	70.0	79.0	34.2	81.4	89.4
Percent of institutional deliveries	12.1	63.8	76.2	25.5	78.9	88.6
Children exclusiveley breastfed (0–5 months)	51.6	34.9	58.9[4]	51.0[1]	54.9	63.7
Children receiving adequate diet (6–23 months)	NA	7.5	10.8	NA	9.6	11.3
Head count ratio	61	34	NA	45.3	21.9	NA
Singulate mean age at marriage	18[6]	19.5	NA	20.0	20.8	NA

Sources:
IIPS (2022), IIPS (2020), IIPS (2016), IIPS (1993), IIPS (2021), IIPS (2016),, IIPS (1993)
Notes:
1. For children aged 0–12 months.
2. For children aged 0–4 years of age.
3. From NFHS 2 (1998–99).
4. For children aged 0–6 months.
5. Mothers who had at least four ANC visits.
6. Singulate mean age at marriage for 1992–93 pertains to women aged 13–49, while for 2015–16, it pertains to women aged 15–49 years.

Analysis of these outcomes over time (Table 1.2) reveals substantial progress between 2005–06 and 2019–21 in both India and Bihar. However, the progress has been less satisfying at the all-India level with respect to the usage of modern contraceptive methods, availing ANC services and complementary feeding. In Bihar, the MCH outcomes have been lower than that of the all-India figures. It holds for all the indicators studied. The gap between the all-India and Bihar outcomes is marked by the utilisation of ANC and PNC services.

Further, India has experienced worsening inequities and widening disparities between the rich and the poor, across social groups, and between geographic regions (Bango & Ghosh, 2022; Målqvist et al., 2011; Uthman et al., 2012). Progress on this front has been uneven and inequitable, and many women and children still lack access to adequate care (Sanneving et al., 2013). Further, despite significant improvements in maternal and child health (MCH) outcomes at the national level during the last three decades, India narrowly missed MDG 4 and 5 (Table A2.1). Supply-side factors are a major reason underlying the slow progress and growth of regional inequities and social disparities in health outcomes (Kumar & Dansereau, 2014; Singh, 2016). Several researchers found that various health outcome dissimilarities occur primarily from disparities in availability, accessibility, affordability, quality, and utilisation of healthcare services (Balarajan et al., 2011; Baru & Bisth, 2010). It has been argued that the inequalities in healthcare services led to overall health disparities across regions and states of the population (Balarajan et al., 2011).

Apart from the supply-side factors, micro-level studies have recognised five demand-side structural factors such as economic status, gender, education, social group status (caste or tribe), and age (adolescents) that are associated with inequity in MCH in India (Balarajan et al., 2011). Among the supply-side factors "quality" and "continuum" of availability of MCH services are found to be important among underserved population even if they reach the facilities to obtain such services (Ghosh et al., 2015). Owing to such "quality" issues out-of-pocket expenditure (OOPE) has been increasing as demand for services shifted from public to private (Issac et al., 2016; Mohanty & Kastor, 2017). These factors, in turn, have critical implications for finishing the "unfinished agenda" of MDG 4 and 5 and moving towards Universal Health Coverage (UHC) as a part of sustainable development goals (SDGs). The disparities have persisted even after the implementation of the National Rural Health Mission (NRHM) in 2005 as a policy response to develop the health system by providing universal access to equitable, affordable, and quality maternal and child healthcare services. However, some regions showed much progress in reducing maternal and child mortality and increasing access to MCH care, while others lagged behind. As a result, progress has not been equitable and many women from deprived groups still lack access to maternal and child healthcare (Sanneving et al., 2013). A recent study by Bango and Ghosh (Bango & Ghosh, 2022) have argued that though the magnitude of intrastate and socio-economic inequalities has reduced, people from deprived social groups and poor developing states are still experiencing inequality.

Table 1.2 MCH outcomes in India and Bihar

Indicators	India			Bihar		
	2005–06	2015–16	2019–21	2005–06	2015–16	2019–21
Controlling fertility:						
Use of modern contraception methods after marriage	48.5	47.8	56.5	28.9	23.3	44.4
ANC services:						
First ANC visit in the first trimester of pregnancy	43.9	58.6	70.0	18.7	34.6	52.9
Availed at least four ANC check-ups	37.0	51.2	58.1	11.2	14.4	25.2
Protection against neonatal tetanus (through tetanus toxoid Injections)	76.3	89.0	92.0	73.2	89.6	89.5
Took 100 IFA tablets/syrup for anaemia during pregnancy	15.2	30.3	44.1	6.3	9.7	18.0
Availed full ANC services	11.6	21.0	27.0	4.2	3.3	7.0
Institutional delivery and PNC services:						
Delivered in an institution	38.7	78.9	88.6	19.9	63.8	76.2
Home delivery assisted by a skilled person	8.2	4.30	3.2	9.7	8.2	6.1
Availed post-partum check-ups within 48 hours of delivery	34.6	62.4	78.0	13.4	42.3	57.3
Child health outcomes:						
Children aged 12–23 months fully immunised	43.5	62.0	76.4	32.8	61.7	71.0
Exclusively breastfeeding a child at least up to six months of birth	46.4	54.9	63.7	28.0	53.4	58.9
Children aged 6–8 months receiving solid or semi-solid food and breastmilk	52.6	42.7	45.9	54.5	30.8	39.0

Source: Fact sheets of NFHS.

1.4.3 Behaviour change through information diffusion and social networks

Apart from conventional demand–supply and contextual variables, the provision of tailored information on MCH and contraceptione-related information may also play a very important role in utilisation of MCH care and contraceptive services. In recent years, such demand-side strategies have emerged to complement investment in health facilities. These strategies consist of Behaviour Change Communication (BCC) measures. BCC is the use of communication strategies (like individual counselling, group-based educational sessions, mass media, messages through mobile phones, self-help groups (SHGs), etc.) for improving targeted outcomes (Barnett et al., 2022). Given that attitudes are learned, they are thought to predispose individuals to choose certain actions over others; effective and persuasive communication is, therefore, considered capable of providing individuals with internal cues to engage in healthier behaviour (Cassell et al., 1998; O'Keefe, 1990).

In the last two decades, community-based interventions have been recognised as key to achieving the health-related targets under the sustainable development goals, particularly with respect to maternal and child health outcomes (Desai et al., 2020b), by inducing health behavioural change through information dissemination and awareness generation. It has been argued that interventions to improve women's and children's health should engage with groups to strengthen the capabilities of individuals, groups, and communities to accelerate the adoption of health practices and shape the social determinants of health (Kuruvilla et al., 2016; Marston et al., 2016). An important component of such community-driven approach is the utilisation of the platform provided by the establishment of women's groups formed to empower women and enhance livelihoods (Bhandari et al., 2003; Rosato et al., 2008; Saggurti et al., 2019). Such groups bring women from a socio-economically homogenous background, sharing common goals and facing similar constraints together to discuss topics that are of concern to them and help them devise their own solutions (Saggurti et al., 2019). The interventions implemented through such groups are based on:

> a participatory process and action cycle approach, in which group members identify and prioritize maternal and new-born health problems in the community, collectively select strategies to address these problems, implement the strategies, and assess the results.
>
> (Saggurti et al., 2019, p. 990)

The effectiveness of such groups stems from their nature and functioning. The commonality of the background of SHG members and their frequent interaction creates solidarity and social capital (Putnam et al., 1994). Such social capital can take three inter-related forms: bonding social capital,[5] bridging social capital,[6] and linking social capital[7] (Woolcock, 1998). The SHGs are able to draw on this social capital to promote their shared goals (Beeker et al., 1998; Saha et al., 2013).

The call for "health layering" of SHGs and utilise them as tools for community-focused health interventions based on behavioural change (Mehta et al., 2020a) complements the interventions within the health systems being implemented at the state and national levels (Government of India, 2017). Evidence around the role of community participation and/or SHGs on maternal and newborn healthcare is evolving (Rosato et al., 2008; Schurmann & Johnston, 2009). Studies have shown that community participation particularly through SHG mechanisms provides a platform for women to express their concerns and create solidarity through shared visions and strive to attain such goals by utilising the synergy generated from the collective strength and social capital (Saha et al., 2013). Further, SHGs are effective in reaching marginalised and economically disadvantaged sections, as collective action is scalable, cost-effective, and capable of producing diverse effects over a long period (Mozumdar et al., 2018; Perry et al., 2014).

The role of front-line health workers has been reported to have led to improved MCH outcomes (Rammohan et al., 2021; Sserwanja, Turimumahoro, et al., 2022). Similarly, sources of information like radio and television (Aboagye et al., 2022; Fatema & Lariscy, 2020; Ghosh et al., 2021; Igbinoba et al., 2020; Nguyen et al., 2016; Sserwanja, Mutisya, et al., 2022) and messages spread over mobile phones (Rajkhowa & Qaim, 2022) have led to an increase in awareness among the general population, particularly women, and accelerated the adoption of recommended MCH practices. Health layering of self-help groups (SHGs) has also resulted in an improvement of MCH outcomes, reduction of newborn mortality while working to strengthen health systems in India (Darmstadt et al., 2005; Desai et al., 2020a; Gichuru et al., 2019; Hazra et al., 2020; Husain & Dutta, 2022; Mehta et al., 2020b; Mozumdar et al., 2018; Murshid & Ely, 2019; Saggurti et al., 2018; Saha et al., 2013; Walia et al., 2020) and in other developing countries (Bhutta et al., 2013, 2014; El Arifeen et al., 2013; Kuruvilla et al., 2014; Mangham-Jefferies et al., 2014; McClure et al., 2007). The role of women-led collectives in bridging development deficits aggravated by the COVID-19 pandemic has been reported by various sources (Kant & Hazra, 2023).[8] Studies point out the contribution of women SHGs in rural India in supporting vulnerable groups and migrant workers during the pandemic (Mahato & Jha, 2022; Yadav, 2021).

Peer support through social networks has also emerged as a policy intervention for promoting effective and sustainable MCH delivery over the last two decades. Peer support broadly refers to:

ongoing social and practical assistance provided by non-professionals to help people manage their health conditions, respond to particular healthcare needs, and/or contribute to overall well-being. It includes recurring interactions between people such as family members, neighbours, friends, or other associates but excludes incidental interactions and formal relationships like contacts between patients and service providers.

(Dugle et al., 2023, p. 2)

Peer support takes different forms, like one-to-one, group discussion, and online and telephone support sessions (Grant et al., 2021). It can be informal or more formalised, with trained peer supporters. Peer support in healthcare settings can be standardised by content or function (Boothroyd & Fisher, 2010; Fisher et al., 2015) . This is very important as "people often find themselves left on their own to enact and manage a complex set of factors to start and continue behaviour change" (Boothroyd & Fisher, 2010, p. i63). Peer effects can, in such situations, provide timely and optimal levels of support (Boothroyd & Fisher, 2010) and provide the individual with the encouragement to persist with the desirable behavioural pattern (Fisher et al., 2014). Those from "hardly reached" populations have also been found to benefit from peer support interventions, suggesting that peer support is a viable strategy for reaching socially marginalised groups that health services often fail to cover (Sokol & Fisher, 2016). Studies have reported the importance of peer support in the health sector (Perry et al., 2014). Peer effects have been found to play a major role in reducing obesity (Christakis & Fowler, 2007) and depression (Maselko et al., 2020); improving the health of patients affected by cancer (Sokol & Fisher, 2016), post-myocardial infarction (Berkman et al., 1992; Ebrahimi et al., 2021), and stroke (Sokol & Fisher, 2016); and promoting breastfeeding (Cameron et al., 2010), lifestyle education (Mohammadpourhodki et al., 2019), mental health during pregnancy (Fang et al., 2022; Rice et al., 2022), and utilisation of antenatal services (Hodnett et al., 2010; Thapa et al., 2019).

Despite the growing importance of BCC in improving MCH outcomes (Bernhardt, 2004; Mildon & Sellen, 2019) and reducing disparities in such outcomes between socio-economic groups (Hazra et al., 2020; Horii et al., 2016), there are few empirical assessments of the dissemination of information through the media, internet and front-line health workers to improve members' adoption of the provided health services undertaken in an integrated manner in India. Studies on the role of peer networks in improving health outcomes in the Indian context are also limited. For instance, to the best of our knowledge, there has been only one study on peer effects in the Indian context (Brooks et al., 2020). The studies, particularly those on JEEViKA (Gangadharan et al., 2014; Gupta et al., 2019; Husain & Dutta, 2022; JEEViKA, 2019; Kathuria, 2019; The World Bank, 2016), have used exploratory and econometric analysis to assess whether SHGs and media have improved the adoption of MCH practices. However, they have not explored the nature of peer networks. Nor have they examined the societal context in which the actors (i.e., women) are embedded and how this context constraints the formation of social capital, links between members, and the flow of information and peer effects. The present study is an attempt to address this deficiency.

1.5 Research questions

The present study analyses MCH outcomes in India and Bihar. Focusing on the demand for health, it seeks to examine whether networks (viz. links existing between members of formal institutions), individual counselling by front-line health workers, and information channels in the form of mass media can be used to disseminate knowledge about best practices in maternal health-seeking behaviour, leading to changes in health-seeking behaviour. The analysis is undertaken using the nationally representative National Family Health Survey (NFHS) data. In the absence of data on networks and information channels, we have relied on proxy indicators in our analysis. However, such indirect measures have limitations; further, aggregative analysis does not reveal the grass-roots realities. Specifically, we cannot identify the obstacles to the adoption of recommended MCH practices.

The study commences with an analysis of all-India data to examine the role of information through formal and informal ties and connections in improving MCH outcomes. It is followed by a detailed assessment of the efficacy of health communication through self-help group (SHG) bodies in Bihar. Such communication, however, targets only a specific group of women who may potentially limit the reach of such BCC strategies. We argue that spill-over effects from the SHG members may generate a peer effect in the village, leading to behavioural change among the non-SHG members also. Increasing the effectiveness of the BCC strategy requires us to compare the relative effectiveness of such peer effects and direct counselling by front-line health workers. Finally, we examine the nature of networks in which women are embedded. Using social network analysis and qualitative data we analyse the socio-cultural context of the women and how familial relations existing in a patriarchal society shape and restrict the nature of peer effects and information diffusion.

The research questions of the proposed study are as follows:

- What is the role of information networks and channels (like mass media, contacts with front-line health workers, SHG membership, etc.) in improving MCH practices? (Chapter 3)
- What are the factors that determine the breadth of such networks? (Chapter 3)
- How effective are SHGs in creating social capital and network to improve MCH outcomes? (Chapter 4)
- Are there any peer effects from SHG members to non-members? Are they exogenous or endogenous? Are they more effective than direct counselling by ASHAs? (Chapter 5)
- What are the family and community-level obstacles to such information diffusion at the grass-roots level? (Chapter 6)

This study has focused on 13 MCH outcomes that may be clubbed into three broad categories:

1.   **Outcome indicators related to uptake of maternal healthcare**

- Whether pregnancy was registered in the first trimester?
- Whether at least four ANC visits were made?
- Whether at least 100 IFA tablets/syrup were consumed?
- Whether two tetanus toxoid (TT) injections were taken to prevent neonatal tetanus?
- Whether full ANC (as defined by pregnancy registration in the first trimester of pregnancy, at least four ANC visits, at least 100 IFA tablets/syrup, and at least one TT) was received?
- Whether delivery was conducted in an institution?
- Whether delivery was conducted by a skilled birth attendant?
- Whether received a postnatal check-up within 48 hours of delivery?

2.   **Outcome indicators related to contraceptive use**

- Whether currently using modern methods of contraception?
- Whether received advice on post-partum contraception methods after the last birth?

3.   **Outcome indicators related to child health**

- Whether received vaccine at birth (OPV0) for the indexed child?
- Given exclusive breastfeeding for six months to the indexed child.
- Started complementary feeding after six months.

1.6 Data

To answer these questions, we have used two sources of data. The first two research questions are answered using unit-level data from the fifth round of National Family Health Survey data (2019–21). It is a nationally representative data base on reproductive health, that is part of the Demographic Health Survey programme covering over 90 countries. Starting in 1984, the Demographic Health Survey has undertaken over 400 surveys till date. In India there have been five surveys undertaken so far. The survey covers 7,24,115 women aged 15–49 years from 6.37 lakh households from 707 districts. The subsequent questions are answered using data from a mixed-method study in six districts of Bihar between January to March 2020, and December 2020. Details of the survey design, data collection method, and analytical methods are given in Chapter 3.

1.7 Structure

The book is structured as follows. Chapter 2 describes the data sources used in the study. In addition to a brief introduction to the NFHS data set, the chapter states the sampling strategy and data collection instruments used in collecting the primary data. This chapter also analyses the sample profile and village-level characteristics. Chapter 3 analyses the National Family Health Survey data (2019–21) to find out the role of access to information and networks on the adoption of different MCH practices; it also examines variations in access to channels of information across socio-economic groups. It enables us to contextualise why social networks can serve as important conduits for diffusion of information and improve the utilisation rates of maternal and child healthcare services, particularly in underdeveloped settings. Results of primary data analysis are presented and discussed in Chapters 4–6. Chapter 4 analyses the reported behaviour of respondents, examines differences in adoption rates between JEEViKA members and non-members, and discusses issues relating to spill-over and bandwagon effects. Chapter 5 examines the process underlying behavioural changes. We start by examining whether peer effects exist. Although there is evidence to show that village outcomes affect individual outcomes, such peer effects are endogenous and do not reflect the exogenous impact of peers. The effects are due to the presence of Government programmes. We examine the role of different information channels in generating the behavioural changes, focussing on the role of front-line health workers (ASHAs and community mobilisers). Chapter 6 uses methods borrowed from social network analysis to analyse the nature of information dissemination. It enables us to examine the flow of information from the source to the target recipents to identify the obstacles to information diffusion at the grass-roots level. Finally, in Chapter 7, we summarise the main findings of the study and discuss possible intervention strategies.

1.8 Relevance of the study

Experience with public health interventions has demonstrated that changing the knowledge, attitudes, and practices of target population groups is possible. However, research has also shown that such effects are typically modest and short-lived. We argue that the network-based strategy to improve MCH outcomes may have more long-lasting effects and be replicable.

The proposed study, based on social network analysis, is expected to address the challenge of permanently modifying behavioural changes as follows:

- In India, a few women in the locality are utilised as core members to form MFIs/SHGs. Such women are typically more empowered, have

sound knowledge of Government schemes, have contacts with local officers, serve as officials in several MFIs/SHGs, and have access to multiple
egocentric networks (such members are located at the hub of a wheel,
with the rim delineating other members, and spokes connecting the links
between them). Educational intervention through such dominant members will enable a large number of women to be targeted simultaneously,
increase the acceptability of the message, and ensuring that the information provided is considered to be authoritative. Further, members of the
network could support and reinforce the woman in her efforts to integrate
the recommendations of the healthcare provider into her daily routine.
Finally, providers could assess whether the woman is receiving conflicting
information or recommendations from other members of her daily environment and take necessary steps. This makes it more likely that the intervention will be accepted in the short run and sustained in the long run.

- Understanding specific mechanisms causing the behavioural change:
  Social networks provide the means to understand mechanisms for behaviour change. Our study is based on the assumption that people learn, contemplate, acquire information, try, and ultimately adopt new behaviours
  in the context of their interpersonal relationships. The more complex or
  challenging the behaviour changes are, the more people tend to rely on
  their social networks at each stage of change. So analysing social networks
  and their role in disseminating information about maternal healthcare
  practices will help us to understand the mechanisms underlying behavioural change.

- Sustaining change after the resources are withdrawn, or the programme
  ends: Generally, funding for the services and the change-agent training
  disappears or gets reduced over time. Withdrawal of external support sig-
  nals to the community that the problem is no longer important, and the
  effort in sustaining the change need not be continued anymore. Further,
  it is difficult for people to sustain their own personal behaviour change,
  and many people revive to their original behaviours after completing a
  behaviour change intervention. By deploying social network techniques
  in the behaviour change program, sustainability can be achieved because
  the change is based on local members who remain embedded in the community even after the program is over. The process of change, therefore, is
  independent of external interest and support and can be maintained based
  on local efforts.

- Scaling interventions to have more pervasive social impacts, and/or allow
  the intervention to be replicated in other backward regions: If MFI/
  SHG-based peer effects can be used to modify health-related choices and
  decision-making, policymakers may also contemplate scaling up such
  intervention strategies to modify behaviour in other domains. Broader
  social issues related to women empowerment and social change can be better addressed. On the other hand, if the mechanism of behavioural change

can be identified, social engineering can be employed in other regions to introduce appropriate transformative components into the community structure. This will allow the replication of intervention strategies in other regions.

Notes

1 Defined as having a body mass index of less than 18.5 kg/m²
2 Kerala, Andhra Pradesh, Tamil Nadu, Karnataka, and Punjab continue to be better performing states, while Assam, Bihar, Uttar Pradesh, and Nagaland are found to be the worst performers. Further, it can be noted that Uttar Pradesh with the highest population ranks the lowest in Health Index with a score of 28.6 while Kerala is on top of the table with a score of 74.01.
3 ASHAs are local women aged between 25 and 40 years. Every village/large habitat is to have an ASHA chosen by and accountable to the Panchayat. She is to serve as a bridge between Anganwadi workers, auxiliary nurse midwives, and the community. As a link between the community and the health facility schemes, the ASHAs are expected to be the first person to be called for any health-related demand. The NRHM envisages a large scale transfer of health-related skill and information to the ASHAs, enabling effective grass-root level intervention.
4 The continuum of care (CoC) in maternal healthcare refers to the continuation of care during the maternal period – provided in the form of antenatal care, delivery care, and post-partum care for the appropriate number of visits. CoC emphasizes two key dimensions, i.e., time and place. The time dimension highlights the continuity of care over time at different stages of pregnancy, childbirth, and post-partum. The place dimension links various levels of services provided at home, communities, and health facilities. According to NFHS 4 data, CoC in maternal healthcare was found to be quite unsatisfactory and hardly any improvement is noticeable. Although 70% of the births were assisted by skilled birth attendance, only 14.4% had at least four antenatal check-ups and more importantly, only 3.3% had full antenatal check-ups. It may also be noted that only 42.3% had postnatal check-ups within two days of delivery.
5 Ties between immediate family members, neighbours, and close friends.
6 Ties between people from different ethnic, geographical, and occupational backgrounds.
7 Ties between poor people and those in positions of influence in formal organizations such as banks and schools.
8 SHGs used wall paintings and *rangolis* to generate awareness about COVID and the importance of distancing, manufactured sanitizers, masks and PPE kits, ran community kitchens and provided dry rations. JEEViKA used the VAANI app to spread messages about the pandemic (Kant & Hazra, 2023).

References

Aboagye, R. G., Seidu, A.-A., Ahinkorah, B. O., Cadri, A., Frimpong, J. B., Hagan, J. E., Kassaw, N. A., & Yaya, S. (2022). Association between frequency of mass media exposure and maternal health care service utilization among women in sub-Saharan Africa: Implications for tailored health communication and education. *Plos One, 17*(9), e0275202. https://doi.org/10.1371/journal.pone.0275202

Ali, B., & Chauhan, S. (2020). Inequalities in the utilisation of maternal health Care in Rural India: Evidences from National Family Health Survey III &; IV. *BMC Public Health*, 20(1), 369. https://doi.org/10.1186/s12889-020-08480-4

Awasthi, A., Pandey, C. M., Chauhan, R. K., & Singh, U. (2016). Disparity in maternal, newborn and child health services in high focus states in India: A district-level cross-sectional analysis. *BMJ Open*, 6(8), e009885. https://doi.org/10.1136/bmjopen-2015-009885

Balarajan, Y., Selvaraj, S., & Subramanian, S. (2011). Health care and equity in India. *The Lancet*, 377(9764), 505–515. https://doi.org/10.1016/S0140-6736(10)61894-6

Bango, M., & Ghosh, S. (2022). Social and regional disparities in utilization of maternal and child healthcare services in India: A study of the post-national health mission period. *Frontiers in Pediatrics*, 10. https://doi.org/10.3389/fped.2022.895033

Barnett, I., Meeker, J., Roelen, K., & Nisbett, N. (2022). Behaviour change communication for child feeding in social assistance: A scoping review and expert consultation. *Maternal and Child Nutrition*, 18(3), 1–14. https://doi.org/10.1111/mcn.13361

Barro, R. J. (1998). *Determinants of economic growth: A cross-country empirical study*. MIT Press.

Baru, R. V., & Bisth, R. (2010). *Health service inequities as a challenge to health security*. http://hdl.handle.net/10546/346634

Beeker, C., Guenther-Grey, C., & Raj, A. (1998). Community empowerment paradigm drift and the primary prevention of HIV/AIDS. *Social Science & Medicine*, 46(7), 831–842. https://doi.org/10.1016/S0277-9536(97)00208-6

Berkman, L. F., Leo-Summers, L., & Horwitz, R. I. (1992). Emotional support and survival after myocardial infarction. *Annals of Internal Medicine*, 117(12), 1003–1009. https://doi.org/10.7326/0003-4819-117-12-1003

Bernhardt, J. M. (2004). Communication at the core of effective public health. *American Journal of Public Health*, 94(12), 2051–2053. https://doi.org/10.2105/ajph.94.12.2051

Bhandari, N., Bahl, R., Mazumdar, S., Martines, J., Black, R. E., & Bhan, M. K. (2003). Effect of community-based promotion of exclusive breastfeeding on diarrhoeal illness and growth: A cluster randomised controlled trial. *The Lancet*, 361(9367), 1418–1423. https://doi.org/10.1016/S0140-6736(03)13134-0

Bhutta, Z. A., Das, J. K., Bahl, R., Lawn, J. E., Salam, R. A., Paul, V. K., Sankar, M. J., Blencowe, H., Rizvi, A., Chou, V. B., Walker, N., Lancet Newborn Interventions Review Group, & Lancet Every Newborn Study Group. (2014). Can available interventions end preventable deaths in mothers, newborn babies, and stillbirths, and at what cost? *Lancet (London, England)*, 384(9940), 347–370. https://doi.org/10.1016/S0140-6736(14)60792-3

Bhutta, Z. A., Das, J. K., Rizvi, A., Gaffey, M. F., Walker, N., Horton, S., Webb, P., Lartey, A., & Black, R. E. (2013). Evidence-based interventions for improvement of maternal and child nutrition: What can be done and at what cost? *The Lancet*, 382(9890), 452–477. https://doi.org/10.1016/S0140-6736(13)60996-4

Black, R. E., Allen, L. H., Bhutta, Z. A., Caulfield, L. E., de Onis, M., Ezzati, M., Mathers, C., Rivera, J., Onis, M. De, Ezzati, M., Mathers, C., & Rivera, J. (2008). Maternal and child undernutrition: Global and regional exposures and health consequences. *The Lancet*, *371*(9608), 243–260. https://doi.org/10.1016/S0140-6736(07)61690-0

Bloom, D., Canning, D., & Sevilla, J. (2003). *The demographic dividend: A new perspective on the economic consequences of population change*. RAND Corporation. https://doi.org/10.7249/MR1274

Bloom, D. E., Canning, D., & Sevilla, J. (2004). The effect of health on economic growth: A production function approach. *World Development*, *32*(1), 1–13. https://doi.org/10.1016/j.worlddev.2003.07.002

Boothroyd, R. I., & Fisher, E. B. (2010). Peers for progress: Promoting peer support for health around the world. *Family Practice*, *27*(suppl 1), i62–i68. https://doi.org/10.1093/fampra/cmq017

Brooks, S. K., Webster, R. K., Smith, L. E., Woodland, L., Wessely, S., Greenberg, N., & Rubin, G. J. (2020). The psychological impact of quarantine and how to reduce it: Rapid review of the evidence. *The Lancet*, *395*(10227), 912–920. https://doi.org/10.1016/S0140-6736(20)30460-8

Cameron, A. J., Hesketh, K., Ball, K., Crawford, D., & Campbell, K. J. (2010). Influence of peers on breastfeeding discontinuation among new parents: The Melbourne InFANT program. *Pediatrics*, *126*(3), e601–e607. https://doi.org/10.1542/peds.2010-0771

Cassell, M. M., Jackson, C., & Cheuvront, B. (1998). Health communication on the internet: An effective channel for health behavior change? *Journal of Health Research*, *3*(4), 71–79.

Christakis, N. A., & Fowler, J. H. (2007). The spread of obesity in a large social network over 32 years. *New England Journal of Medicine*, *357*(4), 370–379. https://doi.org/10.1056/NEJMsa066082

Dandona, R., Majumder, M., Akbar, M., Bhattacharya, D., Nanda, P., Kumar, G. A., & Dandona, L. (2022). Assessment of quality of antenatal care services in public sector facilities in India. *BMJ Open*, *12*(12), e065200. https://doi.org/10.1136/bmjopen-2022-065200

Darmstadt, G. L., Bhutta, Z. A., Cousens, S., Adam, T., Walker, N., & de Bernis, L. (2005). Evidence-based, cost-effective interventions: How many newborn babies can we save? *The Lancet*, *365*(9463), 977–988. https://doi.org/10.1016/S0140-6736(05)71088-6

Dasgupta, S., Roy, S., & Wheeler, D. (2021). Explaining regional variations in mother-child health: Additional identified determinants in India and Bangladesh. *Health Policy OPEN*, *2*, 100038. https://doi.org/10.1016/j.hpopen.2021.100038

Desai, S., Misra, M., Das, A., Singh, R. J., Sehgal, M., Gram, L., Kumar, N., & Prost, A. (2020a). Community interventions with women's groups to improve women's and children's health in India: A mixed-methods systematic review of effects, enablers and barriers. *BMJ Global Health*, *5*(12). https://doi.org/10.1136/bmjgh-2020-003304

Desai, S., Misra, M., Das, A., Singh, R. J., Sehgal, M., Gram, L., Kumar, N., & Prost, A. (2020b). Community interventions with women's groups to improve women's and children's health in India: A mixed-methods systematic review of effects, enablers and barriers. *BMJ Global Health*, *5*(12), e003304. https://doi.org/10.1136/bmjgh-2020-003304

Dugle, G., Antwi, J., & Quentin, W. (2023). Peer support interventions in maternal and child healthcare delivery in sub-Saharan Africa: Protocol for a realist review. *Systematic Reviews*, 12(1), 199. https://doi.org/10.1186/s13643-023-02366-3

Ebrahimi, H., Abbasi, A., Bagheri, H., Basirinezhad, M. H., Shakeri, S., & Mohammadpourhodki, R. (2021). The role of peer support education model on the quality of life and self-care behaviors of patients with myocardial infarction. *Patient Education and Counseling*, 104(1), 130–135. https://doi.org/10.1016/j.pec.2020.08.002

El Arifeen, S., Christou, A., Reichenbach, L., Osman, F. A., Azad, K., Islam, K. S., Ahmed, F., Perry, H. B., & Peters, D. H. (2013). Community-based approaches and partnerships: Innovations in health-service delivery in Bangladesh. *The Lancet*, 382(9909), 2012–2026. https://doi.org/10.1016/S0140-6736(13)62149-2

Every Woman Every Child. (2016). *The global strategy for women's, children's and adolescent's health (2016–2030)*. United Nations. https://www.who.int/life-course/publications/global-strategy-2016-2030/en/

Fang, Q., Lin, L., Chen, Q., Yuan, Y., Wang, S., Zhang, Y., Liu, T., Cheng, H., & Tian, L. (2022). Effect of peer support intervention on perinatal depression: A meta-analysis. *General Hospital Psychiatry*, 74, 78–87. https://doi.org/10.1016/j.genhosppsych.2021.12.001

Fatema, K., & Lariscy, J. T. (2020). Mass media exposure and maternal healthcare utilization in South Asia. *SSM - Population Health*, 11, 100614. https://doi.org/10.1016/j.ssmph.2020.100614

Fisher, E. B., Ayala, G. X., Ibarra, L., Cherrington, A. L., Elder, J. P., Tang, T. S., Heisler, M., Safford, M. M., Simmons, D., & Peers for Progress Investigator Group. (2015). Contributions of peer support to health, health care, and prevention: Papers from peers for progress. *Annals of Family Medicine*, 13(Suppl 1), S2–8. https://doi.org/10.1370/afm.1852

Fisher, E. B., Coufal, M. M., Parada, H., Robinette, J. B., Tang, P. Y., Urlaub, D. M., Castillo, C., Guzman-Corrales, L. M., Hino, S., Hunter, J., Katz, A. W., Symes, Y. R., Worley, H. P., & Xu, C. (2014). Peer support in health care and prevention: Cultural, organizational, and dissemination issues. *Annual Review of Public Health*, 35(1), 363–383. https://doi.org/10.1146/annurev-publhealth-032013-182450

Fogel, R. W. (2004). Health, nutrition, and economic growth. *Economic Development and Cultural Change*, 52(3), 643–658. https://doi.org/10.1086/383450

Gandhi, S., Dash, U., & Suresh Babu, M. (2022). Horizontal inequity in the utilisation of Continuum of Maternal Health care Services (CMHS) in India: An investigation of ten years of National Rural Health Mission (NRHM). *International Journal for Equity in Health*, 21(1), 7. https://doi.org/10.1186/s12939-021-01602-3

Gangadharan, L., Jain, T., Maitra, P., & Vecci, J. (2014). *The behavioural response to women's empowerment programs experimental evidence from JEEViKA in Bihar* (Issue December), Policy brief. New Delhi: The Inernational growth Centre.

Ghosh, R., Mozumdar, A., Chattopadhyay, A., & Acharya, R. (2021). Mass media exposure and use of reversible modern contraceptives among married women in India: An analysis of the NFHS 2015–16 data. *PLoS One*, 16(7 July), 1–23. https://doi.org/10.1371/journal.pone.0254400

Ghosh, S., & Husain, Z. (2019). Has the national health mission improved utilisation of maternal healthcare services in Bihar? *Economic & Political Weekly*, *54*(31), 44–51.

Ghosh, S., Siddiqui, M. Z., Barik, A., & Bhaumik, S. (2015). Determinants of skilled delivery assistance in a rural population: Findings from an HDSS site of rural West Bengal, India. *Maternal and Child Health Journal*, *19*(11), 2470–2479.

Gichuru, W., Ojha, S., Smith, S., Smyth, A. R., & Szatkowski, L. (2019). Is microfinance associated with changes in women's well-being and children's nutrition? A systematic review and meta-analysis. *BMJ Open*, *9*(1), 1–17. https://doi.org/10.1136/bmjopen-2018-023658

Gordillo-Tobar, A., Quinlan-Davidson, M., & Mills, S. L. (2017). *Maternal and child health: The World Bank group's response to sustainable development goal 3—target 3.1 and 3.2* (Discussion Paper). https://openknowledge.worldbank.org/server/api/core/bitstreams/c19d8334-113a-55a6-84e7-34134b5b34cf/content

Government of India. (2005). *Millennium Development Goals (MDGs): India country report*. New Delhi: Government of India.

Government of India. (2017). *Bihar: Roadmap for development of health sector. A report of special task force of Bihar*. New Delhi: Government of India.

Grant, E., Johnson, L., Prodromidis, A., & Giannoudis, P. V. (2021). The impact of peer support on patient outcomes in adults with physical health conditions: A scoping review. *Cureus*, *13*(8), e17442. https://doi.org/10.7759/cureus.17442

Grossman, M. (1972). On the concept of health capital and the demand for health. *Journal of Political Economy*, *80*(2), 223–255. https://doi.org/10.1086/259880

Gupta, S., Kumar, N., Menon, P., Pandey, S., & Raghunathan, K. (2019). *Engaging women's groups to improve nutrition: Findings from an evaluation of the Jeevika multisectoral convergence pilot in Saharsa, Bihar*. The World Bank.

Haacker, M. (2004). HIV/AIDS: The impact on the social fabric and the economy. In M. Haacker (Ed.), *The Macroeconomics of HIV/AIDS*. International Monetary Fund.

Hazra, A., Atmavilas, Y., Hay, K., Saggurti, N., Verma, R. K., Ahmad, J., Kumar, S., Mohanan, P. S., Mavalankar, D., & Irani, L. (2020). Effects of health behaviour change intervention through women's Self-Help Groups on maternal and newborn health practices and related inequalities in rural india: A quasi-experimental study. *EClinicalMedicine*, *18*(xxxx). https://doi.org/10.1016/j.eclinm.2019.10.011

Hiwale, A. J., & Chandra Das, K. (2022). Geospatial differences among natural regions in the utilization of maternal health care services in India. *Clinical Epidemiology and Global Health*, *14*, 100979. https://doi.org/10.1016/j.cegh.2022.100979

Hodnett, E. D., Fredericks, S., & Weston, J. (2010). Support during pregnancy for women at increased risk of low birthweight babies. *The Cochrane Database of Systematic Reviews*, *6*, CD000198. https://doi.org/10.1002/14651858.CD000198.pub2

Horii, N., Habi, O., Dangana, A., Maina, A., Alzouma, S., & Charbit, Y. (2016). Community-based behavior change promoting child health care: A response to socio-economic disparity. *Journal of Health, Population, and Nutrition*, *35*, 12. https://doi.org/10.1186/s41043-016-0048-y

Horton, R. (2008). Maternal and child undernutrition: An urgent opportunity. *Lancet*, *371*(9608), 179. https://doi.org/10.1016/S0140-6736(07)61869-8

Husain, Z., & Dutta, M. (2022). Impact of Self Help Group membership on the adoption of child nutritional practices: Evidence from JEEViKA's health and nutrition strategy programme in Bihar, India. *Journal of International Development*, 26(4), 422–437. https://doi.org/10.1002/jid.3703

Husain, Z., Ghosh, S., & Dutta, M. (2022). *Discontinuity in uptake of Ante-Natal care services in Rural India: Identifying local and global influences using spatial statistical techniques*. OP-78. Occasional Papers. Institute of Development Studies Kolkata.

Igbinoba, A. O., Soola, E. O., Omojola, O., Odukoya, J., Adekeye, O., & Salau, O. P. (2020). Women's mass media exposure and maternal health awareness in Ota, Nigeria. *Cogent Social Sciences*, 6(1). https://doi.org/10.1080/23311886.2020.1766260

India State-Level Disease Burden Initiative Malnutrition Collaborators, & Collaborators. (2019). The burden of child and maternal malnutrition and trends in its indicators in the states of India: The global burden of disease study 1990 – 2017. *The Lancet Child & Adolescent Health*, 3(12), 855–870. https://doi.org/10.1016/S2352-4642(19)30273-1

Indian Council of Medical Research, Public Health Foundation of India, & Institute for Health Metrics and Evaluation. (2017). *Health of the Nation's States—The India State-Level Disease Burden Initiative*.

International Institute for Population Sciences. (1993). *National Family Health Survey (NFHS-1), 1992*. International Institute for Population Sciences.

International Institute for Population Sciences. (2000). *National Family Health Survey (NFHS-2), 1998–99*. International Institute for Population Sciences.

International Institute for Population Sciences. (2007). *National Family Health Survey (NFHS-3), 2005–06*. International Institute for Population Sciences.

International Institute of Population Sciences. (2015). *National Family Health Survey -4 State Fact Sheet Bihar*. International Institute for Population Sciences.

International Institute of Population Sciences. (2017). *National Family Health Survey -4, State Fact Sheet Bihar*. International Institute for Population Sciences.

International Institute of Population Sciences. (2018). *National Family Health Survey -4, India*. International Institute for Population Sciences.

International Institute of Population Sciences. (2022). *National Family Health Survey -5, India*. International Institute for Population Sciences.

International Institute of Population Sciences. (2020). *National Family Health Survey -5, State Fact Sheet Bihar*. International Institute for Population Sciences.

Issac, A., Chatterjee, S., Srivastava, A., & Bhattacharyya, S. (2016). Out of pocket expenditure to deliver at public health facilities in India: A cross sectional analysis. *Reproductive Health*, 13(1), 99. https://doi.org/10.1186/s12978-016-0221-1

Jamison, D. (2006). Investing in Health. In M. C. D. Jamison, J. Berman, A. Meacham, G. Alleyne, D. Evans, P. Jha, A. Mills, & P. Musgrove (Eds.), *Disease control an dpriorities in developing countries* (2nd editio). The World Bank.

JEEViKA. (2019). *Proposal on JEEViKA as National Resource Organization (NRO) for integration Food, Nutrition, Health and WASH (FNHW) interventions*. Patna: Government of Bihar.

Kant, A., & Hazra, A. (2023). Bridge over troubled waters: Women-led response to maternal and child health services in India amidst the COVID-19 pandemic. In S. Pachauri & A. Pachauri (Eds.), *Global perspectives of COVID-19 pandemic* on health, education, and role of media (pp. 63–83). Springer Nature Singapore. https://doi.org/10.1007/978-981-99-1106-6_4

Kathuria, A. K. (2019). JEEViKA multisectoral convergence initiative in Bihar: Engaging women's groups to improve nutrition. https://documents1.worldbank .org/curated/en/286621572412901383/pdf/India-Impact-Evaluation-of-JEEViKA -Multisectoral-Convergence-Initiative-in-Bihar-Engaging-Women-s-Groups-to -Improve-Nutrition-Summary-Report.pdf

Kochar, P. S., Dandona, R., Kumar, G. A., & Dandona, L. (2014). Population-based estimates of still birth, induced abortion and miscarriage in the Indian state of Bihar. BMC Pregnancy and Childbirth, 14(1), 413. https://doi.org/10.1186/ s12884-014-0413-z

Kumar, G. A., Dandona, R., Chaman, P., Singh, P., & Dandona, L. (2014). A population-based study of neonatal mortality and maternal care utilization in the Indian state of Bihar. BMC Pregnancy and Childbirth, 14(1), 357. https://doi.org /10.1186/1471-2393-14-357

Kumar, S., & Dansereau, E. (2014). Supply-side barriers to maternity-care in India: A facility-based analysis. PLoS One, 9(8), e103927. https://doi.org/10.1371/journal .pone.0103927

Kuruvilla, S., Bustreo, F., Kuo, T., Mishra, C. K., Taylor, K., Fogstad, H., Gupta, G. R., Gilmore, K., Temmerman, M., Thomas, J., Rasanathan, K., Chaiban, T., Mohan, A., Gruending, A., Schweitzer, J., Dini, H. S., Borrazzo, J., Fassil, H., Gronseth, L., ... Costello, A. (2016). The global strategy for women's, children's and adolescents' health (2016–2030): A roadmap based on evidence and country experience. Bulletin of the World Health Organization, 94(5), 398–400. https:// doi.org/10.2471/BLT.16.170431

Kuruvilla, S., Schweitzer, J., Bishai, D., Chowdhury, S., Caramani, D., Frost, L., Cortez, R., Daelmans, B., de Francisco, A., Adam, T., Cohen, R., Alfonso, Y. N., Franz-Vasdeki, J., Saadat, S., Pratt, B. A., Eugster, B., Bandali, S., Venkatachalam, P., Hinton, R., ... Success Factors for Women's and Children's Health Study Groups. (2014). Success factors for reducing maternal and child mortality. Bulletin of the World Health Organization, 92(7), 533–44B. https://doi.org/10.2471/BLT .14.138131

Mahato, T., & Jha, M. K. (2022). Women's Self-Help Groups and COVID-19 pandemic: Resilience and sustenance BT - Inclusive businesses in developing economies: Converging people, profit, and corporate citizenship (Rajagopal & R. Behl (Eds.), pp. 323–342). Springer International Publishing. https://doi.org/10 .1007/978-3-031-12217-0_16

Mâlqvist, M., Nga, N. T., Eriksson, L., Wallin, L., Hoa, D. P., & Persson, L. Å. (2011). Ethnic inequity in neonatal survival: A case-referent study in northern Vietnam. Acta Paediatrica, 100(3), 340–346. https://doi.org/10.1111/j.1651-2227 .2010.02065.x

Mangham-Jefferies, L., Pitt, C., Cousens, S., Mills, A., & Schellenberg, J. (2014). Cost-effectiveness of strategies to improve the utilization and provision of maternal and newborn health care in low-income and lower-middle-income countries: A systematic review. BMC Pregnancy and Childbirth, 14(1), 243. https://doi.org/10 .1186/1471-2393-14-243

Mankiw, N. G., Romer, D., & Weil, D. N. (1992). A contribution to the empirics of economic growth. *The Quarterly Journal of Economics*, *107*(2), 407–437. https://doi.org/10.2307/2118477

Marston, C., Hinton, R., Kean, S., Baral, S., Ahuja, A., Costello, A., & Portela, A. (2016). Community participation for transformative action on women's, children's and adolescents' health. *Bulletin of the World Health Organization*, *94*(5), 376–382. https://doi.org/10.2471/BLT.15.168492

Maselko, J., Sikander, S., Turner, E. L., Bates, L. M., Ahmad, I., Atif, N., Baranov, V., Bhalotra, S., Bibi, A., Bibi, T., Bilal, S., Biroli, P., Chung, E., Gallis, J. A., Hagaman, A., Jamil, A., LeMasters, K., O'Donnell, K., Scherer, E., ... Rahman, A. (2020). Effectiveness of a peer-delivered, psychosocial intervention on maternal depression and child development at 3 years postnatal: A cluster randomised trial in Pakistan. *The Lancet Psychiatry*, *7*(9), 775–787. https://doi.org/10.1016/S2215-0366(20)30258-3

Mathers, C. D., Lopez, A. D., & Murray, C. J. L. (2006). The burden of disease and mortality by condition: Data, methods, and results for 2001. In A. D. Lopez, C. D. Mathers, M. Ezzati, D. T. Jamison, & C. J. L. Murray (Eds.), *Global Burden of Disease and Risk Factors*. The World Bank.

McArthur, J. W., Rasmussen, K., & Yamey, G. (2018). How many lives are at stake? Assessing 2030 sustainable development goal trajectories for maternal and child health. *BMJ*, k373. https://doi.org/10.1136/bmj.k373

McClure, E. M., Carlo, W. A., Wright, L. L., Chomba, E., Uxa, F., Lincetto, O., & Bann, C. (2007). Evaluation of the educational impact of the WHO essential newborn care course in Zambia. *Acta Paediatrica*, *96*(8), 1135–1138. https://doi.org/10.1111/j.1651-2227.2007.00392.x

Mehta, K. M., Irani, L., Chaudhuri, I., Mahapatra, T., Schooley, J., Srikantiah, S., Abdalla, S., Ward, V., Carmichael, S. L., Bentley, J., Creanga, A., Wilhelm, J., Tarigopula, U. K., Bhattacharya, D., Atmavilas, Y., Nanda, P., Weng, Y., Pepper, K. T., Darmstadt, G. L., & Ananya Study Group. (2020a). Health layering of Self-Help Groups: Impacts on reproductive, maternal, newborn and child health and nutrition in Bihar, India. *Journal of Global Health*, *10*(2), 021007. https://doi.org/10.7189/jogh.10.021007

Mehta, K. M., Irani, L., Chaudhuri, I., Mahapatra, T., Schooley, J., Srikantiah, S., Abdalla, S., Ward, V., Carmichael, S. L., Bentley, J., Creanga, A., Wilhelm, J., Tarigopula, U. K., Bhattacharya, D., Atmavilas, Y., Nanda, P., Weng, Y., Pepper, K. T., Darmstadt, G. L., & Ananya Study Group. (2020b). Health layering of Self-Help Groups: Impacts on reproductive, maternal, newborn and child health and nutrition in Bihar, India. *Journal of Global Health*, *10*(2), 021007. https://doi.org/10.7189/jogh.10.021007

Mildon, A., & Sellen, D. (2019). Use of mobile phones for behavior change communication to improve maternal, newborn and child health: A scoping review. *Journal of Global Health*, *9*(2). https://doi.org/10.7189/jogh.09.020425

Mohammadpourhodki, R., Bagheri, H., Basirinezhad, M. H., Ramzani, H., & Keramati, M. (2019). Evaluating the effect of lifestyle education based on peer model on anxiety in patients with acute myocardial infarction. *Journal of Complementary and Integrative Medicine*, *16*(3). https://doi.org/10.1515/jcim-2018-0132

Mohanty, S. K., & Kastor, A. (2017). Out-of-pocket expenditure and catastrophic health spending on maternal care in public and private health centres in India: A comparative study of pre and post national health mission period. *Health Economics Review*, 7(1), 31. https://doi.org/10.1186/s13561-017-0167-1

Mozumdar, A., Khan, M. E., Mondal, S. K., & Mohanan, P. S. (2018). Increasing knowledge of home based maternal and newborn care using Self-Help Groups: Evidence from rural Uttar Pradesh, India. *Sexual & Reproductive Healthcare*, 18, 1–9. https://doi.org/10.1016/j.srhc.2018.08.003

Murshid, N. S., & Ely, G. E. (2019). Microfinance participation and contraceptive use and intention in Bangladesh. *International Social Work*, 62(4), 1274–1285. https://doi.org/10.1177/0020872818774089

Mushkin, S. J. (1962). Health as an investment. *Journal of Political Economy*, 70(5, Part 2), 129–157. https://doi.org/10.1086/258730

Nath, A. (2011). India's progress toward achieving the millennium development goals. *Indian Journal of Community Medicine*, 36(2), 85. https://doi.org/10.4103/0970-0218.84118

Niti Ayog, The World Bank, and Ministry of Health & Family Welfare. (2019). *Healthy states progressive India: Report on the ranks of states and union territories*. http://social.niti.gov.in/uploads/sample/health_index_report.pdf.

Nguyen, P. H., Kim, S. S., Nguyen, T. T., Hajeebhoy, N., Tran, L. M., Alayon, S., Ruel, M. T., Rawat, R., Frongillo, E. A., & Menon, P. (2016). Exposure to mass media and interpersonal counseling has additive effects on exclusive breastfeeding and its psychosocial determinants among Vietnamese mothers. *Maternal and Child Nutrition*, 12(4), 713–725. https://doi.org/10.1111/mcn.12330

O'Keefe, D. J. (1990). *Persuasion*. Sage.

Panda, B. K., & Mohanty, S. K. (2019). Progress and prospects of health-related sustainable development goals in India. *Journal of Biosocial Science*, 51(3), 335–352. https://doi.org/10.1017/S0021932018000202

Perry, H. B., Zulliger, R., & Rogers, M. M. (2014). Community health workers in low-, middle-, and high-income countries: An overview of their history, recent evolution, and current effectiveness. *Annual Review of Public Health*, 35, 399–421. https://doi.org/10.1146/annurev-publhealth-032013-182354

Putnam, R. D., Leonardi, R., & Nanetti, R. Y. (1994). *Making democracy work:civic traditions in modern Italy*. Princeton University Press.

Rahman, M. M., Rouyard, T., Khan, S. T., Nakamura, R., Islam, M. R., Hossain, M. S., Akter, S., Lohan, M., Ali, M., & Sato, M. (2023). Reproductive, maternal, newborn, and child health intervention coverage in 70 low-income and middle-income countries, 2000–30: Trends, projections, and inequities. *The Lancet Global Health*, 11(10), e1531–e1543. https://doi.org/10.1016/S2214-109X(23)00358-3

Raina, N., Khanna, R., Gupta, S., Jayathilaka, C. A., Mehta, R., & Behera, S. (2023). Progress in achieving SDG targets for mortality reduction among mothers, newborns, and children in the WHO South-East Asia Region. *The Lancet Regional Health - Southeast Asia*, 18, 100307. https://doi.org/10.1016/j.lansea.2023.100307

Rajkhowa, P., & Qaim, M. (2022). Mobile phones, women's physical mobility, and contraceptive use in India. *Social Science and Medicine*, 305(January), 115074. https://doi.org/10.1016/j.socscimed.2022.115074

Rammohan, A., Goli, S., Saroj, S. K., & Jaleel, C. P. A. (2021). Does engagement with frontline health workers improve maternal and child healthcare utilisation and outcomes in India? *Human Resources for Health*, 19(1), 1–21. https://doi.org/10.1186/s12960-021-00592-1

Rice, C., Ingram, E., & O'Mahen, H. (2022). A qualitative study of the impact of peer support on women's mental health treatment experiences during the perinatal period. *BMC Pregnancy and Childbirth*, 22(1), 689. https://doi.org/10.1186/s12884-022-04959-7

Rosato, M., Laverack, G., Grabman, L. H., Tripathy, P., Nair, N., Mwansambo, C., Azad, K., Morrison, J., Bhutta, Z., Perry, H., Rifkin, S., & Costello, A. (2008). Community participation: Lessons for maternal, newborn, and child health. *The Lancet*, 372(9642), 962–971. https://doi.org/10.1016/S0140-6736(08)61406-3

Saggurti, N., Atmavilas, Y., Porwal, A., Schooley, J., Das, R., Kande, N., Irani, L., & Hay, K. (2018). Effect of health intervention integration within women's Self-Help Groups on collectivization and healthy practices around reproductive, maternal, neonatal and child health in rural India. *PLoS One*, 13(8), e0202562. https://doi.org/10.1371/journal.pone.0202562

Saggurti, N., Porwal, A., Atmavilas, Y., Walia, M., Das, R., & Irani, L. (2019). Effect of behavioral change intervention around new-born care practices among most marginalized women in Self-Help Groups in rural India: Analyses of three cross-sectional surveys between 2013 and 2016. *Journal of Perinatology*, 39(7), 990–999. https://doi.org/10.1038/s41372-019-0358-1

Saha, S., Annear, P., & Pathak, S. (2013). The effect of Self-Help Groups on access to maternal health services: Evidence from rural India. *International Journal for Equity in Health*, 12(1), 36. https://doi.org/10.1186/1475-9276-12-36

Sanneving, L., Trygg, N., Saxena, D., Mavalankar, D., & Thomsen, S. (2013). Inequity in India: The case of maternal and reproductive health. *Global Health Action*, 6(1), 19145. https://doi.org/10.3402/gha.v6i0.19145

Schultz, T. P. (1999). Health and schooling investments in Africa. *Journal of Economic Perspectives, American Economic Association*, 13(3), 67–88.

Schurmann, A. T., & Johnston, H. B. (2009). The group-lending model and social closure: Microcredit, exclusion, and health in Bangladesh. *Journal of Health, Population, and Nutrition*, 27(4), 518–527. https://doi.org/10.3329/jhpn.v27i4.3398

Singh, A. (2016). Supply-side barriers to maternal health care utilization at health sub-centers in India. *PeerJ*, 4, e2675. https://doi.org/10.7717/peerj.2675

Sokol, R., & Fisher, E. (2016). Peer support for the hardly reached: A systematic review. *American Journal of Public Health*, 106(7), e1–8. https://doi.org/10.2105/AJPH.2016.303180

Sserwanja, Q., Mutisya, L. M., & Musaba, M. W. (2022). Exposure to different types of mass media and timing of antenatal care initiation: Insights from the 2016 Uganda Demographic and Health Survey. *BMC Women's Health*, 22(1), 1–8. https://doi.org/10.1186/s12905-022-01594-4

Sserwanja, Q., Turimumahoro, P., Nuwabaine, L., Kamara, K., & Musaba, M. W. (2022). Association between exposure to family planning messages on different mass media channels and the utilization of modern contraceptives among young women in Sierra Leone: Insights from the 2019 Sierra Leone Demographic Health

Survey. *BMC Women's Health*, 22(1), 1–10. https://doi.org/10.1186/s12905-022 -01974-w

State Health Society. (2011). *Meeting people's health needs in rural areas: Programme implementation plan, 2010–11.* http://statehealthsocietybihar.org/pip2010-11/ statepip-2010-11/statepip-2010-11.pdf

Strauss, J., & Thomas, D. (1998). Health, nutrition, and economic development. *Journal of Economic Literature*, 36(2), 766–817. http://www.jstor.org/stable /2565122

Thapa, P., Bangura, A. H., Nirola, I., Citrin, D., Belbase, B., Bogati, B., Nirmala, B. K., Khadka, S., Kunwar, L., Halliday, S., Choudhury, N., Ozonoff, A., Tenpa, J., Schwarz, R., Adhikari, M., Kalaunee, S. P., Rising, S., Maru, D., & Maru, S. (2019). The power of peers: An effectiveness evaluation of a cluster-controlled trial of group antenatal care in rural Nepal. *Reproductive Health*, 16(1), 150. https://doi.org/10.1186/s12978-019-0820-8

The World Bank. (2006). *Population and the World Bank: Background paper prepared for the HNP sector strategy* (Health, Nutrition, and Population Working Paper).

The World Bank. (2016). *Livelihoods and nutrition: A women's empowerment and convergence initiative.* http://documents1.worldbank.org/curated/ pt/109401572440521978/pdf/Livelihoods-and-Nutrition-A-Women-s -Empowerment-and-Convergence-Initiative-JEEViKA.pdf.

UN Inter-Agency Group for Child Mortality Estimation. (2019). *Levels and trends in child mortality 2019.* UNICEF.

UN Interagency Group for Child Mortality Estimation. (2017). *Levels and trends in child mortality: Report 2017.* http://childmortality.org/files_v21/download/IGM Ereport2017childmortality final.pdf

UNDP. (2015). Sustainable development goals. In *UNDP.* https://www.undp.org/ content/undp/en/home/sustainable-development-goals.html

Uthman, O. A., Aiyedun, V., & Yahaya, I. (2012). Exploring variations in under-5 mortality in Nigeria using league table, control chart and spatial analysis. *Journal of Public Health*, 34(1), 125–130. https://doi.org/10.1093/pubmed/fdr050

Victora, C. G., Adair, L., Fall, C., Hallal, P. C., Martorell, R., Richter, L., & Sachdev, H. S. (2008). Maternal and child undernutrition: Consequences for adult health and human capital. *Lancet*, 371(9609), 340–357. https://doi.org/10.1016/S0140 -6736(07)61692-4

Walia, M., Irani, L., Chaudhuri, I., Atmavilas, Y., & Saggurti, N. (2020). Effect of sharing health messages on antenatal care behavior among women involved in microfinance-based Self-Help Groups in Bihar India. *Global Health Research and Policy*, 5(1), 3. https://doi.org/10.1186/s41256-020-0132-0

WHO. (2017). *Trends in maternal mortality: 2000 to 2017: Estimates by WHO, UNICEF, UNFPA, World Bank Group and UN Population Division.*

Woolcock, M. (1998). Social capital and economic development: Toward a theoretical synthesis and policy framework. *Theory and Society*, 27(2), 151–208. https://doi .org/10.1023/A:1006884930135

Yadav, S. K. (2021). Self-Help Group (SHG) and COVID-19: Response to migrant crisis in Haryana, India during the pandemic. *Social Work with Groups*, 44(2), 152–158. https://doi.org/10.1080/01609513.2020.1805974

Chapter 2

Introducing the data

Secondary and primary sources

2.1 Introduction

The analysis of the study is based on two sources of data. The first part of the analysis is undertaken using the National Family Health Survey (NFHS) data set. Given the limits on the information available in the data set, we have supplemented the analysis with a field survey undertaken in six districts of Bihar. A mixed-method design was employed to collect information about networks at the grass-roots level.

2.2 Secondary data source

2.2.1 National Family Health Survey data

The secondary data for the analysis undertaken in Chapter 3 was obtained from the fifth round of NFHS, an Indian variant of the Demographic and Health Survey (DHS), which was conducted between 2019 and 2021 in all the Indian states and Union Territories. DHS has been conducting surveys to provide estimates of various socio-demographic and population health indicators in over 90 countries in regular intervals since 1984. In India, various rounds of NFHS have been collecting data on different indicators of fertility, mortality, nuptiality, maternal and child health, and nutritional status based on a nationally representative sample since 1992-93. The fifth round of the survey collected information from 636,699 households, 724,115 women aged 15–49 years (out of which 512,408 women were currently married at the time of survey), and 232,920 children under five years. In the state module, the sample sizes were 76,910 for current women and 35,622 for children born during the five years preceding the survey. The data set is accessible after obtaining requisite permission and approval from the MEASURE-DHS archive (www.dhsprogram.com).

DOI: 10.4324/9781003499251-2

2.2.2 Profile of the respondents

The sample profile of the study population is given in Table 2.1. The mean age of the respondents was similar in the all-India sample and the sample of Bihar. However, the mean years of schooling were nearly three years higher for the respondents representing all-India compared to those from Bihar. Women's wage-earning sector activities were found to be substantially lower in Bihar (10.37%) compared to their counterparts representing overall India (17.14%). The proportion of Muslims was somewhat higher in Bihar (19.94%) compared to overall India (78.67%), proportion of respondents who reported other religious affiliations (than Hindu or Muslim) was found to be higher in the all-India sample (4.59%) compared to Bihar (0.30%). The percentage of respondents belonging to OBC was observed to be higher in Bihar (54.20%) compared to all-India, while percentages of SC/ST and General castes were higher. As expected, being an economically underdeveloped state, the normalized mean wealth score of the respondent's households (on a scale of 0–100) was 36.26, while for overall India it was 49.12. Further, respondents in Bihar were predominantly from rural areas (about 85%) compared to overall India (about 72%).

Table 2.1 Sample profile of women who have delivered their last child during five years preceding the survey, NFHS-5, 2019–21

Background characteristics	India	Bihar
Mean age of respondents	27.11 (±5.04)	26.40 (±5.23)
Mean completed years of schooling of respondents	8.05 (±5.19)	5.25 (±5.25)
Respondents were working in any wage-earning sector preceding 12 months of the survey (in percent)	17.14	10.37
Religious affiliation (in percent)		
Hindu	78.67	79.76
Muslim	16.73	19.94
Others	4.59	0.30
Affiliation to social group (in percent)		
General caste	18.08	15.94
SC/ST	32.35	29.85
OBC	49.57	54.20
Normalised mean wealth Score (0–100)	49.12 (±19.57)	36.26 (±16.62)
Type of place of residence (in percent)		
Urban	27.73	15.09
Rural	72.27	84.91
Total number of cases	**26.552**	**2,036**

Source: Estimated from unit-level data of NFHS-5 by the authors.
Note: Values in parenthesis indicate standard deviation.

2.3 Primary data source

2.3.1 Sampling strategy

A multi-stage sampling design was adopted in the present study. In the first stage, we selected 13 districts out of 38 districts of Bihar, where the JEEViKA Technical Support Programme (JTSP) and Health and Nutrition Strategy Programme (HNS) were in place during the last five years preceding the survey. In the second stage, these 13 districts were classified into three tercile groups based on a composite index of human development indicators, namely, percentages of non-SC/ST population, female literacy, and male non-agricultural labourers – using data from the 2011 census. In the third stage, two districts from each tercile group were selected randomly. The selected districts are arranged accordingly – Nalanda and Saharsha for the bottom tercile; Begusarai and Muzaffarpur from the middle tercile; and Purba Champaran and Katihar from the upper tercile (see Figure 2.1). Thus, a total of six districts were selected for the study (Table 2.2).

After the selection of the study districts, i.e., at the fourth stage, four community development blocks were selected in each district based on the implementation of the JTSP and HNS programme. Two blocks were selected randomly where JTSP and HNS programme had been implemented during the last five years, while another two blocks were also selected randomly

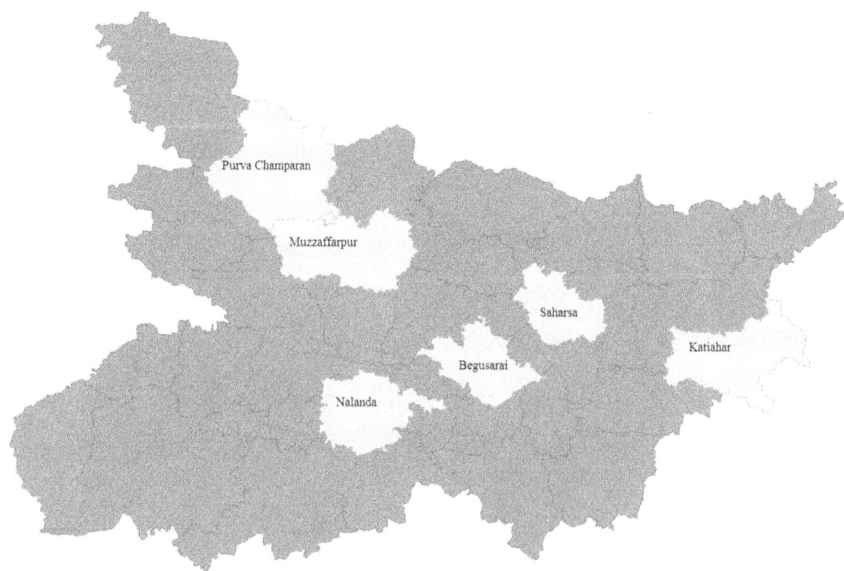

Figure 2.1 Map of Bihar showing survey districts.

Table 2.2 Selection of districts

Rank	District	FLIT[a]	FCPOP[b]	MALENONAG[c]	Index
1	Nawada	46.70	72.95	41.23	53.63
2	Saharsa	39.20	82.21	42.75	54.72
3	Gopalganj	53.99	84.84	29.39	56.07
4	Patna	51.04	79.95	43.91	58.30
5	Nalanda	50.24	77.01	48.58	58.61
6	Samastipur	50.63	81.02	46.99	59.55
7	Muzaffarpur	52.27	83.52	44.09	59.96
8	Begusarai	52.68	84.50	42.85	60.01
9	Pashchim Champaran	42.46	78.25	60.18	60.29
10	Khagaria	48.30	84.73	49.30	60.78
11	Purba Champaran	43.41	86.70	55.30	61.80
12	Purnia	39.28	83.57	63.93	62.26
13	Katihar	41.59	85.51	63.51	63.54

Source: Calculated from Office of the Registrar General and Census Commissioner, India (2011), by the authors.
Notes:
a. FLIT (Percent of females who are literate): 100 × (Literate female/Female pop aged above 7 years).
b. FCPOP (Percentage of non-SC and ST population): 100 * (Population − SC and ST population)/ population.
c. MALENONAG (Percentage of male non-agricultural workers in male workforce): 100 − Male Agricultural Main & Marginal workers as percentage of Total Male Main workers.

from the rest of the blocks. Thus, altogether 24 (= 6 × 4) blocks were selected from the study districts.

In the fifth stage, five villages from each block were selected by employing the probability proportional to size sampling (PPS) method. As the name suggests, in the PPS method, the likelihood of selecting large villages is higher, compared to relatively smaller villages. This ensures capturing adequate socio-economic variations in the study samples and helps in the generalisation of results from the study. Thus, a total of 120 villages (= 6 districts × 4 blocks × 5 villages) were selected. In the last stage, 20 women comprising ten JEEViKA members and ten non-members were selected from each village. Thus, the total sample size of the study stands at 2400 (= 6 districts × 4 blocks × 5 villages × 20 respondents). The final list of blocks and districts is given in Table A2.1. As some villages may "vanish" over time – due to changes in the flow of the river, dwindling population, renaming, etc. – an additional village was identified for each block.

During the pilot study, we found that some women were averse to admit that they are associated with any JEEViKA in the presence of other family members. Such behaviour may be attributed to social restrictions on mobility outside the domain of the household and barriers to engage in community-based activities by housewives. Identifying JEEViKA members through a process of house listing is likely to magnify the self-selection problem. As a result, we dropped the idea of house listing and had to choose JEEViKA members and non-members randomly. The recruitment criterion was that the respondent had at least one living child aged below three years, and was a permanent resident of the village.

2.3.2 Survey instruments

Data were collected by a trained group of field investigators (Figure 2.2) using three questionnaires:

(i)   *Village questionnaire*: Used to collect information about the demographic profile and health facilities of the village.
(ii) *Individual questionnaire*: This was the main survey instrument. The questionnaire elicited information on the individual characteristics of the respondent, adoption of maternal and child best practices, persons motivating the adoption of such practices, and consumption practices of the respondent and her children aged below three years.
(iii) *Informant questionnaire*: A third questionnaire recorded information on the motivator and the person who motivated the motivator. This was originally undertaken to devise an instrument for resolving the endogeneity issues related to identifying peer effects (Manski, 2013), and follows the method adopted by recent studies (Bramoullé et al., 2009; Lin, 2010; Hoffman, 2017).

The questionnaires were pre-tested on 100 respondents at Vaishali village, in Vaishali district on 23 December 2019, followed by a feedback session.

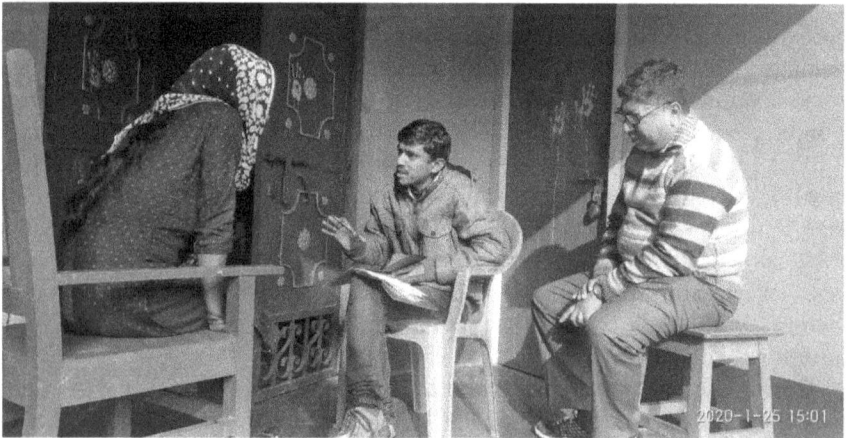

Figure 2.2 Interviewing respondents in Muzaffarpur.
Source: Author.

Before administering the questionnaires, investigators obtained verbal informed consent from the study participants by reading out a statement explaining why the study was being conducted and guaranteeing that the information provided by the participants would be kept confidential and used only for research purposes. Moreover, the voluntary nature of participation in the study was emphasised in the statement of informed consent (Figure 2.3).

In order to control data quality, the Principal and Co-Investigators monitored and cross-checked data collection activities during the field survey through periodic field visits. The data was edited at the field level by Supervisors.

The entered data was cleaned by identifying mismatched and unmatched entries and verified from the original questionnaire. In some cases, where responses were incomplete or inconsistent, a telephonic resurvey was undertaken from June to July 2020.

2.3.3 Revisions in sampling strategy and data collection

As mentioned before, the pilot survey was undertaken in the last week of December 2019. The main survey was initiated in the first week of January 2020 and was progressing smoothly. The qualitative data collection was planned for the last week of March 2020.

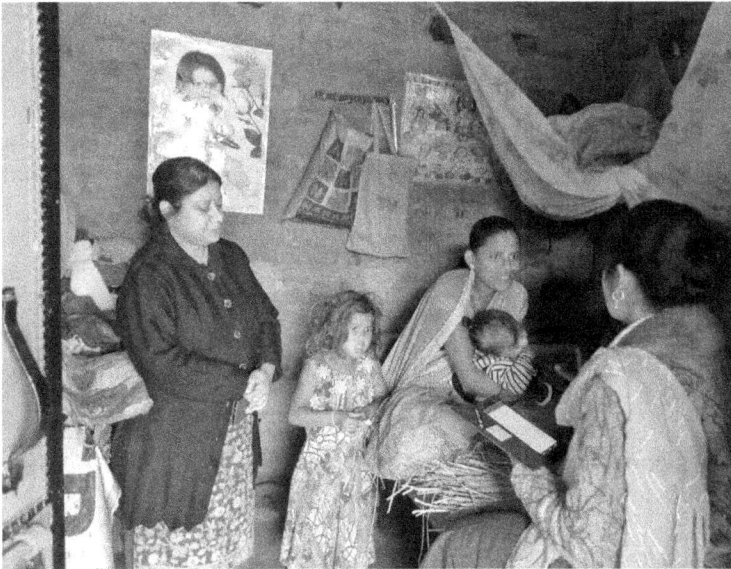

Figure 2.3 Interviewers were supervised by investigators.

Source: Author.

Unfortunately, in March, the outbreak of COVID-19 in India disrupted the survey schedule. The announcement of the national-level lockdown forced us to abandon the quantitative data collection before it could be completed. After cleaning the data and resurveying some respondents we had information on 2250 out of a planned 2400 respondents (i.e., 93.75% of the survey had been completed). As a resumption of the field survey would entail retraining, and lead to a delay in completion of the study, we decided not to resume the survey but analyse the data collected so far.

2.4 Sample profile

2.4.1 About the villages

The health situation is, in general comparatively better in Nalanda and Begusarai, and poor in Purva Champaran (Table A2.2). The sptial distribution of health infrastructure and personnel has been analysed using choropleth maps (Appendices A2.1–A2.4).The maps reveals that the per capita availability of health institutions and auxiliary nurse midwives (ANMs) is highest in Nalanda and lowest in Purva Champaran. The presence of Accredited Social Health Activists (ASHAs) is highest in Katiahar. Despite its proximity to Patna, Nalanda has low per capita ASHA and poor coverage under the Janani Suraksha Yojana (JSY).

Table A2.3 represents the characteristics of the villages in the study districts of Bihar. The table documents the religion, caste membership, occupational profile, educational attainments, and mean age at first marriage of females of the villages in the six districts of Saharsa, Nalanda, Muzaffarpur, Begusarai, Purba Champaran, and Katihar.

Hinduism is the largest religious tradition followed in the state, with 92.11% of the villages having Hinduism as the majority religion, followed by Islam (7.02%) and *Others* (0.88%). Among the study districts, Hinduism is the most followed religion in all of the villages of Saharsa and Nalanda, and Hindus dominate in a majority of the villages in the other four districts as well. Religions falling within the *Others* category are dominant only in Katihar, in 5.56% of the villages.

More than half of the villages have the Other Backward Classes as the majority caste, with a total of 56.14%, followed by SCs (at 23.68%), the General category (at 18.42%), and STs at (1.75%). The presence of STs is predominant in the district of Katihar (11.11% of the villages), whereas, villages having the General category as the majority caste are concentrated in the district of Nalanda (45%).

The study found that the households in the state were engaged in different kinds of occupations, which have been clubbed under four categories – cultivators, agricultural labourers, non-agricultural wage earners, and persons employed in petty businesses or self-employed. The highest percentage of villages in the state has cultivators as the main occupational category (46.49%).

The presence of agricultural labourers as the majority occupational category is highest in the district of Purba Champaran (77.78% villages), and that of non-agricultural wage labourers is highest in Muzaffarpur (55% villages). The self-employed category is concentrated in Purba Champaran district only, in 5.56 of the villages.

In terms of female literacy, only 0.88% of the villages have "no education" among females on average, and only the district of Saharsa has some villages (5%) falling under this category. Almost two-thirds (63.16%) of the villages have the average level of completed education of females at the secondary or madhyamik level, with Purba Champaran district having the highest (94.44%) and Katihar district having the lowest (5.56%) proportion of villages at this level. The percentage of villages with average female educational qualification of Class 12 and above is not very high in any of the districts, with Katihar having no such village.

The mean age at first marriage for females is at the legal age of marriage, that is 18 years, for two-thirds (66.67%) of the villages in the state, with the highest concentration being in Begusarai district (94.44%). The highest percentage of villages with females having their mean age at first marriage between 15 and 17 years can be observed in Saharsa (70%), whereas in Katihar, the mean age at first marriage is between 19 and 22 years in 38.89% of the villages.

The average mean age at marriage for the state is 18.04 years. Awareness-generating health camps on maternal and neonatal care were not held in 94.74% of the villages in the six months preceding the survey. The mean number of such camps in this period in and around the villages is 0.11.

Table A2.4 shows the percentage of villages within the study districts which have different types of childcare centres, hospitals, and healthcare centres, such as Integrated Child Development Services or ICDS and Anganwadi centres, primary health centres, community and rural healthcare centres, government hospitals, government dispensaries, private clinics, private nursing homes, and AYUSH centres. This table also represents the issue of accessibility of the villages to these healthcare facilities and the average distance to each of these facilities from the villages.

It can be observed that almost all the villages (99.12) have ICDS or Anganwadi centres, and 0.88% of villages have year-round access to such centres. All the villages either have APHC centres or have access to them. It is the same scenario with regard to private clinics, private hospitals, or nursing homes, and AYUSH centres. No village has a district or government hospital; however, almost all of them (98.25%) have access to these. The presence of government dispensaries is also quite low in the villages, with 7.02% of the villages having such subsidised dispensaries.

The mean distance from the villages to district or government hospitals is the highest, at 28.42 km. ICDS or Anganwadi centres are the nearest to the villages, within an average of 1 km.

Table 2.3 Availability of front-line health workers (FLHWs)

Health provider	Percentage of village with FLHWs	Mean number in village
ICDS/Anganwadi	99.12	5.04
ASHA	100.00	4.85
Trained birth attendant (TBA)	7.02	1.50
Auxiliary nurse midwife (ANM)	88.60	1.13
Lady doctor	10.53	1.00
Private doctor	7.02	2.13

Source: Calculated from primary survey data.

2.4.2 Healthcare facilities and availability of front-line health workers (FLHWs) in survey sites

Table 2.3 represents the provisions for different types of healthcare providers in the study villages. The coverage of ICDS and Anganwadi workers is almost full, with 99.12% of the villages having such workers. With Accredited Social Health Activist or ASHA workers it is a similar situation, with all of the villages having ASHA workers. The percentage of villages having auxiliary nurse midwives (ANM) is also quite high, at 88.60%. This is followed by the presence of female doctors (in 10.53% of the villages), and trained birth attendants and private doctors (both in 7.02% of the villages).

Among the different healthcare personnel, the average number of ICDS or Anganwadi workers is the highest (5.04), the second highest being that of ASHA workers (4.85), followed by private doctors (2.13).

2.4.3 Respondent profile

Table A2.5 shows the mean for various socio-demographic characteristics of the respondents in the six study districts. The total sample size is 2250. Out of them, 1124 respondents are SHG members and 1126 respondents are non-members.

From the table, we can observe that the SHG members group is associated with estimated mean years of age of 26.91. By comparison, the non-members group is associated with numerically lesser mean years of age, that is, 24.11. The table shows that the mean number of children ever born for respondents who are SHG members is 3.37, and it is 2.31 for non-members. The mean number of living children of the respondents is 3.19 and 2.22 for SHG members and non-members, respectively. The mean of completed years of schooling of the respondents is 4.29 years for SHG members and 5.73 years for non-members. The SHG group is associated with an asset index score of 0.002, and the non-SHG group is by comparison associated with a numerically higher asset index score of 0.03. We can therefore observe that SHG members are older, have given birth to more children, have more living children, have studied less, and are less affluent in terms of asset holding than non-members. However, after conducting the respective *t*-tests, we can say that such differences are significant at a 5% level only for age, number of children, number of living children, and years of education. There is no statistically significant difference between the asset index scores of SHG members and non-members, even at a 10% level.

Table A2.6 attempts to understand the association of the socio-economic profile of the respondents with the incidence of them being SHG members or non-members.

The table shows that the share of respondents who are part of SHGs is the highest for the age group 26–30 years, at 43.87%, whereas, the share of respondents who are non-members is the highest for the age group 21–25 years, at 52.14%. Almost half of the respondents (44.80%) from the total sample fall within the 21–25 age group as well.

With regard to the household size of the sample, we can observe that the share of respondents belonging to 5–7 member households is the highest for both SHG members (89.25%) and non-members (83.63%). The percentage of respondents belonging to households with eight members or more is quite low for both SHG members and non-members, and the total percentage of such respondents is also low (0.40%).

As far as literacy is concerned, the table shows that almost half of the SHG members (41.65%) are non-literate and more than one-third (38.52%) of the non-members have 6–10 years of education as the highest educational level.

The occupational profile of the respondents shows that the highest percentage (85.47%) of the respondents are unemployed, and 2.09% have reported themselves as house workers. The percentage of unemployed respondents who are SHG members is 80.02, and it is 90.93 for non-members. Agricultural labour is the second most common occupation of the respondents, with 5.02% of the respondents falling under this category. For SHG members, the percentage is higher, at 7.19%, whereas, for non-members, it is 2.85%.

If we look at the occupational profile of the respondents' husbands, the highest percentage is that of non-agricultural wage labour (38.12%), followed by wage and salaried employees (17.65%). Among SHG members, 39.54% of the respondents reported that their husbands worked as non-agricultural wage labourers, whereas it is 36.70% for non-members.

On the basis of their asset index, the respondents have been grouped under low, middle, and high asset index groups. The table shows that there is not much difference in the share of SHG members and non-members within the three groups.

The respondents from our sample have been grouped into four socio-religious categories, that is, SC/ST-Hindu, OBC-Hindu, UC-Hindu, and Muslims/others. From the table, we can observe that the share of respondents belonging to the OBC-Hindu category is the highest for both SHG members (53.37%) and non-members (55.78%). It is also the highest for the total sample (54.58%), followed by UC-Hindus (31.24%), Muslims/others (7.96%), and SC/ST-Hindus (6.22%).

The table also shows the proportion of SHG members and non-members from each of the six study districts. The share of SHG members is the same, that is, 15.54%, for the districts – Purba Champaran, Katihar, and Begusarai. The share of non-members is also the same for these three districts, at 15.57%. Again, the districts Muzaffarpur, Nalanda, and Saharsha have an almost similar share of SHG members, at 17.76% each for Muzaffarpur and Saharsha and 17.85% for Nalanda. The percentage of non-members is also similar for these districts – that is, 17.79 for both Muzaffarpur and Saharsha, and 17.70 for Nalanda.

In order to understand whether there is any statistically significant association between the above characteristics of the respondents and their membership or non-membership to SHGs, respective chi-square tests were conducted. From the results, we can conclude that, at a 5% level of significance, the age groups of respondents, household size, educational levels, occupational profiles of both respondents and their husbands, and socio-religious categories have statistically significant associations with the respondents being SHG members or non-members. There is no statistically significant association between SHG membership and asset index groups as well as with being residents of the six districts.

2.5 Qualitative information

The quantitative data analysis was supplemented by a qualitative survey. Originally planned for March to April 2020, it was rescheduled to December 2020 due to COVID-19. The qualitative survey had three components:

- Focus group discussions (FGDs),
- Social network analysis (SNA), and
- Short interviews with Accredited Social Health Activists (ASHAs) in survey sites.

Details of FGDs and SNA are discussed in Sections 2.5.1 and 2.5.2.

2.5.1 Focus group discussions

FGDs involve gathering 8–12 people from similar backgrounds or experiences together to discuss a specific topic of interest, while the discussion is moderated by the researcher (Kitzinger, 1994; Cornwall & Jewkes, 1995; Morgan, 1996; Israel et al., 1998; Hayward, Simpson, and Wood, 2004). FGDs are loosely structured discussions where questions are asked about the perceptions, attitudes, beliefs, opinions, or ideas of participants. Unlike other research methods, FGDs encourage discussion and interactions between participants. FGDs allow participants to agree or disagree with each other. It provides an insight into how a group thinks about the research issue, sheds light on the range of opinions and ideas within the community being studied, and highlights the inconsistencies and variations in beliefs, experiences, and practices of the members. Thus, FGDs allow researchers to supplement quantitative data analysis by exploring the meanings of results that cannot be explained statistically.

Participant identification is an important issue when conducting FGDs. Recruitment can be expensive, difficult, and continues to be a source of contentious debate (Krueger & Casey, 2000). Although approaches to participant recruitment are contested, the underlying consideration should be the impact on the discussion. Researchers can use different methods to recruit suitable participants, including recruitment questionnaires and telephone, or door-to-door canvassing. Furthermore, participants can be recruited by offering incentives or through local networks and contacts (Krueger, 1994). However, the use of local contacts has been criticised for its dependence on the availability, willingness, and accessibility of the local contact and the loss of control and direction of the researcher in the recruitment process. This can lead to convenience sampling by selecting participants based on their accessibility (Krueger, 1994), leading to volunteer bias. Purposive sampling is widely recommended since focus group discussion relies on the ability and capacity of participants to provide relevant information (Morgan, 1988).

Another important consideration is the number of respondents to be invited for discussion. Although it is generally accepted that between six and eight participants are sufficient (Krueger and Casey, 2000), some studies have reported as few as four and as many as 15 participants (Fern, 1982; Nyumba et al., 2018). One potential drawback in a focus group discussion is the lack of guarantee that all those recruited will attend the discussion. To overcome this, Rabiee (2004) recommends that researchers may over-recruit by 10–25%. Ten participants are therefore considered large enough to gain a variety of perspectives and small enough not to become disorderly or fragmented (Krueger, 1994). With more than 12 members, the group becomes difficult to manage and may disintegrate into two or even three smaller groups, each having their own independent discussion.

FGDs were held in the first week of December 2020. Given constraints on safe travelling, we did not undertake FGDs in Saharsha and Katihar. Three FGDs were held in each of the remaining four districts. Details are given in Table 2.4. Given the need to maintain social distancing, we restricted the number of participants to eight members. Participants were recruited from married women who had children. There was no age criterion but at least two participants in each group had children below three years. Field staff was also instructed to ensure that at least two participants were JEEViKA members. Although some researchers suggest that a series of FGDs with the same group should be held till the discussion gets exhausted, this was not

Table 2.4 Details of FGDs held

District	Block	Village	Participants	JEEViKA
Purba Champaran	Mehsi	Jhitkaiya	8	3
		Rajepur	8	4
	Tetariya	Mohammadpur Sagar	8	4
		Bahuragopisingh	8	4
Muzaffarpur	Gaighat	Kanta Piraucha	8	4
		Lachman Nagar	8	4
Begusarai	Barauni	Singhdaha	8	3
		Jamina	8	4
Nalanda	Chandi	Sartha	8	3
		Birnawan	8	3
	Bihar Sharif	Meghi	8	3
		Tetrawan	8	4

Source: Primary survey data.

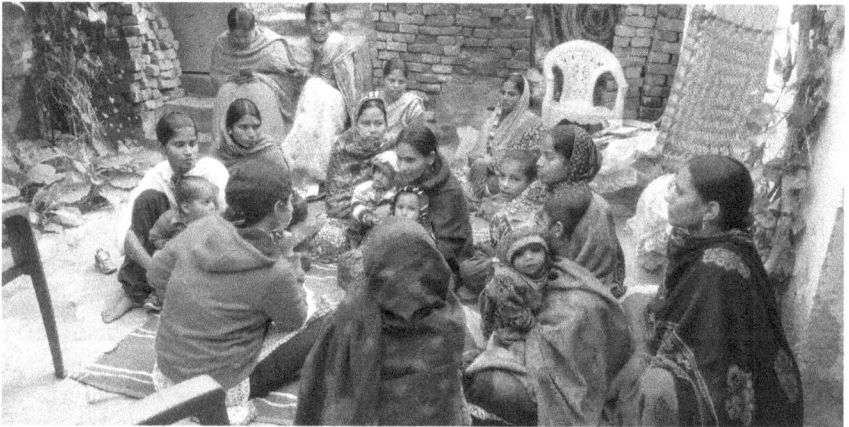

Figure 2.4 Focus group discussion at Nalanda.

feasible at the time of the survey. We held only one meeting with each group; in keeping with standard practice, it was held within the village in normal and familiar settings where participants would be psychologically comfortable (Figure 2.4). The details of FGDs are reported in Table 2.4.

2.5.2 Social network analysis

Finally, in order to understand the social relationships leading to information flow about MCH practices being studied, the structure of such relationships, and identify key players in such information flow we have used SNA.

It comprises preparing sociograms disclosing patterns of inter-relationships, examining their structural properties, and analysing implications for social implications (Scott, 2017). To understand the nature of information flows, we prepared 12 network maps in the four districts where qualitative interviews were undertaken.

In planning a network study, issues of sampling, population, and network boundary are to be considered. In general, two types of network analysis may be performed – complete networks, or ego networks. When studying complete networks, all possible links between members belonging to a population are identified. This is often a complex and time-consuming task, involving the delineation of the network boundary. However, it enables the analysis of network features like centralization and density.

As the network mapping had to be done during the COVID-19 pandemic, we opted to trace ego networks. In this case, a starting node (ego) is randomly identified, and alters (connecting nodes) are identified. Snowball sampling (Bryman, 2008) is often used to identify the starting nodes, with the first person approached being asked to identify other starting nodes. Normally, ego networks are continued using snowballing, until saturation occurs, with names being repeated (Bryman, 2008). There are several limitations of snowball sampling, with the bias being an important issue (Scott, 2017). It implies that the network structure depends upon the choice of the ego. Further, time and resource constraints limit the "rolling of the snowball" till the complete network is uncovered. Alternately, several individuals may be asked to define the population boundary, and networks between all the identified members traced (Laumann et al., 1989; Wasserman & Faust, 1994). Using actors to trace out the network boundaries crucially depends upon identifying people with a comprehensive understanding of the network, and who can offer a reliable picture of the network members (Prell, 2012). Given the limited mobility and low levels of awareness of women in rural Bihar, the adoption of this approach is fraught with risks. We, therefore, adopted a nominalist approach (Prell, 2012), using our research questions to define the population of egos. Given our focus on MCH outcomes, the population was defined as currently married women with at least one child aged below three years. We randomly selected 12 egos (three from each of the four districts where FGDs were undertaken) from this population. The geographical variation in starting nodes enabled us to compare networks and their characteristics, facilitating generalisation of our conclusions.

Although the egos were clearly defined, the alters could be any person in the village, or even outside it. So using a roster to identify links with the ego (Prell et al., 2008) was not feasible. In such cases, the free-recall method is widely used – particularly when studying ego networks where the boundary is not known. This method asks the respondent to identify alters based on the recall method (Wellman & Wortley, 1990).[1] In such cases, limits may be imposed on the number of alters that may be identified; it is referred to as the fixed-choice approach (Coleman et al., 1966). A problem with this method is that we end with incomplete or inaccurate data that offers a limited view of the network, leading to measurement errors (Wasserman & Faust, 1994). We, therefore, decided to allow respondents to list as many alters as they wanted – the free choice approach.

A schedule was used to collect the network data. Respondents were asked, "From whom did you obtain information about …". In four cases, the information was with respect to antenatal care (ANC) services, in four cases it was with respect to institutional delivery and postnatal care (PNC) services, and in four cases, information related to child immunization and nutrition. After the name-generating question – to identify persons with whom the respondent had the link – we sought information on attributes (gender, caste, education, whether JEEViKA member, and nature of the relationship). We collected data on directed ties that considered the direction of information flow between actors. It provides information on both the existence of ties between actors, but also on who initiated the link. It is, therefore, a richer form of data than undirected ties that trace only the existence of links. Further, directed data has the advantage that it may be used to generate both directed and undirected network maps. The data is recorded in a binary format (= 0 for no tie, = 1 for a tie). It is also possible to assign values to the strength of ties, by getting respondents to rank actors. This method, however, leads to measurement-related errors and was avoided.[2]

An important decision is whether to trace the complete network, or to draw a sample and use it to make inferences about the entire network. While complete enumeration is viable in the case of small networks, it may not be a feasible option when studying large-scale networks. For instance, a village with a population of 500 persons would generate 124,750 links – making analysis extremely computer-intensive. In the case of quantitative data, it is possible to draw a random sampling through methods satisfying certain statistical properties and use it to draw inferences about the general population. Analogously, studying part of a complete network – by drawing a representative sample of individuals and mapping links between them – and generalising findings to the complete system may appear a reasonable strategy. Unfortunately, relational sampling may not always work with network data – a representative sample of actors may not always yield an accurate "partial" network capturing the entire system (Alba, 1982). One reason is the huge loss of data, making the identification of most structural features difficult. Burt (1987) estimates that the data lost through relational sampling is 100 – k, where k is the sample as a proportion of the population. The problem gets magnified in the presence of non-response and missing data. In such cases, snowball sampling to generate egocentric networks has been suggested as a viable alternative (Frank, 1978, 1979). Although the structure revealed through snowball samples is "inbuilt" into the sampling method, Frank (2011) shows that such partial networks may reveal important properties of the original network. Such sampling is suitable when the connected segment traced is representative of other segments of the network.

Given field-level constraints, the network was followed up to four levels, including the starting level. As a result, the complete network was not revealed. Apart from the need to complete the survey without much travelling and interaction, our decision may also be justified on empirical grounds. When data on ego networks were collected, we found that grass-roots health workers played a major role in information dissemination; any attempt to trace the network quickly ended with such persons, so that the network structure was very sparsely populated, and terminated within three layers. In such cases, even a partial view of the network may reveal its underlying nature, as all segments of the system are similar in nature.

The resulting network information was entered as adjacency matrices. It is a case-by-case binary matrix, indicating the existence of ties between egos (in rows) and alters (in columns). A particular cell (ij) gives the tie between the ith alter and jth ego. The presence of a tie is indicated by a value of one, with all diagonal cells being zero. As we are using directed data, the matrix will not be symmetrical; in the case of undirected data, the adjacency matrix is symmetrical. We had 12 such matrices from four districts. The three networks from each district collected data on information dissemination for ANC services, institutional delivery, PNC services, and child health, respectively.

Given the practical limitations of studying the complete network present in a village during the pandemic, we randomly identified starting nodes (egos) in 12 villages and identified their ego networks using snowball sampling. The egos were recruited from currently married women who had children aged below three years, and who were permanent residents of the village after their marriage. Data collection was constrained by:

(i) The low literacy levels of respondents and their reluctance to provide information about sources of information,
(ii) In most cases saturation was reached as ego identified grass-roots health workers as their source of information,
(iii) Difficulties of tracking an alter because his/her mobile number was not known to the ego,
(iv) The alter was not present in the village at the time of the survey, and
(v) The alter resided outside the village being surveyed.

As a result, some networks, which were too sparse, had to be discarded. Other networks were followed up to four levels (alter of alter of alter of starting node). Table 2.5 provides details of the eight networks that were retained for analysis.

Information was collected on relational data (which provided information about MCH practices to the agent) and attributes like age, gender, caste,

Table 2.5 Details of egocentric networks

District	Block	Village	Information about	Map no.
Purba Champaran	Mehsi	Jhitkaiya	ANC services	1
		Rajepur	Institutional delivery (ID) and PNC services	*
	Tetariya	Mohammadpur Sagar	Child immunization and nutrition	*
		Bahuragopisingh	ANC services	2
Muzaffarpur	Gaighat	Kanta Piraucha	ID and PNC services	3
		Lachman Nagar	Child immunization and nutrition	4
Begusarai	Barauni	Singhdaha	ANC services	*
		Jamina	ID and PNC services	5
Nalanda	Chandi	Sartha	Child immunization and nutrition	6
		Birnawan	ANC services	7
	Bihar Sharif	Meghi	ID and PNC services	*
		Tetrawan	Child immunization and nutrition	8

Source: Primary survey data.
Note: Maps marked with * were not analysed formally due to their sparse nature.

education, whether JEEViKA member, and relation with ego. The adjacency matrices were mapped using attribute matrices, and their features analysed using UCINET (Borgatti et al., 2002).

2.6 Short interviews with ASHAs

In six of the villages where FGDs were conducted, we also spoke to the ASHAs about their experience in communicating with the villagers and the constraints faced by them. This discussion was in the form of unstructured interviews.

Notes

1 Use of recall method often leads to noise as respondents may not recall with same degree of accuracy; there may also be differences in perceptions about who constitutes the alter. Such errors are likely to be negligible given the nature of our research question. However, missing data may be a problem if a node cannot be traced because he/she resides in a different village, or because he/she is temporarily absent from the survey site.
2 Participants are forced into dividing actors into exclusive categories, when she would prefer to place several actors in the same rank category (Prell, 2012).

References

Alba, R. (1982). Taking stock of network analysis: A decade's results. In *Research in the sociology of organizations*. New Emerald[MS1] Insight.

Borgatti, S.P., Everett, M.G., & Freeman, L. C. (2002). *Ucinet for windows: Software for social network analysis*. Analytic Technologies.

Bramoullé, Y., Djebbari, H., & Fortin, B. (2009). Identification of peer effects through social networks. *Journal of Econometrics*, *150*(1), 41–55. http://doi.org.10.1016/j.jeconom.2008.12.021

Bryman, A. (2008). *Social research methods*. Oxford University Press.

Burt, R. S. (1987). A note on missing network data in the general social survey. *Social Networks*, *9*(1), 63–73. http://doi.org.10.1016/0378-8733(87)90018-9

Coleman, J. S., Katz, E., & Menzel, E. (1966). *Medical innovations: A diffusion study*. Bobs-Merrill Company Inc.

Cornwall, A., & Jewkes, R. (1995). What is participatory research? *Social Science & Medicine*, *41*(12), 1667–1676. http://doi.org.10.1016/0277-9536(95)00127-S

Fern, E. F. (1982). The use of focus groups for idea generation: The effects of group size, acquaintanceship, and moderator on response quantity and quality. *Journal of Marketing Research*, *19*(1), p. 1. http://doi.org.10.2307/3151525

Frank, O. (1978). Sampling and estimation in large social networks. *Social Networks*, *1*(1), 91–101. http://doi.org.10.1016/0378-8733(78)90015-1

Frank, O. (1979). Estimation of population totals by use of snowball samples. In Holland P, and Leinhardt S (eds) *Perspectives on social networks* (pp. 319–347). Academic Press.

Frank, O. (2011). Survey sampling in networks. In J. SCott & P. J. Carrington (Eds.), *The SAGE handbook of social network analysis* (pp. 389–403). Sage Publications Inc.

Hayward, C., Simpson, L., & Wood, L. (2004). Still left out in the cold: Problematising Participatory research and development. *Sociologia Ruralis*, *44*(1), 95–108. http://doi.org.10.1111/j.1467-9523.2004.00264.x

Hoffman, R. (2017). *Following the peers: The role of social networks for health care utilization in the Philippines*. 17/2017. http://hdl.handle.net/10419/184845

International Institute of Population Sciences. (2017). *National family health survey –4, state fact sheet Bihar*. International Institute for Population Sciences.

Israel, B. A. et al. (1998). Review of community-based research: Assessing partnership approaches to improve public health. *Annual Review of Public Health*, *19*(1), 173–202. http://doi.org.10.1146/annurev.publhealth.19.1.173

Kitzinger, J. (1994). The methodology of focus groups: The importance of interaction between research participants. *Sociology of Health and Illness*, *16*(1), 103–121. http://doi.org.10.1111/1467-9566.ep11347023

Krueger, R. A. (1994). *Focus groups: A practical guide for practical research*. Sage Publications Inc.

Krueger, R. A., & Casey, M. A. (2000). *Focus groups: A practical guide for applied research* (4th ed.). Sage Publications Inc.

Laumann, E. O., Marsden, P., & Prensky, D. (1989). The boundary specification problem in network analysis. In L. C. Freeman, D. WHite, & A. K. Romney (Eds.), *Research methods in social network analysis* (pp. 61–88). George Mason University Press.

Lin, X. (2010). Identifying peer effects in student academic achievement by spatial autoregressive models with group unobservables. *Journal of Labor Economics*, *28*(4), 825–860. http://doi.org.10.1086/653506

Manski, C. F. (2013). *Public policy in an uncertain world: Analysis and decisions*. Harvard University Press.

Morgan, D. L. (1988). *Focus group as qualitative research*. Sage Publications Inc.

Morgan, D. L. (1996). Focus groups. *Annual Review of Sociology*, *22*(1), 129–152. http://doi.org.10.1146/annurev.soc.22.1.129

Nyumba, T. O. et al. (2018). The use of focus group discussion methodology: Insights from two decades of application in conservation. *Methods in Ecology and Evolution*, *9*(1), 20–32. http://doi.org.10.1111/2041-210X.12860

Office of the Registrar General and Census Commissioner, India. (2011) *Primary census abstract: India, 2011*. Ministry of Home Affairs, Govt. of India.

Prell, C. et al. (2008). "Who's in the network?" When stakeholders influence data analysis. *Systemic Practice and Action Research*, *21*(6), 443–458. http://doi.org.10.1007/s11213-008-9105-9

Prell, C. (2012). *Social network analysis: History, theory and methodology*. Sage Publications.

Rabiee, F. (2004). Focus-group interview and data analysis. *Proceedings of the Nutrition Society*, *63*(4), 655–660. http://doi.org.10.1079/PNS2004399

Scott, J. (2017). *Social network analysis* (4 ed.). Sage Publications Inc.

Wasserman, S., & Faust, F. (1994). *Social network analysis: Methods and applications*. Cambridge University Press.

Wellman, B., & Wortley, S. (1990). Different strokes from different folks: Community ties and social support. *American Journal of Sociology*, *96*(3), 558–588. http://www.jstor.org/stable/2781064

Appendix

ANM per lakh population

[8 : 11] (11)
[12 : 17] (15)
[18 : 27] (12)

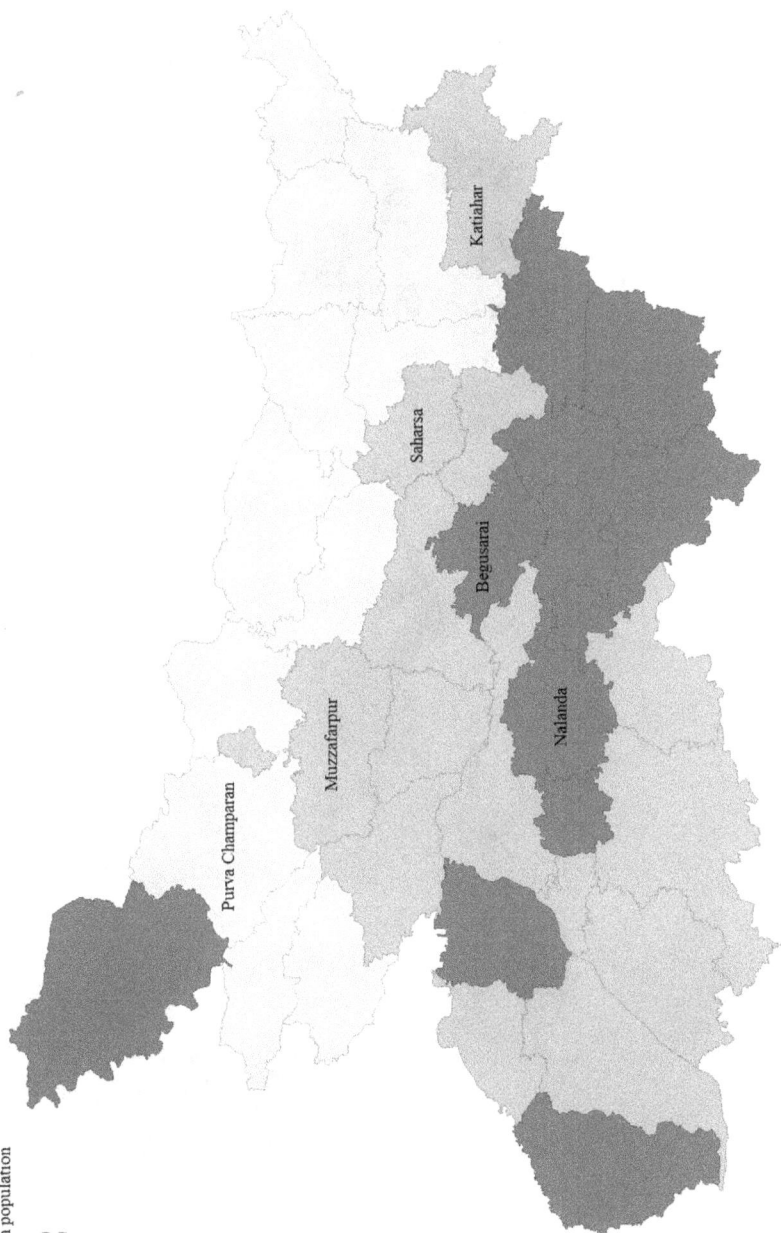

Figure A2.1 ANMs per lakh population.

Sources: Authors.

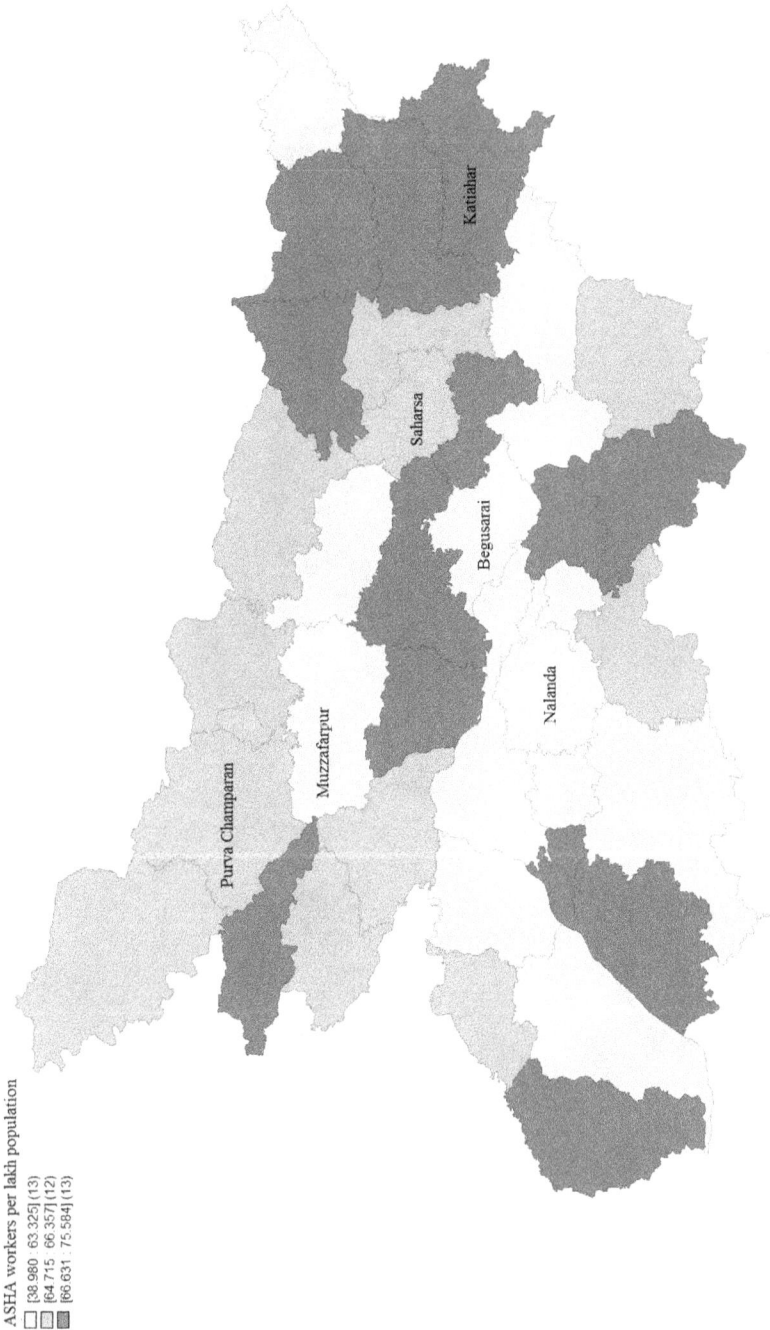

ASHA workers per lakh population

☐ [38.980 63.325] (13)
☐ (64.715 66.357] (12)
■ [66.631 75.584] (13)

Figure A2.2 ASHAs per lakh population.

Sources: Authors.

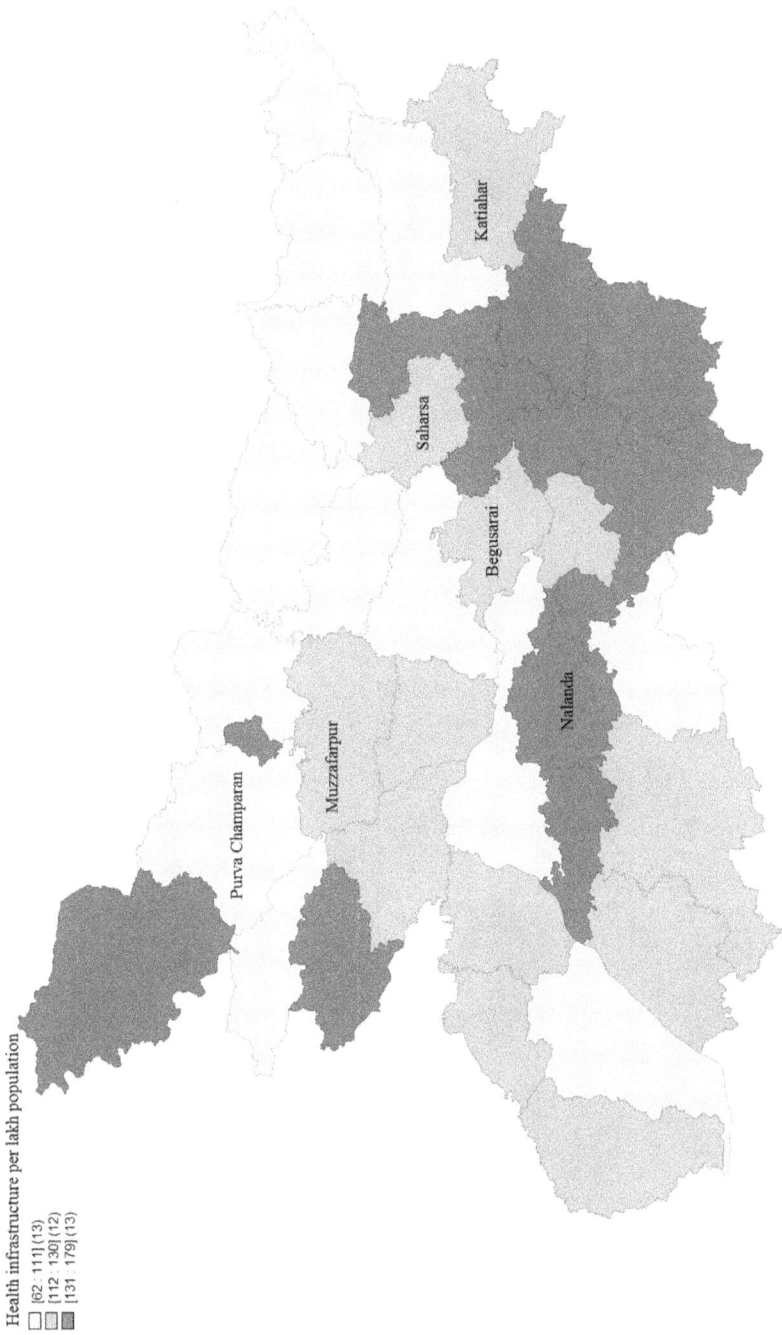

Health infrastructure per lakh population

☐ [62 : 111] (13)
☐ [112 : 130] (12)
■ [131 : 179] (13)

Katiahar

Saharsa

Begusarai

Nalanda

Purva Champaran

Muzzafarpur

Figure A2.3 Health infrastructure per lakh population.

Sources: Authors.

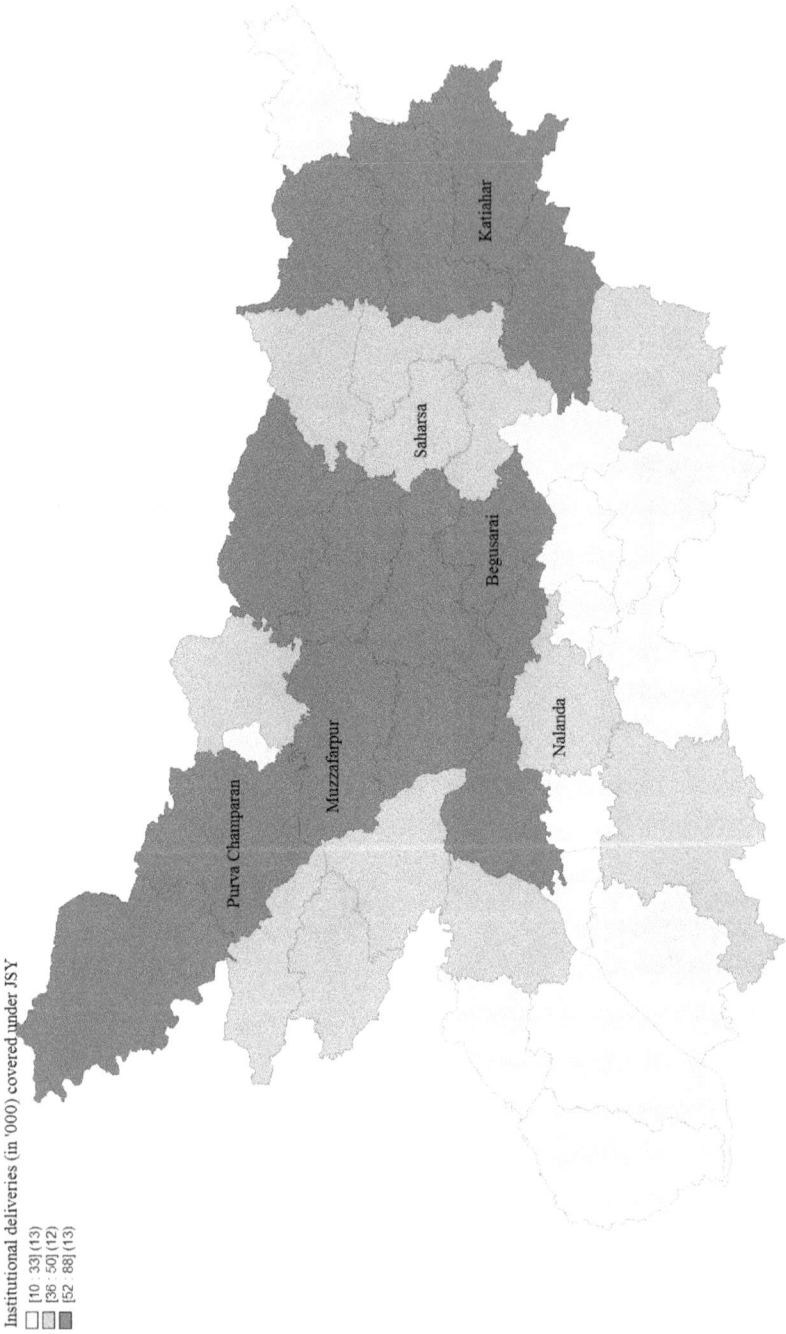

Institutional deliveries (in '000) covered under JSY

[10   33] (13)
[36   50] (12)
[52   88] (13)

Figure A2.4 Institutional deliveries (per 000) under JSY.

Sources: Authors.

Table A2.1 List of districts, blocks, and villages surveyed

District	Block	Villages to be covered					Extra village
Nalanda	Biharsarif	Pachauri	Biskurwa	Mohiuddinpur Utra	Tetranwan Mubarakpur	Meghi Nongawan	Hargawan
	Chandi	Sartha	Birnawan	Saidi	Katauna (Part in Giriak)	Chandi	Araut
	Katrisarai	Maira Barith	Katri			Dewaspura	Patria
Muzaffarpur	Silao	Surajpur	Mahuri	Bindidih	Dharampura	Kamal Bigha	Narharbigha
	Musahri	Khabra urf Kiratpur Gurdas	Chak Ahmad	Barhanpura	Manika Harkishun	Modhopur	Jamalabad
	Baruraj (Motipur)	Pakri	Rampur urf Bishunpur Kesho	Birji	Bariarpur urf Bazidpur	Pagahia Raiti	Senduari Gaj Singh
	Gaighat	Ladaura	Baraila	Maheshwara	Kanta Pirauchha	Lachhman Nagar	Boaridih
	Minapur	Khemaipatti	Minapur	Dubaha Rani Khaira urf Benua	Tengrahan Gosaipur	Majlis Madho urf Chhapra	Harsher
Saharsa	Sour Bazar	Baijnathpur	Tiri	Chanaur	Dhamsena	Suhath	Kanp
	Sattar Katiya	Bara	Patori	Pachgachhia	Ulkahi	Baghi urf Bhaluasukhasan	Agwanpur
	Salkhua	Kabira	Mamarkha(Mobarakpur)	Utesra	Kotwalia	Samhar Khurd	Gaurdah
	Sonbarsa	Agma	Paita	Khasurha	Bhaura	Mahuapatti Uttarwari	Manguar
Begusarai	Barauni	Singdaha	Sahuri	Zamira	Bishunpur Chand	Narayanpur	Gangasagar
	Naokothi	Chhatauna	Begampur	Pahsara	Bahadurpur	Samsa	Hasanpur
	Sahebpur Kamal	Sanha	Sabdalpur	Raghunathpur Barari	Shahpur Kamal	Pachmir	Phulmalik
	Begusarai	Bandwar	Ajhaur	Kaith	Lakho	Pachmma	Dhobauli

(Continued)

Table A2.1 (Continued)

District	Block	Villages to be covered					Extra village
Purba Champaran (Motihar)	Tetaria	Balbhadarpur	Narha Panapur	Bahuara Gopi Sinh	Mohammadpur Sagar	Tajpur	Kadma
	Ghorasahan	Ghorasahan urf Kotwa	Jamunia Kawaia	Bagahi Bhelwa	Laukhan	Singhrahiya	Nonaura
Katihar	Mehsi	Rajepur	Harpurnag	Tajpur Bara	Kothia Hariram	Jhitkahia	Kash Pakri
	Kalyanpur	Kaleyanpur	Barharwa Mahanad	Rajpur	Gawandri	Dilawarpur	Hajipur
	Hasangunj	Jagarnathpur	Ramnagar Bansi	Kalsar	Dherwa	Balua	Rampur
	Sameli	Mothoria	Dumar	Bakia	Chandpur	Muradpur (Part in Kursela)	Maula Nagar Chakla
	Falka	Chatar	Sohtha	Gobindpur	Bharsia	Amol	Baretha
	Amdabad	Karimullahpur	Ahmadabad	Gobindpur	Bhawanipur	Par Diara	Dumaria

Source: Primary survey data.
Note:
The village of Barhanpura could not be located and had to be replaced by Jamalabad in Musahri block of Muzaffarpur district.

Table A2.2 Demographic indicators for selected districts

Indicators	Begusarai	Muzaffarpur	Katihar	Nalanda	Purba Champaran	Saharsa
Population (female) age 6 years and above who ever attended school (%)	54.60	56.50	49.00	54.40	50.30	46.00
Population below age 15 years (%)	40.40	38.20	41.90	40.40	43.10	41.30
Sex ratio of the total population (females per 1000 males)	1050.00	1074.00	1045.00	1058.00	1054.00	1051.00
Sex ratio at birth for children born in the last 5 years (females per 1000 males)	1016.00	924.00	892.00	885.00	864.00	976.00
Women who are literate (%)	47.30	51.70	36.40	44.80	44.00	36.50
Women aged 15–19 years who were already married or pregnant at the time of the survey (%)	17.90	13.00	15.80	16.30	18.00	12.60
Any modern method (%)	33.50	9.10	25.60	30.80	5.70	27.30
Mothers who had antenatal check-ups in the first trimester (%)	32.10	23.80	31.50	37.50	22.20	33.50
Mothers who had at least four antenatal care visits (%)	7.90	10.10	8.60	8.50	12.10	9.30
Mothers whose last birth was protected against neonatal tetanus (%)	85.50	89.70	92.20	94.50	80.00	86.80
Mothers who consumed iron folic acid for 100 days or more when they were pregnant (%)	6.20	4.00	6.80	6.50	3.40	11.80
Mothers who had full antenatal care (%)	1.10	1.30	2.00	1.20	1.00	3.20
Institutional birth (%)	77.10	61.70	49.10	78.80	46.80	58.80
Home delivery conducted by skilled health personnel (out of total deliveries) (%)	4.90	6.70	6.00	4.60	14.30	4.30
Children under age 6 months exclusively breastfed (%)	25.50	77.70	65.90	36.70	49.00	61.10
Children aged 6–8 months receiving solid or semi-solid food and breastmilk (%)	29.50	33.70	24.20	30.00	41.20	11.00
Total children aged 6–23 months receiving an adequate diet (%)	3.10	7.70	6.50	6.00	8.00	2.00

Source: IIPS (2017)

Table A2.3 Profile of districts studied

Variables	Saharsa	Nalanda	Muzzaffarpur	Begusarai	Purba Champaran	Katihar	Total
Religion							
Hindu	100.00	100.00	95.00	88.89	94.44	72.22	92.11
Muslim	0.00	0.00	5.00	11.11	5.56	22.22	7.02
Others	0.00	0.00	0.00	0.00	0.00	5.56	0.88
Caste							
SC	40.00	25.00	25.00	16.67	27.78	5.56	23.68
ST	0.00	0.00	0.00	0.00	0.00	11.11	1.75
OBC	60.00	30.00	60.00	50.00	72.22	66.67	56.14
General	0.00	45.00	15.00	33.33	0.00	16.67	18.42
Occupation							
Cultivator	65.00	85.00	10.00	83.33	11.11	22.22	46.49
Agricultural labourer	25.00	15.00	35.00	0.00	77.78	61.11	35.09
Non-agricultural wage	10.00	0.00	55.00	16.67	5.56	16.67	17.54
Petty self-employed	0.00	0.00	0.00	0.00	5.56	0.00	0.88
Education							
No education	5.00	0.00	0.00	0.00	0.00	0.00	0.88
(Class 1–4)	0.00	0.00	20.00	0.00	0.00	44.44	10.53
(Class 5–7)	10.00	0.00	0.00	0.00	0.00	44.44	8.77
(Class 8–9)	30.00	5.00	15.00	5.56	0.00	5.56	10.53
Secondary/Madhyamik	50.00	85.00	60.00	83.33	94.44	5.56	63.16
(Class 12 and above)	5.00	10.00	5.00	11.11	5.56	0.00	6.14
Mean age at first marriage (years)							
Aged between 15 and 17 years	70.00	10.00	5.00	5.56	0.00	5.56	16.67
Aged 18 years	30.00	80.00	75.00	94.44	66.67	55.56	66.67
Aged between 19 and 22 years	0.00	10.00	20.00	0.00	33.33	38.89	16.67

Source: Primary survey data

Table A2.4 Health facilities in districts studied

Health facilities	Percentage of villages with facility (A)	Percentage of villages with accessible health facilities (B)	Total of A and B (in percentage)	Total health facility	Mean distance to health facility
ICDS/Anganwadi	99.12	0.88	100.00	114	1.00
Sub-centre	54.39	44.74	99.12	113	3.41
APHC	8.77	91.23	100.00	114	7.83
Block PHC	6.14	92.98	99.12	113	7.89
CHC/RH	6.14	92.98	99.12	113	12.19
District/Govt. hospital	0.00	98.25	98.25	112	28.42
Govt. dispensary	7.02	92.10	99.12	113	15.36
Private clinic	13.16	86.84	100.00	114.00	9.78
Private hospital/ Nursing home	2.63	97.37	100.00	114.00	13.15
AYUSH	8.77	91.23	100.00	114.00	19.50

Source: Primary survey data.

Table A2.5 Mean of current age, ever borne children, living children. Years of schooling and asset index scores – SHG members and non-members

Background characteristics	SHG Members (1124)	Non-members (1126)	Total (2250)
Mean years of age of the respondent	26.91	24.11	25.51
Std. Dev.	0.13	0.11	0.09
Upper limit	26.66	23.89	25.33
Lower limit	27.16	24.32	25.68
t-ratio	-16.59 (0.00)		
Mean number of children ever born	3.37	2.31	2.84
Std. Dev.	0.05	0.04	0.03
Upper limit	3.28	2.23	2.78
Lower limit	3.46	2.39	2.90
t-ratio	-17.22 (0.00)		
Mean number of living children	3.19	2.22	2.70
Std. Dev.	0.04	0.04	0.03
Upper limit	3.11	2.14	2.64
Lower limit	3.28	2.29	2.76
t-ratio	-17.15 (0.00)		
Mean years of completed years of schooling	4.29	5.73	5.01
Std. Dev.	0.14	0.14	0.10
Upper limit	4.02	5.45	4.81
Lower limit	4.55	6.01	5.20
t-ratio	7.31 (0.00)		
Asset index score	0.002	0.03	0.02
Std. Dev.	0.03	0.03	0.02
Upper limit	-0.05	-0.02	-0.02
Lower limit	0.05	0.08	0.05
t-ratio	0.78 (0.43)		

Source: Primary survey data.

Table A2.6 Socio-demographic characteristics of SHG members and non-members

Background characteristics	SHG Members (1124)	Non-members (1126)	Total (2250)
Age of the respondent (%)			
17–20	4.44	17.08	10.76
21–25	37.48	52.14	44.80
26–30	43.87	25.98	34.93
31 and above	14.21	4.80	9.51
chi-square	214.42 (0.00)		
Household size (%)			
3–4 members	10.39	15.93	13.16
5–7 members	89.25	83.63	86.44
8 members and more	0.36	0.44	0.40
chi-square	15.27 (0.00)		
Educational attainment (%)			
Non-literate	41.65	32.21	36.93
1–5 years	22.38	14.95	18.67
6–10 years	27.00	38.52	32.76
More than ten years	8.97	14.32	11.64
chi-square	66.90 (0.00)		
Occupation of respondent (%)			
Unemployed	80.02	90.93	85.47
House worker	3.11	1.07	2.09
Cultivator	0.71	1.07	0.89
Livestock	0.44	0.18	0.31
Agricultural labour	7.19	2.85	5.02
Non-agricultural wage labour	2.93	2.05	2.49
Petty self-employed	3.11	1.25	2.18
Construction	0.36	0.27	0.31
Wage and salaried	2.13	0.36	1.24
chi-square	67.42 (0.00)		
Occupation of respondents' husband (%)			
Unemployed	0.98	3.84	2.41
Cultivator	6.23	6.07	6.15
Livestock	0.36	0.45	0.40
Agricultural labour	10.86	12.68	11.77
Non-agricultural wage labour	39.54	36.70	38.12
Petty self-employed	13.71	14.55	14.13
Construction	5.52	5.00	5.26
Transport	4.19	4.02	4.10
Wage and salaried	18.61	16.70	17.65
chi-square	23.71 (0.00)		

(Continued)

Table A2.6 (Continued)

Background characteristics	SHG Members (1124)	Non-members (1126)	Total (2250)
Asset index classes (%)			
Low	33.13	33.54	33.33
Middle	34.55	32.21	33.38
High	32.33	34.25	33.29
chi-square	1.58 (0.45)		
Caste and religion (%)			
SC/ST-Hindu	4.97	7.47	6.22
OBC-Hindu	53.37	55.78	54.58
UC-Hindu	33.30	29.18	31.24
Muslims/others	8.35	7.56	7.96
chi-square	9.74 (0.02)		
Districts (%)			
Purba Champaran	15.54	15.57	15.56
Muzaffarpur	17.76	17.79	17.78
Nalanda	17.85	17.70	17.78
Katihar	15.54	15.57	15.56
Begusarai	15.54	15.57	15.56
Saharsha	17.76	17.79	17.78
chi-square	0.01 (1.00)		

Source: Primary survey data.

Chapter 3

Networks and information diffusion

Evidence from national family health survey

3.1 Introduction

In recent years a consensus has emerged that creating demand for the use of MCH services is necessary to improve MCH outcomes. Policymakers are gradually realising that microfinance institutions (MFIs) and self-help groups (SHGs) – originally established with the objective to mobilise women from poor households to improve their economic conditions – may also be used as an instrument for improving MCH outcomes (Gichuru et al., 2019; Murshid & Ely, 2019; Walia et al., 2020). Similarly, studies have reported on the effectiveness of front-line health workers (Rammohan et al., 2021; Sserwanja, Turimumahoro, et al., 2022), mass media (Aboagye et al., 2022; Fatema & Lariscy, 2020; R. Ghosh et al., 2021; Igbinoba et al., 2020; Nguyen et al., 2016; Sserwanja, Mutisya, et al., 2022) and the use of mobile phones (Rajkhowa & Qaim, 2022) to increase awareness about health practices and encourage the adoption of recommended MCH practices. Peer effects have also been reported to have played a major role in improving health outcomes (Bouckaert, 2014; Fletcher, 2014; Webel et al., 2010) through information dissemination (Katz & Lazarsfeld, 2005).

This chapter, therefore, examines the role of different channels for the diffusion of information on the adoption levels of MCH services. The analysis is undertaken using National Family Health Survey (NFHS) data for the fifth round (2019–21). It is undertaken at an all-India level, and also for the state of Bihar. The specific research questions addressed in this chapter are:

(i) Does the flow of information and greater contacts facilitate the adoption of MCH practices?
(ii) What are the determinants of access to information and networks?

The analysis is undertaken at the all-India level. Further, as an empirical assessment of such aspects is required particularly in the resource-constrained and demographically backward state of Bihar having a history of poor MCH

DOI: 10.4324/9781003499251-3

outcomes and a high unmet need for contraception (Ghosh & Husain, 2019), the analysis is also undertaken for Bihar.

As mentioned above, the earlier attempts were made separately for each of the predictor variables such as exposure to media/internet or knowledge and engagement with microfinance institutions or contact with front-line health workers or exposure to family planning messages in media or women's mobility. To the best of our knowledge there are no studies so far which have analysed these channels of information dissemination together in an integrated manner. The present chapter has made an attempt to find out the role of these sources of information on measures of MCH outcomes and adoption of modern contraceptive methods.

3.2 Materials and methods

3.2.1 Data

The analysis was undertaken using unit-level data from the fifth round of National Family Health Survey (NFHS), conducted between 2019 and 2021 in all the Indian states and union territories. The survey covered 724,115 women aged 15–49 years (out of which 512,408 women were currently married at the time of survey) and 232,920 under-five children from 636,699 households. The present analysis consists of 26,552 currently married women from the state module who delivered their last birth during the five years preceding the survey (i.e., for whom maternal health-seeking behavioural indicators were available) and 35,622 under-five children for whom data of our interest were collected. For the state of Bihar, these figures were 2,036 and 3,147, respectively.

3.2.2 Outcome indicators

The present analysis used the following binary outcome indicators belonging to three different domains, namely, outcome regarding uptake of maternal healthcare, outcome regarding contraceptive usage, and outcome regarding child healthcare. These are as follows:

(1) **Outcome indicators related to uptake of maternal healthcare**
    (a) Outcome related to antenatal care
        (i) Whether pregnancy was registered in the first trimester (no/yes)
        (ii) Whether at least four ANC visits were made (no/yes)
        (iii) Whether at least 100 IFA tablets/syrup were consumed (no/yes)
        (iv) Whether two tetanus toxoid (TT) injections were taken to prevent neonatal tetanus (no/yes)
        (v) Whether full ANC (as defined by pregnancy registration in the first trimester of pregnancy, at least 4 ANC visits, at least 100 IFA tablets/syrup, and at least one TT) was received (no/yes)

(b) Outcome indicators related to delivery care
  (vi) Whether delivery was conducted in an institution (no/yes)
  (vii) Whether delivery was conducted by a skilled birth attendant (no/yes)
(c) Outcome indicator related to post-partum care
  (viii) Whether received postnatal check-up within 48 hours of delivery (no/yes)
(2) **Outcome indicators related to contraceptive usage**
  (ix) Whether currently using modern methods of contraception (no/yes)
  (x) Whether received advice on post-partum contraceptive methods after last birth (no/yes)
(3) **Outcome indicators related to child health**
  (xi) Whether received vaccine at birth (OPV0) for the indexed child (no/yes)
  (xii) Given exclusive breastfeeding for six months to the indexed child (no/yes)
  (xiii) Started complementary feeding after six months (no/yes).

3.2.3 Sources of information

It may be noted that NFHS does not contain any direct information on the network of a household or women which can enhance the uptake of the aforesaid outcome indicators. However, the said dataset does contain five domains of information, which can suitably be used as proxies indicating facilitating factors of having network with others. These domains are – exposure to media and internet; freedom of movement (or mobility); knowledge of microfinance activities and obtaining loans in such organisations; meeting with front-line workers such as ANM, ASHA, and *Anganwadi* Worker (AWW); and exposure to family planning messages in different media. A detailed description of the variables with their categorisation has been given in the Table 3.1.

3.2.4 Control variables

It is well-established that apart from the variables facilitating the possibility of having a network (as given in the Table 3.1), earlier literature on maternal and child healthcare utilisation suggests that they have been determined by a host of other socio-demographic, economic, and cultural factors. For this reason, a number of control variables representing these domains were included in the study. These variables are: current age of the mother (continuous), completed years of schooling (continuous), work status (whether working in any wage-earning sector activities at the time of survey or not), religious affiliation (Hindu, Muslim, Others), caste membership (scheduled castes (SC)/

Table 3.1 Indicators of access to information in NFHS-5

Domains	Variables	Coding
Exposure to media and internet (MEDIA)	Frequency of reading newspaper or magazines	Not at all = 0
		Less than once a
	Frequency of listening to radio	week = 1
	Frequency of watching television	At least once a
		week = 2
	Owns a mobile telephone	No = 0
	Use internet	Yes = 1
Freedom of movement (MOBILITY)	Usually allowed to go to the market	Not at all = 0
	Usually allowed to go to the health facility	With someone else only = 1
	Usually allowed to go to places outside this village	Alone = 2
Knowledge of microfinance (MFIN)	Do not have any knowledge	No = 0
	Knew or taken loan	Yes = 1
Contact with front-line health workers (FLHW)	Meet ASHA/ANM in the last three months	No = 0
		Yes = 1
	Meet AWW in the last three months	
Exposure to family planning messages (FPEXP)	Heard family planning on radio in last few months	No = 0
		Yes = 1
	Heard family planning on tv in last few months	
	Heard family planning in newspaper/ magazine in last few months	

Source: Categorised from unit-level data by the authors.

scheduled tribes (ST), other backward caste (OBC), general caste), and place of residence (rural, urban). Apart from these variables, state and district fixed effects were also incorporated into the models (states in the all-India models and districts in the state models).

3.2.5 Methods

First, polychoric principal component analyses (PCA)[1] were carried out for the variables representing each domain of the predictor variables as mentioned in the Table 3.1 to obtain a single index for each domain (except knowledge of microfinance because it is a single dummy variable). For instance, polychoric PCA was conducted by taking into account five variables indicating exposure to media/internet (Table 3.1) and a single value was obtained. Secondly, for the sake of comparison across indices, all the indices were normalised on a scale of 0–100. Then descriptive statistics were produced and exploratory analyses were carried out to find out the bivariate association between outcome variables and main predictor variables by using t-test. Finally, multivariate binary probit regression models were conducted for all the outcome variables to find out the strength and direction of association between main predictor variables (i.e., the indices derived from the polychoric PCA) and outcome variable after controlling a range of potentially confounding variables as mentioned in the earlier section. Probit models were used because all the outcome variables were dichotomous (yes/no). The regression specification was:

$$Y_{ij} = \beta_0 + \beta_1 FLHW_i + \beta_2 MOBILITY_i + \beta_3 MFIN_i + \beta4MEDIA_i + \beta_5 X_i \qquad [3.1]$$

Where

Y_{ij}: is a binary variable indicating whether the ith respondent has adopted j^{th} health practice or availed of the jth health service.
FLHW is the normalised score indicating contacts of the ith respondent with the front-line health worker.
MFIN is a categorical ordered variable indicating contacts with self-help groups (SHGs) of the ith respondent.
MEDIA is the normalised score of exposure to media like TV, radio, and newspapers of the ith respondent.

When the adoption of modern contraception is considered, MEDIA is replaced by FPEXP (normalised score of exposure to family planning messages through the popular media).

Control variables include: Age, completed years of schooling, work-status, religious affiliation, caste membership, logarithm of wealth score (dropped for maternal health outcome indicators because of multicollinearity with caste membership), place of residence, state fixed-effects (for all India models) and district fixed-effects (for Bihar models).

In addition, we have also identified the determinants of network and information using an econometric model. The model is:

$$Y_{ij} = \beta_0 + \beta_1 FLHW_i \qquad [3.2]$$

Where

Y: Score for the specific information channel/network (i.e. MEDIA, MOBILITY, MFIN, and FLHW).
X is a vector consisting of age, completed years of age, completed years of schooling, work-status, religious affiliation, caste membership, logarithm of wealth score (dropped for maternal health outcome indicators because

of multicollinearity with caste membership), place of residence, state fixed-effects (for all-India models) and district fixed-effects (for Bihar models). Data were analysed using Stata 17.

In this context it may be mentioned that because of high multicollinearity between caste membership and wealth of household in assessing maternal health outcomes, caste was retained and wealth (logarithm of asset scores) was dropped. According to our view, in a caste-based patriarchal society in India, particularly in Bihar, caste membership is a better representation of household economic status. Although we have also carried out alternative regression models by dropping caste and retaining logarithm of asset, we found similar results and thus have not reported in the text for the brevity of space. Also, because of high multicollinearity between exposure to media/internet and exposure to family planning message in media, we have retained exposure to media/internet in all the models except those carried out for usage and advice of family planning message, where exposure to family planning message in media were incorporated and exposure to media/internet was dropped. In the tables we have only reported the results for the main predictor variables; however, results for the control variables were discussed in the text but not reported in the tables.

3.3 Results

3.3.1 Maternal and child health outcomes

Mean with 95% CI of each outcome variables regarding maternal and child health was reported in the Table 3.2 (see also Figure 3.1).

Except the receipt of PNC within 48 hours of delivery, Bihar lags all-India average for all other indicators representing utilisation of maternal healthcare services. The gap in utilisation between overall India and Bihar was more pronounced (more than double) in obtaining four or more ANC visits (0.59 for overall India and 0.24 for Bihar) and 100 or more IFA tablet/syrup (0.52 for overall India and 0.25 for Bihar) and consequently receiving full ANC, in which gap was observed to be nearly four-times (0.27 for overall India and 0,07 for Bihar). Although respondents from Bihar lagged in obtaining at least two TT injection, institutional delivery, and skilled-attendance in delivery, the gap was less pronounced. Such gaps were also not that noticeable regarding child's vaccination with OPV0 at the time of birth and also providing exclusive breastfeeding for six months. More than six-month-old children from Bihar were more likely to start complementary breastfeeding at a higher rate compared to average Indian children. However, current usage of modern contraceptive methods among respondents and receipt of advice on post partum contraception were found to be much higher for overall India (0.47 and 0.83, respectively) compared to their counterparts from Bihar (0.32 and 0.69, respectively).

Table 3.2 Maternal and child health outcomes in India and Bihar, NFHS-5, 2019–21

Outcome variables	India		Bihar	
	Mean	95% CI	Mean	95% CI
Pregnancy registration in the first trimester of pregnancy	0.71	0.70, 0.71	0.53	0.51, 0.55
At least four ANC check-ups	0.59	0.59, 0.60	0.24	0.22, 0.26
Had at least 100 IFA tablet/syrup	0.52	0.51, 0.53	0.25	0.23, 0.28
Had at least two tetanus	0.83	0.83, 0.84	0.76	0.74, 0.78
Received full ANC	0.27	0.26, 0.27	0.07	0.05, 0.08
Delivered in an institution	0.90	0.89, 0.90	0.76	0.75, 0.78
Received skilled-attendance during delivery	0.91	0.90, 0.91	0.80	0.79, 0.82
Received PNC within 48 hours of delivery	0.22	0.22, 0.23	0.24	0.22, 0.25
Using modern contraceptive methods	0.47	0.47, 0.48	0.32	0.30, 0.34
Received advice on post-partum contraception	0.83	0.82, 0.83	0.69	0.66, 0.71
Received vaccine at birth (OPV0) for the indexed child	0.85	0.85, 0.85	0.81	0.81, 0.81
Given exclusive breastfeeding for six months to the indexed child	0.64	0.64, 0.64	0.59	0.59, 0.59
Started complementary feeding after six months	0.30	0.30, 0.30	0.35	0.35, 0.35
Total cases	**26, 552**		**2036**	

Source: Estimated from unit-level data by the authors.

3.3.2 Access of respondents to information

Table 3.3 reveals the distribution of normalised scores of main predictor variables with 05% CI. Respondents from Bihar were less likely to be exposed to media/internet compared to overall India according to the index of media exposure/internet (34.91 for overall India vis-à-vis 25.50 for Bihar). However, the index of freedom of movement (or mobility) was comparable between overall India and Bihar (69.46 for overall India, while 70.42 for Bihar). Knowledge and activity regarding microfinance was found to be higher in Bihar compared to overall India (56.47% for Bihar vis-à-vis 49.85% for overall India). Respondents from overall India obtained higher scores in the index of exposure to front-line health workers during three months preceding the survey as well as in the index of exposure to family planning messages in media in the last few months compared to their counterparts in Bihar (46.86 and 40.78 for overall India respectively compared to 38.72 and 25.83 for Bihar respectively).

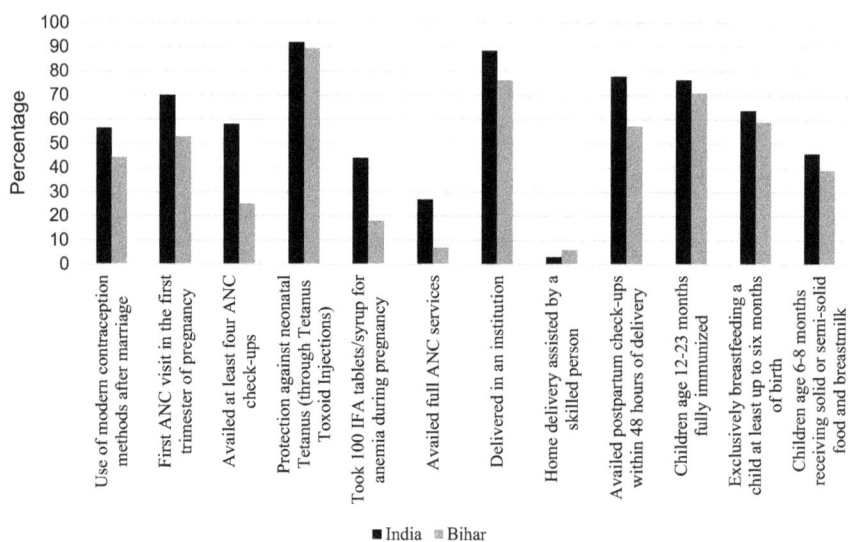

Figure 3.1 Maternal and child health outcomes in India and Bihar, NFHS-5, 2019–21.
Source: IIPS (2020, 2022).

3.3.3 Information and maternal and child health outcomes: An exploratory analysis

Tables A3.1–A3.5 depicted the distribution of different indices (main predictors variables) representing the possibility of having networks across different outcome variables. It can be ascertained that the index of media/internet exposure is positively and significantly associated with utilisation of ANC and delivery services both in overall India and Bihar. Surprisingly, obtaining PNC services within 48 hours of delivery was found to have a negative and significant relationship with the index of exposure to media/internet for overall India; however, not in Bihar. Although contraceptive usage and advice, and receipt of vaccine at birth (OPV0) have a positive and significant association with the index of exposure to media/internet, the association was not significant for Bihar (Table A3.1). Index of freedom of movement (or mobility) has a positive and significant association with utilisation of ANC services, contraceptive usage and advice, and OPV0 for overall India; however, for Bihar only contraceptive advice and OPV0 were found to have a positive and significant association with the index of freedom of movement (Table A3.2). Similarly, except utilisation of PNC services within 48 hours of delivery, providing exclusive breastfeeding for six months to the last child and beginning complementary feeding after six months, all other outcome variables have a positive and significant association with knowledge or activities related to

Table 3.3 Access of respondents to information sources in India and Bihar, NFHS-5, 2019–21

Main predictor variables representing the presence of network	India		Bihar	
	Scores/percentage	95% CI	Scores	95% CI
Index of exposure to media (0–100)	34.91	34.59, 35.23	25.50	24.53, 26.47
Index of freedom of movement (0–100)	69.46	69.10, 69.82	70.42	69.06, 71.78
Knowledge and activity (in percent) of microfinance				
No knowledge	50.15	NA	43.53	NA
Knew or have taken loan	49.85	NA	56.47	NA
Index of exposure to FLWs during three months preceding the survey (0–100)	46.86	46.34, 47.37	38.72	36.88, 40.56
Index of exposure to family planning messages in media in last few months (0–100)	40.78	40.34, 42.22	25.83	24.31, 27.34
Total cases	**26, 552**		**2036**	

Source: Estimated from unit-level data by the authors

microfinance activities in overall India; however, for Bihar only two of the ANC care services, namely, registration of pregnancy in first trimester and at least four ANC check-ups were found to have a positive and significant relationship with knowledge and activity related to microfinance (Table A3.3). Index of exposure to front-line health workers was found to be one of the important predictor variables in availing maternal and child healthcare services for overall India and also for Bihar. It is important to note that all the variables, except current usage of modern contraceptive methods, all other outcome variables have positive and significant association with the index of exposure to front-line health workers. Association was found to be the strongest for availing PNC services within 48 hours of delivery. Opposite to the expectation, the association between the current usage of modern contraceptive methods and the index of exposure to front-line health workers was found to be negative and significant not only for overall India but also for Bihar (Table A3.4). In line with the earlier relationships, the index of exposure to family planning messages in media also has a positive and significant association with almost all the outcome variables relating to maternal and child healthcare and current contraceptive usage and advice (Table A3.5).

3.3.4 Does information matter? Results of econometric analyses

Table 3.4 presents the coefficients obtained from the multivariate binary probit regression models. All the ANC-related response variables, namely, registration of pregnancy within the first trimester, at least four ANC visits, consumption of 100 or more IFA tablets/syrup, at least two TT injections, and uptake of full ANC have a positive and significant relationship with all the main predictor variables, i.e., indices indicating media/internet exposure, mobility outside home, knowledge and activities related to microfinance activities, and exposure to front-line health workers in overall India; however, not always in case of Bihar even after controlling a range of potentially confounding variables. For instance, the index of freedom of movement was observed to be insignificant in obtaining at least four visits and significant negative association with receiving at least two TT injections, while knowledge and activities related to microfinance were found to be negatively and significantly associated with consumption of 100 or more IFA tablets/syrup in case of Bihar. Moreover, contrary to expectation, the index of exposure to front-line health workers also has a significant negative relationship with receiving at least two TT injections. In the case of utilisation of delivery-related services, although institutional delivery has positive and significant relationships with indices of media exposure/internet, mobility, and front-line health workers, it was significantly and negatively associated with knowledge and activities related to microfinance in both overall India and Bihar and it persists for skilled-delivery attendance for Bihar as well. Similarly, knowledge and activities related to microfinance did not help in receiving PNC services within 48 hours for overall India; however, not in the case of Bihar.

Index of exposure to family planning messages in media did significantly enhance the current usage of modern contraception in overall India and in Bihar. Although knowledge and activity related to microfinance positively and significantly increased the current use of modern methods for the respondents from overall India, relationship was not significant for the respondents from Bihar. As obtained in bivariate analysis, the current usage of modern methods declined significantly if exposure to the front-line health workers enhanced even after controlling other potentially confounding variables. Such surprising findings could be due to two reasons. First, it could be due to endogeneity between the predictor and response variable, although we have tried to reduce endogeneity while selecting variables. We have also performed tests for the presence of endogeneity[2]. Secondly, we do not have data on the detailed topic and quality of discussion with the front-line health workers – which could affect the adoption of modern method. At the same time, although all four main predictor variables enhance the likelihood of receiving advice on post-partum contraception for the respondents from overall India, such possibility declined if the respondents knew or had any activity regarding microfinance in the context of Bihar.

The relationship between the indices of possibility of having network and child health outcome indicators was also mixed. For instance, although the likelihood of receiving OPV0 significantly increases with the increase in mobility, knowledge, and activities related to microfinance and exposure to front-line health workers in both overall India and Bihar, it declined significantly with an increase in media/internet exposure. As far as providing exclusive breastfeeding for six months after birth is concerned, the probability of such feeding significantly enhances with an increase in media/internet exposure, knowledge and activities pertaining to microfinance, and exposure to front-line health workers; the likelihood declined significantly with an increase in mobility. The probability of onset of complementary feeding after six months of age although increases significantly with an increase in knowledge and activities related to microfinance and exposure to front-line health workers for both overall India and Bihar, likelihood of such declined significantly with an increase in exposure to media/internet and mobility for overall India. In the case of Bihar, greater mobility among respondents significantly reduces the likelihood of providing complementary feeding to their youngest child at the time of requirement.

The direction of various other socio-demographic, economic, and cultural variables, which potentially affect the outcome variables related to maternal, child health-seeking, and contraceptive behaviour were given in the Tables A3.6 and A3.7. In this case also the results are mixed. In Bihar, the utilisation of all ANC services tends to increase with an increase in age; however, early registration of pregnancy and at least four ANC check-ups decreases with the increase in age. Institutional delivery as well as skilled-attendance in delivery both tend to decline with the increase in age. The likelihood of receiving PNC increases with the increase in age for overall India (Table A3.6). Table A3.6 further reveals that the increase in educational attainment of the respondents is positively and significantly associated with utilisation of maternal healthcare services in general. Working women were generally less likely to utilize the majority of components of maternal healthcare except for some exceptions. Compared to Hindu women Muslim women were significantly more likely to consume 100 or more IFA tablets/syrup but less likely to have skilled-attendance at delivery. However, in most of the components of maternal care utilisation, religious differentials seem to be not that important determinant. Socially marginalised sections of the society that SC/ST and OBCs were generally less likely to utilize maternal care services. There are some exceptions; the utilisation of services by SC/ST and OBCs are high for services such as receiving at least two TT injections (for overall India and Bihar), early registration of pregnancy and PNC services (for Bihar).

Table 3.4 Results of binary probit regression models for India and Bihar, NFHS-5, 2019–21

Variables	All India				Bihar			
	Coefficient	95% CI		Z-statistics	Coefficient	95% CI		Z-statistics
ANC related								
First check-up in the first trimester								
MEDIA	0.0027***	0.0024	0.0029	18.70	0.0020***	0.0011	0.0029	4.47
MOBILITY	0.0004***	0.0003	0.0006	4.63	0.0008***	0.0003	0.0013	3.09
MFIN	0.1839***	0.1728	0.1950	32.52	0.1045***	0.0730	0.1360	6.51
FLHW	0.0009***	0.0008	0.0010	13.44	0.0025***	0.0022	0.0029	13.32
Model statistics								
N (weighted)	2,49,567				28,946			
Pseudo R2	0.0593				0.0820			
At least four ANC check-ups								
MEDIA	0.0039***	0.0036	0.0042	27.35	0.0084***	0.0075	0.0094	17.30
MOBILITY	0.0007***	0.0005	0.0090	7.59	-0.0005	-0.0010	0.0001	-1.77
MFIN	0.2047***	0.1936	0.2158	36.17	0.0420*	0.0070	0.0771	2.35
FLHW	0.0014***	0.0013	0.0015	21.56	0.0019***	0.0015	0.0023	9.00
Model statistics								
N (weighted)	2,45,847				28,767			
Pseudo R2	0.1482				0.1207			
At least 100 IFA Tablets/Syrup								
MEDIA	0.0009***	0.0007	0.0012	6.57	0.0032***	0.0022	0.0043	5.97
MOBILITY	0.0008***	0.0006	0.0010	8.20	0.0034***	0.0027	0.0041	10.07
MFIN	0.0610***	0.0494	0.0724	10.34	-0.0764**	-0.1162	-0.0366	-3.76

FLHW	0.0011***	0.0010	0.0012	15.75	0.0024***	0.0019	0.0029	9.81
Model statistics							
N	2,17,555				21,574			
Pseudo R2	0.1291				0.1018			

At least two tetanus injection

MEDIA	0.0026***	0.0023	0.0029	16.61	-0.0008	-0.0018	0.0002	-1.63
MOBILITY	0.0007***	0.0005	0.0009	6.33	-0.0011***	-0.0016	-0.0005	-3.78
MFIN	0.1106***	0.0983	0.1229	17.61	0.0618***	0.02770	0.0960	3.55
FLHW	0.0005***	0.0004	0.0007	7.18	-.0024***	-0.0028	-0.0020	-11.89
Model statistics							
N	2,49,976				28,981			
Pseudo R2	0.0257				0.0578			

Received Full ANC

MEDIA	0.0026***	0.0023	0.0029	17.81	0.0044***	0.0030	0.0057	6.49
MOBILITY	0.0011***	0.0009	0.0013	10.47	0.0022***	0.0014	0.003	5.26
MFIN	0.2039***	0.1922	0.2157	34.01	0.0238	-0.0264	0.0741	0.93
FLHW	0.0017***	0.0016	0.0019	24.62	0.0027***	0.0021	0.0033	8.62
Model statistics							
N	2,49,976				27,316			
Pseudo R2	0.1438				0.1845			

Delivery related
Obtained institutional delivery

MEDIA	0.0070***	0.0065	0.0074	31.64	0.0105***	0.0094	0.0116	18.42
MOBILITY	0.0003	-0.0002	0.0003	0.20	-0.0004	-0.001	0.0001	-1.58
MFIN	-0.0270**	-0.0425	-0.0116	-3.43	-0.0787***	-0.1146	-0.0428	-4.29
FLHW	0.0017***	0.0015	0.0019	18.81	0.0009***	0.0005	0.0013	4.29
Model statistics							
N	2,43,356				28,981			
Pseudo R2	0.1736				0.1464			

(Continued)

Table 3.4 (Continued)

Variables	All India				Bihar			
	Coefficient	95% CI		Z-statistics	Coefficient	95% CI		Z-statistics
Obtained skilled-attendance at delivery								
MEDIA	0.0053***	0.0048	0.0057	24.65	0.0060***	0.0049	0.0071	10.81
MOBILITY	0.0007***	0.0005	0.0010	5.62	0.0005	-0.0001	0.0011	1.66
MFIN	-0.0031	-0.0184	0.0121	-0.40	-0.1575***	-0.1943	-0.1207	-8.39
FLHW	0.0015***	0.0013	0.0017	16.25	0.0011***	0.0006	0.0015	4.84
Model statistics								
N	2,43,552				28,981			
Pseudo R2	0.1263				0.1097			
Received PNC within 48 hours of delivery								
MEDIA	0.0016***	0.0013	0.0019	10.65	0.0004	-0.0005	0.0013	0.84
MOBILITY	-0.0002	-0.0004	0.0000	-1.17	0.0008**	0.0003	0.0014	3.03
MFIN	-0.0277**	-0.0393	-0.0160	-4.64	0.0393*	0.0047	0.0739	2.23
FLHW	0.0041	0.0039	0.0042	59.02	0.0030***	0.0026	0.0034	15.05
Model statistics								
N	2,49,927				28,981			
Pseudo R2	0.0541				0.0688			

Contraceptive related

Using modern contraceptive methods

MOBILITY	0.0000	-0.0002	0.0001	-0.75	-0.0001	-0.0001	0.0001	-1.59
MFIN	0.8760***	0.0021	0.0025	28.57	0.0262	-0.0068	0.0591	1.56
FLHW	-0.0012***	-0.0013	-0.0010	-18.62	-0.0025***	-0.0029	-0.0021	-12.68
FPEXP	0.0023***	0.0021	0.0025	28.57	0.0036***	0.0031	0.0041	13.26
Model statistics								
N	2,49,976				28,981			
Pseudo R2	0.0463				0.0794			

Received advice on post-partum contraception

MOBILITY	0.0027***	0.0024	0.0029	20.68	0.0029***	0.0021	0.0037	7.53
MFIN	0.0100***	0.0849	0.1150	13.05	-0.2081***	-0.2567	-0.1594	-8.38
FLHW	0.0035***	0.0034	0.0037	39.45	0.0003	-0.0003	0.0008	0.97
FPEXP	0.0061***	0.0059	0.0063	51.96	0.0106***	0.0098	0.0114	26.26
Model statistics								
N	1,74,598				14,463			
Pseudo R2	0.0883				0.1359			

Child related

Received vaccine at birth (OPV0) for the indexed child

MEDIA	-0.0021***	-0.0027	-0.0016	-7.48	-0.0031**	-0.0047	-0.0016	-3.94
MOBILITY	0.0018***	0.0014	0.0022	7.85	0.0035***	0.0024	0.0047	6.14
MFIN	0.1338***	0.1069	0.1608	9.74	0.2685***	0.1987	0.3384	7.54
FLHW	0.0023***	0.0020	0.0026	14.37	0.0020***	0.0011	0.0028	4.54
Model statistics								
N	59,123				7,664			
Pseudo R2	0.0870				0.1376			

(Continued)

Table 3.4 (Continued)

Variables	All India			Bihar		
	Coefficient	95% CI		Z-statistics	Coefficient	95% CI		Z-statistics

Given exclusive breastfeeding for six months to the indexed child

Variables	Coefficient	95% CI		Z-statistics	Coefficient	95% CI		Z-statistics
MEDIA	0.0017***	0.0011	0.0024	5.20	0.0085***	0.0061	0.0109	6.94
MOBILITY	-0.0007**	-0.0012	-0.0002	-2.75	-0.0054**	-0.0071	-0.0036	-6.02
MFIN	0.0911***	0.0603	0.1218	5.80	0.1369*	0.0270	0.2468	2.44
FLHW	0.0020***	0.0016	0.0024	10.06	0.0042***	0.0029	0.0054	6.58
Model statistics								
N	31,208				3,473			
Pseudo R2	0.0513				0.1474			

Started complementary feeding after six months

Variables	Coefficient	95% CI		Z-statistics	Coefficient	95% CI		Z-statistics
MEDIA	-0.0012***	-0.0014	-0.0010	-9.39	0.0020***	0.0012	0.0028	5.06
MOBILITY	-0.0016***	-0.0018	-0.0009	-15.71	-0.0013***	-0.0019	-0.0007	-4.55
MFIN	0.0840***	0.0721	0.0958	13.85	0.0799***	0.0452	0.1146	4.51
FLHW	0.0046***	0.0045	0.0048	66.59	0.0044***	0.0040	0.0049	20.89
Model statistics								
N	2,16,538				24,863			
Pseudo R2	0.0629				0.0923			

Source: Estimated from unit-level data by the authors.
Note: Control variables include: Age, completed years of schooling, work-status, religious affiliation, caste membership, logarithm of wealth score (dropped for maternal health outcome indicators because of multicollinearity with caste membership), place of residence, state fixed-effects (for all-India models), and district fixed-effects (for Bihar models).

Respondents from rural areas are less likely to utilize different components of maternal care except PNC care.

According to Table A3.7, usage of modern contraception and post-partum contraceptive advice significantly increases with age. Although the current usage of modern method tends to be higher for working women, such relationship does not hold for receiving advice. Contrary to expectation, usage of modern contraception as well as the likelihood of receiving post-partum contraception decreases with enhancement of women's educational attainment. Muslim women were significantly less likely to use modern methods compared to their Hindu counterparts in the case of overall India as well as Bihar, but such a negative relationship holds for Bihar in receiving advice on post-partum contraception. Marginalised sections of the society (SC/ST) were significantly more likely to use modern methods in Bihar (but not in overall India), though they tend to receive advice on post-partum contraception compared to general caste women. However, for OBC women, such a relationship is generally found to be negative. Household economic status was found to have a positive and significant relationship with the usage of modern methods but not with receipt of advice. Rural women were significantly less likely to receive advice on post-partum contraception compared to their urban counterparts.

Table A3.7 further revealed that the higher educational attainment of the respondents did not help to comply with exclusive breastfeeding for six months for their youngest child in overall India as well as in Bihar. Although better-educated respondents started commentary feeding after six months for overall India, the relationship was just the opposite in the case of Bihar. Women's workforce participation is generally found to be negatively associated with all the measures of child health outcomes. Although Muslim respondents were significantly not likely to have OPV0 and exclusive breastfeeding for six months for their youngest child, they were significantly more likely to start complementary feeding after six months. Respondents from socially marginalised communities (SC/ST) from Bihar were less likely to receive OPV0 for their youngest child, but more likely to start complementary feeding after six months. Household economic status generally helps in comply with recommended child health measures.

3.4 Determinants of information flow

The analysis reveals the efficacy of network and information channels in encouraging adoption of the MCH practices. A related question is what are the determinants of the network and information scores?

The mean scores for different network mediators are given in Figure 3.2 for India and Bihar. It may be seen that the scores are, in general, lower in Bihar vis-à-vis scores at the all-India level, with the differences being quite

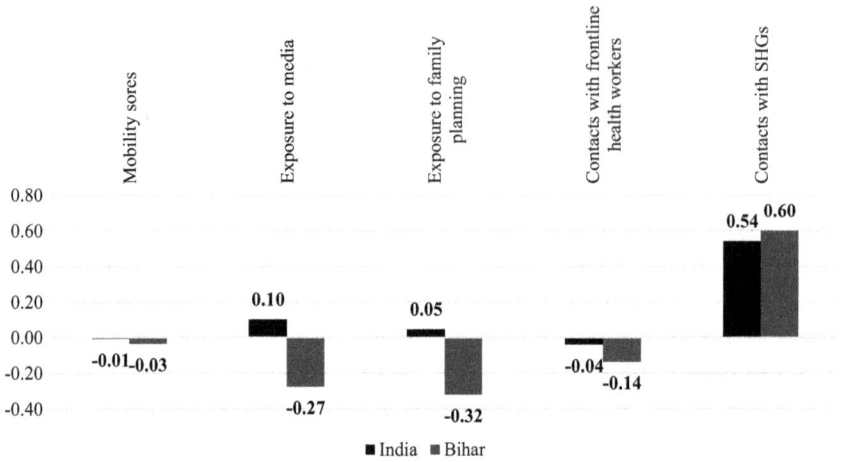

Figure 3.2 Mean scores for network mediators in India and Bihar, NFHS-5, 2019–21.

Note: Normalised scores are reported for mobility, exposure to media, exposure to family planning information, and contacts with front-line health workers. In case of the last indicator (contact with SHGs), the proportion reporting any such contact is shown in the figure.

Source: Estimated from unit-level data by the authors.

high for exposure to mass media, exposure to family planning messages, and contacts with front-line health workers. It implies the possibility of regional variations in the ability to access information – a theme that needs to be explored in greater detail. The only exception is with respect to SHGs. Economic empowerment of women through SHGs is a major component of women development programmes in Bihar; it has facilitated health layering through SHGs. Another point to note is that mobility scores are very low even at the all-India level. It is a major area of concern.

Table 3.5 reports the mean scores for the information and network variables across socio-economic correlates. It may be seen that, for the all-India sample, educated women, and respondents from general caste groups have better access to information, while Muslims are disadvantaged. It holds for all sources of information. In general respondents from affluent households have better contacts and access to information; the only exception is the extensive contacts of front-line health workers and women belonging to less affluent households older or more educated women, and those from affluent households and from SC groups are more likely to have contacts with SHGs. Exposure to media and family planning messages is relatively higher among women aged 20–39 years. Expectedly front-line health workers are observed to target younger women, aged 15–29 years; it is because they belong to the reproductive age group. Older women are observed to be more mobile. It may be due to the patriarchal nature of Indian society, where restrictions on the movements of younger women are used to control the perceived sexuality of women.

The situation is broadly similar in Bihar with some exceptions. Younger women are better placed with respect to information; however, their mobility is restricted. More educated women have better contacts and information; however, they are less connected to front-line health workers. Women from affluent families have higher levels of exposure to media and family planning messages. Women from both the poorest and richest families have higher mobility scores. Hindu women have better sources of information and are also mobile; however, it is Muslim women who have more contacts with front-line health workers. Respondents belonging to non-advantaged social groups have higher levels of exposure to media and family planning messages. Front-line health workers target disadvantaged social groups (SCs and OBCs), while SC and ST women are more mobile. With respect to contacts with SHGs, there does not appear to be systematic variations across the socio-economic correlates.

The results of the econometric model identifying determinants of sources of information and contacts are reported in Table 3.6. The results reveal that access to information is easier for older and more educated women. However, front-line health workers expectedly target younger and less educated women. Access to media is also higher for younger women, while less educated women have more SHG contacts in Bihar. Access to information is higher for general caste groups and less for SCs, STs, and OBCs; however, it does not depend systematically on religion. At the all-India level, Muslim women are less mobile, are exposed less to public media, and have less contacts with SHGs. In Bihar, on the other hand, Muslim women have more contacts with SHGs but are disadvantaged so far as other sources of information are considered, like contacts with front-line health workers. Women from other minority communities have more contacts with front-line health workers, more exposure to media (all-India level), and have more contacts with SHGs (in Bihar). In general information is easier to access in urban areas. However, expectedly, rural women have more contacts with front-line health workers and (at the all-India level) through SHGs.

3.5 Discussion

The present study brings out two important issues. First, all the indices pertaining to possibility of having network, namely, exposure to media/internet, mobility, knowledge and activities of microfinance, relationship with front-line health workers, and exposure to family planning knowledge from media could enhance the utilisation of maternal, childcare, and contraceptive

Table 3.5 Variations in information and network scores across socio-economic correlates for India and Bihar, NFHS-5, 2019–21

Correlates	India					Bihar				
	Exposure to media	Exposure to family planning messages	Contact with front-line health workers	SHG contacts	Mobility	Exposure to media	Exposure to family planning messages	Contact with front-line health workers	SHG contacts	Mobility
Age group										
15–19 years	29.03	31.87	36.80	47.49	55.95	25	23.4	31.95	62.45	54.19
20–29 years	37.39	41.72	40.19	50.60	67.84	29.5	29.54	35.91	55.57	66.29
30–39 years	36.65	42.22	22.07	55.93	76.67	25.06	28.87	15.35	59.32	78.69
40–49 years	30.42	39.12	16.51	56.02	79.44	17.91	24.52	10.04	65.94	81.9
Education										
No education	14.1	21.56	21.03	48.49	74.34	12.95	12.43	20.75	60.72	76.93
Primary	21.94	30.45	25.32	53.79	73.76	19.64	21.77	23.84	56.61	71.34
Secondary	40.67	47.53	30.45	55.40	72.39	35.66	43.01	27.07	59.85	67.94
Higher	67.28	64.82	28.78	59.07	77.66	63.3	65.91	21.49	55.62	73.6
Wealth index quantile										
Poorest	13.4	18.95	29.38	49.55	72.17	14.26	12.68	26.63	60.06	74.25
Poorer	21.88	31.27	29.48	51.55	71.89	22.72	24.7	25.02	59.68	71.79
Middle	31.45	40.38	28.99	55.70	72.48	31.58	40.35	19.38	62.62	70.77
Richer	42.16	46.76	27.03	56.17	73.7	44.77	54.89	21.86	59.77	70.8
Richest	60.66	62.19	21.14	55.65	78.34	61.73	68.41	5.63	47.78	79.2
Religion										
Hindu	35.39	41.68	26.95	54.70	74.66	25.27	28.48	23.11	60.32	73.49
Muslim	29.35	35.04	28.91	47.60	68.3	24.7	24.33	24.33	55.99	71.04
Others	46.22	45.86	22.52	60.98	77.32	14.68	9.01	0.00	11.11	39.68

Caste

Others	43.54	48.82	22.61	52.26	76.06	37.25	42.7	19.18	54.75	70.65
SC	29.32	36.77	28.26	55.32	75.13	19.86	20.71	23.60	61.65	75.1
ST	22.7	29.84	26.65	48.05	73.49	21.93	21.88	20.51	54.70	75.8
OBC	35.34	40.73	28.41	54.66	72.38	24.02	26.71	24.46	60.30	72.73

Source: Estimated from unit-level data by the authors.

Table 3.6 Socio-economic determinants of access to information in India and Bihar, NFHS 5, 2019–21

Mobility index	India			Bihar		
	Coef.	[95% Conf. Interval]		Coef.	[95% Conf. Interval]	
Age	0.61***	0.60	0.62	0.74***	0.69	0.79
Education	0.46***	0.44	0.48	0.04	-0.05	0.12
Employed	5.95***	5.75	6.15	8.44***	7.15	9.72
Religion (Ref: Hindu)						
Muslim	-5.70***	-5.96	-5.44	-1.46**	-2.57	-0.35
Others	-0.26	-0.65	0.14	-33.75***	-47.64	-19.85
Caste (Ref: General)						
OBC	-1.01***	-1.23	-0.79	-1.70**	-2.91	-0.49
Others	-0.51***	-0.76	-0.26	-3.05***	-4.42	-1.69
Log of wealth index	0.26***	0.16	0.35	0.86***	0.48	1.23
Rural	-5.37***	-5.55	-5.19	-7.82***	-8.69	-6.95
State-level fixed effects	Yes					
Intercept	58.24***	56.65	59.84	44.23***	39.20	49.27
Model statistics						
N	422412			18915		
F	1090.77			187.30		
R²	0.10			0.08		

Knowledge of microfinance	Coef.	[95% Conf. Interval]		Coef.	[95% Conf. Interval]	
Age	0.00***	0.00	0.00	0.01***	0.00	0.01
Education	0.00***	0.00	0.00	0.00***	-0.01	0.00
Employed	0.16***	0.16	0.17	0.11***	0.07	0.14
Religion (Ref: Hindu)						
Muslim	-0.06***	-0.07	-0.05	0.08***	0.05	0.10
Others	0.03***	0.02	0.04	0.38**	0.05	0.71
Caste (Ref: General)						
OBC	-0.01***	-0.02	-0.01	-0.05***	-0.08	-0.02
Other	-0.02***	-0.02	-0.01	-0.17***	-0.20	-0.13
Log of wealth index	0.00***	-0.01	0.00	-0.02***	-0.03	-0.02
Rural	0.05***	0.04	0.05	-0.01***	-0.03	0.01
State-level fixed effects						
Intercept	0.09***	0.06	0.13	0.95***	0.83	1.07
Model statistics						
N	422412			18915		
F	1068.520			49.640		
R²	0.100			0.020		

(Continued)

Table 3.6 (Continued)

Mobility index	India			Bihar		
	Coef.	[95% Conf. Interval]		Coef.	[95% Conf. Interval]	
Front-line health worker	Coef.	[95% Conf. Interval]		Coef.	[95% Conf. Interval]	
Age	-1.03***	-1.05	-1.02	-1.09***	-1.15	-1.03
Education	0.39***	0.36	0.41	0.20***	0.10	0.30
Employed	0.06	-0.20	0.33	6.56***	5.11	8.01
Religion (Ref: Hindu)						
Muslim	0.91***	0.57	1.26	-0.27	-1.52	0.98
Others	1.69***	1.16	2.21	-0.45	-16.09	15.19
Caste (Ref: General)						
OBC	-0.69***	-0.99	-0.40	-1.16	-2.52	0.20
Others	-2.67***	-3.01	-2.33	-6.59***	-8.13	-5.06
Log of wealth index	-0.95***	-1.08	-0.83	-0.55**	-0.97	-0.12
Rural	6.49***	6.25	6.74	7.69***	6.71	8.67
State-level fixed effects						
Intercept	65.42***	63.28	67.55	55.67***	50.00	61.34
Model statistics						
N	422412			18915		
F	1443.08			231.30		
R²	0.13			0.10		
Exposure to media	Coef.	[95% Conf. Interval]		Coef.	[95% Conf. Interval]	
Age	-0.02***	-0.03	-0.01	-0.16***	-0.20	-0.13
Education	2.83***	2.82	2.85	2.72***	2.66	2.78
Employed	2.17***	2.03	2.31	4.73***	3.87	5.59
Religion (Ref: Hindu)						
Muslim	-3.19***	-3.37	-3.00	-0.95**	-1.69	-0.21
Others	1.80***	1.52	2.08	1.41	-7.84	10.67
Caste (Ref: General)						
OBC	0.55***	0.40	0.71	-1.13**	-1.93	-0.32
Others	2.74***	2.57	2.92	2.98***	2.07	3.89
Log of wealth index	4.40***	4.34	4.47	3.55***	3.30	3.80
Rural	-4.76***	-4.88	-4.63	-5.38***	-5.95	-4.80
State-level fixed effects						
Intercept	-36.90***	-38.03	-35.77	-18.87***	-22.22	-15.51
Model statistics						
N	422412			18915		
F	8940.26			1863.89		
R²	0.47			0.47		

Source: Estimated from unit-level data by the authors.

services, with some exceptions. Secondly, other demand-side socio-demographic, economic, and cultural factors still continue to affect the inequity in the uptake of these services.

Women during the reproductive period require appropriate and adequate information about healthcare services, and mass media (for instances, television, radio, and newspaper/magazines) can disseminate tailored information about maternal healthcare. Mass media plays a crucial role in decision-making for individuals, households, and organisations, in addition to being a source of news and entertainment (Viswanath et al., 2007). In a recent study conducted on the role of media exposure in utilisation of maternal healthcare services in four South Asian countries of India, Bangladesh, Pakistan, and Nepal, it was found that maternal healthcare utilisation was significantly higher among women exposed to mass media across countries, even after controlling a range of confounding variables (Fatema & Lariscy, 2020). The study further found that women exposed to media were 46–86% more likely to receive ANC, 24–53% more likely to obtain skilled birth attendants, and 36–94% more likely to receive PNC across countries. Studies conducted in 28 sub-Saharan African settings from 2010–20 also revealed that listening to radio, watching television, and reading newspapers/magazines at least once a week have a decisive role in obtaining ANC, delivery, and PNC services (Aboagye et al., 2022). Other studies further revealed that internet was the topmost source of maternal health awareness, while advertisement/campaigns in media were the most common means of obtaining maternal health information (Igbinoba et al., 2020); exposure to radio and television was associated with the timing of ANC initiation (Sserwanja, Mutisya et al., 2022; Sserwanja, Turimumahoro et al., 2022). A study conducted in Vietnam found that media exposure along with interpersonal counselling enhanced exclusive breastfeeding. Molla et al., (2017) and Nguyen et al. (2016) also observed that exposure to public media enhanced the likelihood of appropriate timing of complementary feeding to young children. Our results reconfirm these earlier findings.

Apart from the benefit of mass media on maternal and child health outcomes, some of the recent studies conducted in African settings have proven how effective mass media is increasing the uptake of these modern contraceptive methods owing to the fact that information can have a positive influence on people's attitude and actions (Ajaero et al., 2016; Chola et al., 2020). Mass media such as radio, television, newspapers, billboards, magazines, and digital technologies are vital to the promotion of modern contraception. They ought to be considered as major sources of information that can increase the usage of modern methods by providing accurate information, building self-efficacy and promoting attitudes, behavioural change, and social norms that support the use of modern contraceptives (Apanga et al., 2020). A recent study using NFHS 4 data found that exposure to family planning messages through different media such as radio, television, and newspaper/ magazines had a significant positive effect on the use of reversible modern methods even when various individual, district, state, and regional-level factors were controlled (Ghosh et al., 2021). Our study also supports these findings and argues that an increase in coverage of mass media has the potential to increase the use of family planning services among those who are in need.

In many developing countries including India women's physical mobility is restricted by social norms, structural impediments related to poor quality of roads and transport systems, and security issues (Rajkhowa & Qaim, 2022). Arguably, restrictions on female physical mobility and low levels of empowerment can also have negative implications for women's access to healthcare services. In a study conducted in a north Indian city by Bloom et al. (2001b) it was found that women with greater freedom of movement obtained better antenatal care and were more likely to use safe delivery care. The study further argued that women's autonomy was found to be as important as other known determinants like education. Later studies have observed that other dimensions of autonomy, such as decision-making power, have a significant positive effect on the uptake of maternal healthcare (Mondal et al., 2020). Other studies found that low maternal freedom of movement was associated with increased odds of incomplete immunisation of the child and for not seeking treatment for the child's acute respiratory infection (Malhotra et al., 2014). However, greater maternal freedom may not help in adequate time allocation for exclusive breastfeeding and complementary feeding practices and thus results in suboptimal feeding practices (Irenso et al., 2022; Shroff et al., 2011). The present findings also support these findings. Our analyses also suggest that greater mobility does help in acquiring post-partum contraceptive advice though, it does not help in utilisation of modern methods of family planning. Earlier studies have found that women's mobile phone use is positively associated with their physical mobility range and use of non-surgical contraceptives, whereas it is negatively associated with surgical contraceptive methods (Rajkhowa & Qaim, 2022). This implies that negative or insignificant relationship between women's physical mobility and contraceptive usage as observed in our study as a result of higher use of sterilisation methods among women in overall India and Bihar.

Microfinance is the provision of financial services, including savings, deposit, and credit services, to the poor (Ledgerwood, 2013). Although it was designed to reduce household poverty and an increase in annual household expenditure, particularly among females, microfinance institutions were later engaged with health and nutrition intervention in various LMICs. A meta-analysis of 27 studies carried out in different LMICs between 1990 and 2018 found that microfinance was associated with a 64% increase in the number of women using contraceptives (Gichuru et al., 2019). Additionally, some positive changes were also noted in female empowerment and child nutritional outcomes in the study. In a recent study conducted by using the NFHS 4 dataset, it was found that both microfinance program awareness and participation are associated with higher odds of antenatal care, postnatal checkups, as well as the use of a modern method of contraceptive within 12 months of childbirth (Dehingia et al., 2019). Studies conducted in Bangladesh found that microfinance enhances the likelihood of usage of modern contraception (Murshid & Ely, 2019). A study in Bihar shows that sharing health messages in microfinance-based SHGs is associated with a significant increase in ANC practice. The results suggest the potential of microfinance-based SHGs for improved maternal health service (Walia et al., 2020).

Our study further reconfirms the findings of these studies as we have noticed a positive and significant influence of knowledge and participation in microfinance activities on the uptake of maternal and reproductive health services except delivery care. Why knowledge and participation in microfinance activities do not help in availing institutional delivery or skilled-attendance at delivery needs to be investigated by future studies.

Because of poor maternal and child health outcomes before the current millennium, the Government of India implemented the National Rural Health Mission (NRHM) in 2005 in order to strengthen the existing network of front-line health workers. Subsequently, National Urban Health Mission in 2013 was also started as a strategy to mitigate the shortage of skilled health workers. It is well-established that front-line health workers play an integral role in the supply of MCH services, particularly disseminating information about the government's flagship healthcare programmes among eligible women and their children. A study conducted by using NFHS 4 data revealed that maternal engagement with front-line health workers significantly improves four or more ANC visits, institutional delivery, full immunisation, PNC in 48 hours of delivery, and the likelihood of child survival, particularly among poor and disadvantaged (Rammohan et al., 2021). Almost similar findings were observed in another recent study conducted in the state of Uttar Pradesh (Lyngdoh et al., 2018). Our study also supports these findings. Although earlier studies pointed out that front-line health workers play an important role in disseminating community-based health information including family planning services, our study found that contact with front-line health workers significantly decreases the likelihood of using contraceptive services. Apart from the reasons mentioned in earlier sections (i.e., possibility of endogeneity and quality of discussion during contacts), one can also argue that perhaps the issue of family planning took a back seat because of excessive emphasis on MCH and also due to steady decline of fertility in the recent past. However, to substantiate these arguments, a detailed study seems necessary, which is beyond the scope of the present study.

Apart from these factors, other demand-side factors such as the increase in women's education, focussing employed women in wage-earning sector activities, and targeting socially marginalised and economically disadvantaged living in rural areas are also important to reduce inequity in utilisation of maternal, child care and contraceptive services as many other earlier studies have already pointed out (Ghosh et al., 2015; Ghosh & Siddiqui, 2017).

It is important to note that almost all the studies reviewed in this chapter have used the network variables as predictor variables in a regression model. In contrast, studies identifying correlates of exposure to network are rare. A recent study conducted in African setting has found that higher-aged women (more than 30 years of age), access to mobile phones and internet, belonging to relatively better-off households, and counselling by healthcare providers were facilitating factors for exposure to mass media, while women belonging to younger age brackets and poorer households, and female-headed household were risk factors for the non-exposure of women to mass media. The study argued that empowering household wealth and improving access to ICT could improve women's exposure to mass media (Bloom et al., 2001a). A study conducted sometime back in India asserted that women's educational levels emerged as an important predictor for women's mobility (Gupta & Yesudian, 2006). Earlier studies have found that marginalised social groups, such as SC/ST, come from the economically poorer households, and hence need to move outside the household for work, driven by economic necessity (Deshpande & Kabeer, 2019). General caste households are generally associated with more rigid social norms that constrain women's mobility in the public sphere. It was observed that religious practices, especially in Islam, have also been associated with stricter control over women's public mobility (Chen & Dreze, 1992; Deshpande & Kabeer, 2019; Neff et al., 2012).

3.6 Conclusion

This chapter has established the importance of networks in the form of sources of information and contacts with SHGs and health workers as important determinants of MCH outcomes. Such networks are an important part of behaviour communication change strategies that are being widely used to increase awareness, provide information, and encourage the adaption of MCH practices.

However, it should be acknowledged that the present study has some limitations. First, the study is based on cross-sectional data and thus is not suitable for the analysis of cause–effect relationship. Secondly, none of the community-level variables and supply-side factors were considered in the econometric models because of informational constraints in NFHS data. In the absence of these constraints, the factors are likely to be overestimated. Thirdly, in the absence of information in the NFHS data set, the study does not analyse the pathways through which information and networks change behavioural practices. The latter is important in understanding the impediments embedded in the socio-cultural context to the diffusion of information at the grass-roots level (Barnett et al., 2022).

Nonetheless, in absence of direct indicators representing network, the present study used some proxy indicators though econometrically preparing indices of media/internet exposure, knowledge and participation in microfinance activities, women's mobility outside home, exposure to family planning messages in media, and contact with front-line health workers.

The present study has tried to find out the relationship of these indices with a range of outcome variables representing maternal and child healthcare utilisation, and use of modern contraceptive methods and found that these indices have significant positive influence on outcome indicators in most of the cases. The study has also identified groups with a lack of access to networks and sources of information. These groups may be targeted to improve their access to information and networks, thereby improving their MCH outcomes. Finally, in order to supplement the analysis of the impact of networks and information, we have undertaken a primary study in Bihar, a high-focus state in Eastern India, examining the process of dissemination of information on MCH practices. It will help us to assess the relative effectiveness of different BCC strategies and identify the obstacles in the flow of information to the target recipient.

Notes

1 Polychoric PCA is an alternative form of PCA. Polychoric correlations assume the variables are ordered measurements of an underlying continuum of variables. The variables do not need to be truly continuous and they do not need to be normally distributed.

2 The Wald statistic (24.60) rejects the null hypothesis of exogeneity. The coefficient of FLHW100 turns out to be positive (0.02, 95% CI: .023– .025). This is the expected sign. It was revealed that index of exposure to FLWs is significantly higher for respondents who have adopted modern contraception at the all-India level. In Bihar, a similar result is observed among respondents who adopted modern contraception.

References

Aboagye, R. G., Seidu, A.-A., Ahinkorah, B. O., Cadri, A., Frimpong, J. B., Hagan, J. E., Kassaw, N. A., & Yaya, S. (2022). Association between frequency of mass media exposure and maternal health care service utilization among women in sub-Saharan Africa: Implications for tailored health communication and education. *PLoS One*, *17*(9), e0275202. https://doi.org/10.1371/journal.pone .0275202

Ajaero, C. K., Odimegwu, C., Ajaero, I. D., & Nwachukwu, C. A. (2016). Access to mass media messages, and use of family planning in Nigeria: A spatio-demographic analysis from the 2013 DHS. *BMC Public Health*, *16*(1), 427. https://doi.org/10.1186/s12889-016-2979-z

Apanga, P. A., Kumbeni, M. T., Ayamga, E. A., Ulanja, M. B., & Akparibo, R. (2020). Prevalence and factors associated with modern contraceptive use among women of reproductive age in 20 African countries: A large population-based study. *BMJ Open*, *10*(9), e041103. https://doi.org/10.1136/bmjopen-2020-041103

Barnett, I., Meeker, J., Roelen, K., & Nisbett, N. (2022). Behaviour change communication for child feeding in social assistance: A scoping review and expert consultation. *Maternal and Child Nutrition*, *18*(3), 1–14. https://doi.org/10.1111/mcn.13361

Bloom, S. S., Wypij, D., & Das Gupta, M. (2001a). Dimensions of women's autonomy and the influence on maternal health care utilization in a North Indian city. *Demography*, *38*(1), 67–78.

Bloom, S. S., Wypij, D., & Das Gupta, M. (2001b). Dimensions of women's autonomy and the influence on maternal health care utilization in a North Indian city. *Demography*, *38*(1), 67–78. https://doi.org/10.1353/dem.2001.0001

Bouckaert, N. (2014). Neighborhood peer effects in the use of preventive health care. *SSRN Electronic Journal*. https://doi.org/10.2139/ssrn.2381880

Chen, M., & Dreze, J. (1992). Widows and health in rural north India. *Economic & Political Weekly*, *27*(1), 7–8.

Chola, M., Hlongwana, K., & Ginindza, T. G. (2020). Patterns, trends, and factors associated with contraceptive use among adolescent girls in Zambia (1996 to 2014): A multilevel analysis. *BMC Women's Health*, *20*(1), 185. https://doi.org/10.1186/s12905-020-01050-1

Dehingia, N., Singh, A., Raj, A., & McDougal, L. (2019). More than credit: Exploring associations between microcredit programs and maternal and reproductive health service utilization in India. *SSM - Population Health*, *9*(August), 100467. https://doi.org/10.1016/j.ssmph.2019.100467

Deshpande, A., & Kabeer, N. (2019). *(In)visibility, care and cultural barriers: The size and shape of women's work in India* (4/19; Economics Discussion Paper).

Fatema, K., & Lariscy, J. T. (2020). Mass media exposure and maternal healthcare utilization in South Asia. *SSM - Population Health*, *11*, 100614. https://doi.org/10.1016/j.ssmph.2020.100614

Fletcher, J. M. (2014). Peer effects in health behaviors. In A. J. Culyer (Ed.), *Encyclopedia of health economics* (pp. 467–72, 1st ed.). Elsevier. https://doi.org/10.1016/B978-0-12-375678-7.00311-4

Ghosh, K., Chakraborty, A. S., & Mog, M. (2021). Prevalence of diarrhoea among under five children in India and its contextual determinants: A geo-spatial analysis. *Clinical Epidemiology and Global Health*, *12*, 100813.

Ghosh, R., Mozumdar, A., Chattopadhyay, A., & Acharya, R. (2021). Mass media exposure and use of reversible modern contraceptives among married women in India: An analysis of the NFHS 2015–16 data. *PLoS One*, *16*(7 July), 1–23. https://doi.org/10.1371/journal.pone.0254400

Ghosh, S., & Husain, Z. (2019). Has the national health mission improved utilisation of maternal healthcare services in Bihar? *Economic & Political Weekly*, *54*(31), 44–51.

Ghosh, S., & Siddiqui, M. Z. (2017). Role of community and context in contraceptive behaviour in rural West Bengal, India: A multilevel multinomial approach. *Journal of Biosocial Science*, 49(1), 48–68. https://doi.org/10.1017/S0021932016000080

Ghosh, S., Siddiqui, M. Z., Barik, A., & Bhaumik, S. (2015). Determinants of skilled delivery assistance in a rural population: Findings from an HDSS Site of rural West Bengal, India. *Maternal and Child Health Journal*, 19(11), 2470–2479.

Gichuru, W., Ojha, S., Smith, S., Smyth, A. R., & Szatkowski, L. (2019). Is microfinance associated with changes in women's well-being and children's nutrition? A systematic review and meta-analysis. *BMJ Open*, 9(1), 1–17. https://doi.org/10.1136/bmjopen-2018-023658

Gupta, K., & Yesudian, P. P. (2006). Evidence of women's empowerment in India: A study of socio-spatial disparities. *GeoJournal*, 65(4), 365–380. https://doi.org/10.1007/s10708-006-7556-z

International Institute of Population Sciences. (2020). *National family health survey –5, state fact sheet Bihar*. International Institute for Population Sciences.

International Institute of Population Sciences. (2022). *National family health survey –5, India*. International Institute for Population Sciences.

Igbinoba, A. O., Soola, E. O., Omojola, O., Odukoya, J., Adekeye, O., & Salau, O. P. (2020). Women's mass media exposure and maternal health awareness in Ota, Nigeria. *Cogent Social Sciences*, 6(1). https://doi.org/10.1080/23311886.2020.1766260

Irenso, A. A., Letta, S., Chemeda, A. S., Asfaw, A., Egata, G., Assefa, N., Campbell, K. J., & Laws, R. (2022). Maternal time use drives suboptimal complementary feeding practices in the El Niño-affected eastern Ethiopia community. *International Journal of Environmental Research and Public Health*, 19(7), 3937. https://doi.org/10.3390/ijerph19073937

Katz, E., & Lazarsfeld, P. F. (2005). *Personal Influence the Part Played by People in the Flow of Mass Communications*. Transaction.

Ledgerwood, J. (2013). *The new microfinance handbook ew mfinancial market system perspective*. The World Bank. https://openknowledge.worldbank.org/handle/10986/12272

Lyngdoh, T., Neogi, S. B., Ahmad, D., Soundararajan, S., & Mavalankar, D. (2018). Intensity of contact with frontline workers and its influence on maternal and newborn health behaviors: Cross-sectional survey in rural Uttar Pradesh, India. *Journal of Health, Population and Nutrition*, 37(1), 1–11. https://doi.org/10.1186/s41043-017-0129-6

Malhotra, C., Malhotra, R., Østbye, T., & Subramanian, S. V. (2014). Maternal autonomy and child health care utilization in India: Results from the national family health survey. *Asia-Pacific Journal of Public Health*, 26(4), 401–413. https://doi.org/10.1177/1010539511420418

Molla, M., Ejigu, T., & Nega, G. (2017). Complementary feeding practice and associated factors among mothers having children 6–23 months of age, Lasta District, Amhara Region, Northeast Ethiopia. *Advances in Public Health*, 2017, 1–8. https://doi.org/10.1155/2017/4567829

Mondal, D., Karmakar, S., & Banerjee, A. (2020). Women's autonomy and utilization of maternal healthcare in India: Evidence from a recent national survey. *PLoS One*, 15(12 December), 1–12. https://doi.org/10.1371/journal.pone.0243553

Murshid, N. S., & Ely, G. E. (2019). Microfinance participation and contraceptive use and intention in Bangladesh. *International Social Work*, 62(4), 1274–1285. https://doi.org/10.1177/0020872818774089

Neff, D., Sen, K., & Ling, V. (2012). *Puzzling decline in rural women's labor force participation in India: A reexamination* (No. 196; Working Paper).

Nguyen, P. H., Kim, S. S., Nguyen, T. T., Hajeebhoy, N., Tran, L. M., Alayon, S., Ruel, M. T., Rawat, R., Frongillo, E. A., & Menon, P. (2016). Exposure to mass media and interpersonal counseling has additive effects on exclusive breastfeeding and its psychosocial determinants among Vietnamese mothers. *Maternal and Child Nutrition*, 12(4), 713–725. https://doi.org/10.1111/mcn.12330

Rajkhowa, P., & Qaim, M. (2022). Mobile phones, women's physical mobility, and contraceptive use in India. *Social Science and Medicine*, 305(January), 115074. https://doi.org/10.1016/j.socscimed.2022.115074

Rammohan, A., Goli, S., Saroj, S. K., & Jaleel, C. P. A. (2021). Does engagement with frontline health workers improve maternal and child healthcare utilisation and outcomes in India? *Human Resources for Health*, 19(1), 1–21. https://doi.org/10.1186/s12960-021-00592-1

Shroff, M. R., Griffiths, P. L., Suchindran, C., Nagalla, B., Vazir, S., & Bentley, M. E. (2011). Does maternal autonomy influence feeding practices and infant growth in rural India? *Social Science & Medicine*, 73(3), 447–455. https://doi.org/10.1016/j.socscimed.2011.05.040

Sserwanja, Q., Mutisya, L. M., & Musaba, M. W. (2022). Exposure to different types of mass media and timing of antenatal care initiation: Insights from the 2016 Uganda Demographic and Health Survey. *BMC Women's Health*, 22(1), 1–8. https://doi.org/10.1186/s12905-022-01594-4

Sserwanja, Q., Turimumahoro, P., Nuwabaine, L., Kamara, K., & Musaba, M. W. (2022). Association between exposure to family planning messages on different mass media channels and the utilization of modern contraceptives among young women in Sierra Leone: Insights from the 2019 Sierra Leone Demographic Health Survey. *BMC Women's Health*, 22(1), 1–10. https://doi.org/10.1186/s12905-022-01974-w

Viswanath, K., Ramanadhan, S., & Kontos, E. Z. (2007). Mass media. In *Macrosocial determinants of population health* (pp. 275–294). Springer New York. https://doi.org/10.1007/978-0-387-70812-6_13

Walia, M., Irani, L., Chaudhuri, I., Atmavilas, Y., & Saggurti, N. (2020). Effect of sharing health messages on antenatal care behavior among women involved in microfinance-based self-help groups in Bihar India. *Global Health Research and Policy*, 5(1), 3. https://doi.org/10.1186/s41256-020-0132-0

Webel, A. R., Okonsky, J., Trompeta, J., & Holzemer, W. L. (2010). A systematic review of the effectiveness of peer-based interventions on health-related behaviors in adults. *American Journal of Public Health*, 100(2), 247–253. https://doi.org/10.2105/AJPH.2008.149419

Appendix

Table A3.1 Variations in exposure to media/internet across outcome variables, NFHS-5, 2019–21

Outcome variables	India				Bihar			
	Yes	No	Diff	t-test	Yes	No	Diff	t-test
Pregnancy registration in the first trimester of pregnancy	36.16	28.39	7.76	22.40***	26.18	20.54	5.64	5.93***
At least four ANC check-ups	37.69	28.28	9.41	29.44***	31.49	20.86	10.63	9.86***
Had at least 100 IFA tablet/syrup	39.13	30.69	8.44	24.74***	31.37	22.80	8.57	6.55***
Had at least two tetanus	34.83	29.37	5.46	13.13***	24.24	21.28	2.96	2.62*
Received full ANC	41.74	31.19	10.55	29.26***	38.42	22.52	15.90	8.36***
Delivered in an institution	35.93	19.26	16.86	35.28***	25.67	15.94	9.73	8.55***
Received skilled-attendance during delivery	35.53	20.55	14.98	30.08***	25.05	16.92	8.14	6.67***
Received PNC within 48 hours of delivery	31.91	34.47	-2.56	6.82***	22.92	23.76	-0.84	0.75
Using modern contraceptive methods	35.93	32.14	3.79	11.87***	24.51	23.09	1.42	1.39
Received advice on post-partum contraception	34.22	31.14	3.08	6.02***	23.70	23.23	0.47	0.33
Received vaccine at birth (OPV0) for the indexed child	14.03	10.83	3.20	13.76***	8.71	7.74	0.97	1.57
Given exclusive breastfeeding for six months to the indexed child	13.24	12.82	0.42	1.76	7.97	8.35	-0.38	0.58
Started complementary feeding after six months	13.77	13.84	0.78	0.80	8.75	8.22	0.53	1.94

Source: Estimated from unit-level data by the authors.

Table A3.2 Variations in mobility across outcome variables, NFHS-5, 2019–21

Outcome variables	India				Bihar			
	Yes	No	Diff	t-test	Yes	No	Diff	t-test
Pregnancy registration in the first trimester of pregnancy	70.86	69.63	1.23	3.12**	71.49	70.17	1.31	0.96
At least four ANC check-ups	71.69	68.87	2.82	7.69***	69.06	71.35	-2.29	1.46
Had at least 100 IFA tablet/syrup	72.14	69.29	2.85	7.38***	72.82	70.49	2.33	1.29
Had at least two tetanus	70.77	69.31	1.46	3.11**	70.68	71.44	-0.77	0.48
Received full ANC	72.93	69.69	3.24	7.85***	70.86	70.85	0.01	0.00
Delivered in an institution	70.55	70.25	0.30	0.58	70.73	71.29	-0.56	0.33
Received skilled-attendance during delivery	70.62	69.62	1.00	1.75	70.82	71.00	-0.18	0.10
Received PNC within 48 hours of delivery	70.29	70.58	-0.29	0.69	72.02	70.48	1.54	0.97
Using modern contraceptive methods	71.68	69.63	2.15	5.94***	72.62	70.00	2.62	1.83
Received advice on post-partum contraception	71.28	66.96	4.32	7.44***	74.16	69.13	5.03	2.52***
Received vaccine at birth (OPV0) for the indexed child	70.02	67.61	2.41	2.46*	69.95	63.48	6.47	2.04*
Given exclusive breastfeeding for six months to the indexed child	65.00	66.80	-1.80	1.72	63.22	68.32	-5.10	0.18
Started complementary feeding after six months	69.35	72.05	-2.70	6.63***	68.25	72.61	-4.36	2.93**

Source: Estimated from unit-level data by the authors.

Table A3.3 Variations in involvement in SHG activities across outcome variables, NFHS-5, 2019–21

Outcome variables	India				Bihar			
	Yes	No	Diff	t-test	Yes	No	Diff	t-test
Pregnancy registration in the first trimester of pregnancy	0.50	0.42	0.08	12.14***	0.62	0.56	0.06	2.75**
At least four ANC check-ups	0.51	0.42	0.09	14.58***	0.64	0.57	0.07	2.72**
Had at least 100 IFA tablet/syrup	0.51	0.46	0.05	8.21***	0.57	0.59	-0.02	0.71
Had at least two tetanus	0.49	0.40	0.09	11.40***	0.60	0.56	0.04	1.48
Received full ANC	0.56	0.44	0.12	16.64***	0.64	0.58	0.06	1.25
Delivered in an institution	0.48	0.41	0.07	7.77***	0.59	0.590	0.00	0.93
Received skilled-attendance during delivery	0.48	0.42	0.06	6.22***	0.58	0.62	-0.04	1.59
Received PNC within 48 hours of delivery	0.46	0.47	-0.01	1.33	0.61	0.58	0.03	1.32
Using modern contraceptive methods	0.50	0.45	0.05	8.65***	0.60	0.58	0.02	0.40
Received advice on post-partum contraception	0.52	0.47	0.05	5.09***	0.62	0.64	-0.02	0.57
Received vaccine at birth (OPV0) for the indexed child	0.07	0.06	0.01	2.02*	0.11	0.10	0.01	0.63
Given exclusive breastfeeding for six months to the indexed child	0.07	0.06	0.01	1.79	0.09	0.09	0.00	0.06
Started complementary feeding after six months	0.09	0.09	0.00	0.48	0.09	0.08	0.01	1.58

Source: Estimated from unit-level data by the authors.

Table A3.4 Exposure to front-line health workers across outcome variables, NFHS-5, 2019–21

Outcome variables	India				Bihar			
	Yes	No	Diff	t-test	Yes	No	Diff	t-test
Pregnancy registration in the first trimester of pregnancy	48.12	43.70	4.42	7.61***	43.42	35.20	8.22	4.36***
At least four ANC check-ups	49.85	42.72	7.13	13.21***	43.90	38.23	5.67	2.60**
Had at least 100 IFA tablet/syrup	50.79	46.81	3.98	6.99***	46.68	41.18	5.50	2.17*
Had at least two tetanus	47.35	43.98	3.37	4.87***	38.64	42.60	-3.36	1.77
Received full ANC	52.43	44.83	7.60	12.53***	46.62	39.07	7.55	1.98*
Delivered in an institution	47.71	39.99	7.72	9.63***	40.62	35.78	4.84	2.11*
Received skilled-attendance during delivery	47.55	40.38	7.17	8.54***	40.58	35.07	5.51	2.26*
Received PNC within 48 hours of delivery	56.79	43.64	13.15	21.30***	49.08	36.54	12.54	5.73***
Using modern contraceptive methods	45.69	47.64	-1.96	3.68**	34.35	42.12	-7.77	3.88**
Received advice on post-partum contraception	58.82	46.11	12.71	15.11***	53.61	51.72	1.89	0.66
Received vaccine at birth (OPV0) for the indexed child	52.27	41.47	10.80	18.84***	42.65	35.96	6.69	3.74**
Given exclusive breastfeeding for six months to the indexed child	69.30	63.58	5.72	10.33***	64.77	53.75	11.02	5.65***
Started complementary feeding after six months	52.30	39.47	12.83	53.92***	43.99	30.52	13.47	17.14***

Source: Estimated from unit-level data by the authors.

Table A3.5 Exposure to family planning messages in various media across outcome variables, NFHS-5, 2019–21

Outcome variables	India				Bihar			
	Yes	No	Diff	t-test	Yes	No	Diff	t-test
Pregnancy registration in the first trimester of pregnancy	41.71	34.36	7.35	15.09***	28.89	22.35	6.54	4.29***
At least four ANC check-ups	43.26	34.38	8.88	19.65***	37.24	21.98	15.26	8.82***
Had at least 100 IFA tablet/syrup	44.33	37.52	6.81	14.29***	36.78	25.51	11.27	5.39***
Had at least two tetanus	40.77	33.58	7.19	12.38***	27.18	21.36	5.82	3.23**
Received full ANC	45.94	37.32	8.62	16.94***	45.06	24.49	20.57	6.73***
Delivered in an institution	42.04	21.57	20.47	30.84***	29.16	13.86	15.30	8.40***
Received skilled-attendance during delivery	41.54	23.18	18.36	26.28***	28.34	14.73	13.61	6.99***
Received PNC within 48 hours of delivery	41.03	39.02	2.01	3.84**	26.57	25.60	0.97	0.54
Using modern contraceptive methods	43.11	36.50	6.61	14.85***	29.66	23.95	5.71	3.53**
Received advice on post-partum contraception	43.72	30.41	13.31	18.65***	32.42	17.76	14.66	6.36***
Received vaccine at birth (OPV0) for the indexed child	40.97	30.54	10.43	21.05***	28.75	20.56	8.19	5.39***
Given exclusive breastfeeding for six months to the indexed child	38.81	38.25	0.56	1.07	25.09	28.50	-3.41	2.02*
Started complementary feeding after six months	39.02	40.43	-1.41	6.87***	27.19	27.10	0.09	0.13

Source: Estimated from unit-level data by the authors.

Table A3.6 Direction of the effects of control variables for different outcome variables related to uptake of maternal healthcare, NFHS-5, 2019–21

Control variables	Registration in the first trimester		At least four ANC check-ups		At least 100 or more IFA tablets		At least two TT injections		Full ANC		Institutional delivery		Skilled-attendance in delivery		PNC in 48 hours	
	India	Bihar	India	Bihar	India	Bihar	India	Bihar	India	Bihar	India	Bihar	India	Bihar	India	Bihar
Current age of respondents	-	+	-	+	+	+	NS	+	+	+	-	-	-	-	+	NS
Completed years of schooling of respondents	+	+	+	+	+	+	+	+	+	+	+	+	+	+	+	NS
Whether respondent works	-	NS	-	-	-	+	NS	NS	-	NS	-	-	-	-	+	+
Religious affiliation (Ref: Hindu)																
Muslim	-	NS	NS	NS	+	+	NS	NS	NS	NS	-	NS	-	-	-	NS
Others	+	-	+	NS	NS	NS	NS	-	NS	NS	+	-	-	-	NS	NS
Affiliation to social group (Ref: General Caste)																
SC/ST	-	+	-	-	-	-	+	+	-	-	-	NS	-	NS	-	+
OBC	-	-	-	-	-	NS	NS	+	-	-	-	-	-	NS	-	NS
Rural	-	-	-	-	-	-	-	-	-	-	-	NS	-	-	+	+

Source: Estimated from unit-level data by the authors
NS: Not Significant

Table A3.7 Direction of the effects of control variables for different outcome variables related to uptake of contraceptive services and child healthcare, NFHS-5, 2019–21

Control variables	Current use of modern contraception		Received advice on post-partum contraception		Received OPV0 for the youngest child		Exclusive breastfeeding for six months for the youngest child		Started complementary feeding after six months	
	India	Bihar	India	Bihar	India	Bihar	India	Bihar	India	Bihar
Current age of respondents	+	+	+	+	+	-	NS	NS	-	-
Completed years of schooling of respondents	-	-	-	-	+	NS	-	-	+	-
Whether respondent works	+	+	NS	-	+	-	-	-	-	-
Religious affiliation (Ref: Hindu)										
Muslim	-	-	+	-	-	-	-	-	+	+
Others	+	+	-	NS	+	NS	NS	NS	-	+
Affiliation to social group (Ref: General Caste)										
SC/ST	-	+	+	+	NS	-	+	NS	NS	+
OBC	-	-	NS	-	NS	-	NS	NS	-	+
Normalised mean wealth score (0–100)	+	+	NS	NS	+	+	+	NS	+	-
Rural	-	NS	NS	NS	NS	NS	NS	NS	NS	NS

Source: Estimated from unit-level data by the authors.
NS: Not Significant

Chapter 4

Health communication through SHGs

Assessing the JEEViKA programme in Bihar

4.1 Introduction

In recent years, policymakers are gradually realising that microfinance institutions and self-help groups (SHGs) – originally established to mobilise women from poor households to improve their economic conditions – may also be used as an instrument for improving community health (CH) outcomes sustainably (Mehta et al., 2020). Based on the premise that most health problems emerge due to lack of agency, "health layering" of SHGs has been advocated as they empower women (Wallerstein, 1992; Rosato et al., 2008), and enable them to "develop consciousness to recognise and address the underlying social and political determinants of health. For example, where gender inequity constrains improvements in maternal survival, empowered groups could give women the understanding, confidence, and support to choose a healthy diet in pregnancy, and seek care or advice outside of their homes" (Prost et al., 2013, p. 1737).

In 2006, the Bihar Government and The World Bank initiated an SHG-based programme to empower women and reduce poverty levels; this scheme also attempted to improve health outcomes through an Integrated Health and Nutrition Strategy. The program was initiated under the Bihar Rural Livelihoods Project (BRLP) in six districts and 42 blocks of Bihar. Since then, the program has been scaled up to include all 38 districts of Bihar, replicating the lessons of BRLP in the entire state. The objective of JEEViKA is to enhance the social and economic empowerment of the rural poor in Bihar. The core strategy of the BRLP programme is to build vibrant and bankable women's community institutions in the form of self-help groups (SHGs) that gradually through member savings, internal loaning, and regular repayment become self-sustaining organisations, self-managing their development processes. The project strategy is therefore phased in a manner of first horizontally building up a very large number of primary level women-based SHG groups with the help of rural poor folks, nested under Village Organisations, at the village level.

DOI: 10.4324/9781003499251-4

JEEViKA has thus far mobilised nearly 8.2 million rural women into more than 689,000 SHGs and their federations. These community institutions have emerged as the most effective platforms for linking the poorest to the formal banking system. The JEEViKA programme has been successful in increasing the income level of households under the scheme. A survey in 2016 reported that incomes of about 65% of the households associated with JEEViKA's community investment fund had improved by 30% over the baseline level. However, investments in reducing poverty did not result in commensurate improvements in health and nutrition outcomes.

This led JEEViKA to initiate a pilot study in six blocks in 2012 with the objective of making adoption and utilisation of health, nutrition, and sanitation behaviours and services an integral part of its empowerment strategy (The World Bank, 2016). The Health and Nutrition Strategy is centred on empowering women to bring about a change in health and nutrition practices within their households and the community. The approach focuses on the implementation of a comprehensive behaviour change communication strategy, and includes the following:

(a) ensuring early registration of pregnancy, ante and postnatal check-ups, identification of high-risk cases,
(b) counselling for maternal nutrition (iron folate tablet consumption, dietary diversity during pregnancy),
(c) institutional delivery and birth preparedness,
(d) early initiation and exclusive breastfeeding, complementary feeding practices, and
(e) sanitation and hygiene.

Such behavioural change was sought to be operationalised by JEEViKA's community mobilisers (CMs), Master Resource Persons, and core block and district staff (i.e., district and block programme managers and area and cluster coordinators). The strategy was built around JEEViKA's existing platform of women's community networks. The key facilitators driving the behavioural change were the CMs who impart information to women's SHGs through thematic health, nutrition, and sanitation modules during one of the four weekly SHG meetings held in a month and follow up on actions in the subsequent weekly meeting to reinforce messages. Internal monitoring systems and concurrent monitoring of key outcomes were used to identify "sticky" behaviours that are difficult to change. The sticky behavioural practices were nudged through the design of additional tools (The World Bank, 2016; JEEViKA, 2019). Evaluation of the pilot scheme showed encouraging results, and the strategy was scaled up from 2016 (JEEViKA, 2019).

Studies have reported improvements in institutional delivery, use of contraception methods, utilisation of ante- and postnatal care services, immunisation of children, breastfeeding, and nutritional outcomes (Saha et al., 2013;

Saha et al., 2015; Mozumdar et al., 2018; Saggurti et al., 2018; Hazra et al., 2020; Mehta et al., 2020). There have been studies specifically focussing on the Health and Nutrition Strategy implemented by JEEViKA (The World Bank, 2016; Gupta et al., 2019). Such studies reported promising results:

> Early results, from the progressive implementation of this strategy for over two and half years, are showing positive outcomes, particularly in the key result area of diet diversity. This is evidenced through both ongoing surveys as well as a rigorous impact evaluation to determine the efficacy of the approach. CARE India covered 15,657 children through surveys using the Lot Quality Assurance Sampling (LQAS) methodology, which showed positive trends along with indicators of diet diversity for children in the critical age bracket of 9–11 months. A rigorous impact evaluation of the integrated health, nutrition and sanitation approach by IFPRI in Saharsa District of Bihar further showed small but significant impacts on women's and children's diet diversity, validating the efficacy of the approach".
>
> (The World Bank, 2016)

Another evaluation focussing solely on the district of Saharsa found positive and significant impacts of the intervention on the number of food groups consumed by children (Gupta et al., 2019). Among women, a 30% increase among those consuming at least five out of ten food groups was reported over the baseline levels. Moreover, the consumption of iron-folic acid tablets and calcium tablets increased among pregnant women.

Most of the empirical assessments of attempts to influence SHG members' adoption of the provided health services are localized and may suffer from placement bias. Comparisons of adoption rates of health behaviour between SHG members and non-members may also suffer from endogeneity due to self-selection. Even propensity score matching – used by Mehta et al. (2020) – suffers from this problem, if unobserved characteristics determine assignment to treatment or control group. Thirdly, these studies do not take into account whether respondents are passive members of SHGs, who have enlisted but never attended or participated in meetings, or do so sporadically. This implies that, despite belonging to the treatment group, such members do not receive the treatment. Finally, there may be spill-over effects from SHG members and non-members.

In this chapter we assess the success of the Health and Nutrition Scheme (HNS) in encouraging the adoption of maternal and child health (MCH) practices. Section 4.2 identifies the specific behavioural practices studied. It is followed by a discussion of the methods employed to investigate the research questions. The results are analysed in Section 4.4. This section starts with an analysis of the incidence of adoption of the best practices among JEEViKA members and non-members; it is followed by an examination of the variation in adoption rates across correlates like age and education of respondents, socio-religious groups, and households classified by asset holdings. The exploratory analysis is followed by a discussion of the econometric models testing for significant differences in adoption rates of behavioural practices studied between JEEViKA members and non-members. The section also examines diffusion of the practices within the village – across members and from the members to non-members. A concluding section sums up the main results and discusses the research and policy implications of the study.

4.2 Objectives

In this chapter we will examine the adoption rates of practices that will improve maternal and child health (MCH) outcomes. The practices expected to improve maternal outcomes are:

(i) **Controlling fertility:**
   a. Use of modern contraception methods after marriage,
   b. Advice on post-partum contraception method.
(ii) **ANC services:**
   a. First ANC visit in the first trimester of pregnancy,
   b. Availed at least four ANC check-ups,
   c. Protection against neonatal tetanus (through tetanus toxoid injections),
   d. Took 100 IFA tablets/syrup for anaemia during pregnancy,
   e. Availed full ANC services.[1]
(iii) **Institutional delivery and PNC services:**
   a. Delivered in an institution.
   b. Delivery assisted by a skilled person,
   c. Availed post-partum check-ups within 48 hours of delivery.
(iv) **Child health outcomes:**
   a. Giving polio vaccine at birth (OPV0) to a child,
   b. Exclusively breastfeeding a child at least up to six months of birth,
   c. Complementary feeding after six months of birth.

We obtained information on whether the respondents had adopted the above MCH practices for all the above practices from the respondents with the exception of full ANC services. Whether the respondent had availed full ANC services was determined based on information on practices (ii)–(v); information on whether the respondent had availed this service was not elicited from the respondent directly.

We have examined whether there is any difference in the adoption levels between JEEViKA and non-JEEViKA members. The analysis is followed by an attempt to understand the factors underlying the adoption of the practices. We have also examined whether there is any bandwagon (or peer effects), or whether there is any spill-over of the program effect from JEEViKA members to non-members. The method of analysis is described in detail below.

4.3 Materials and method

4.3.1 Data

The data on which the analysis is based was collected from a primary survey undertaken between January and March 2020. It covered 2,250 respondents aged 15–49 years from six randomly selected districts of Bihar. The details of the survey design, sampling strategy, and survey instruments are given in Section 2.3 in Chapter 2.

4.3.2 Identifying determinants of adopting best practices

The analysis comprises two parts. The first part is exploratory, examining the adoption rates of the best practices, and the second part is to examine its variations across socio-economic correlates like age and education of the respondents, economic status of respondent's family measured using a standard of living index, and socio-religious identity of the respondent.

The exploratory analysis does not control for socio-economic characteristics. To overcome this deficiency, we undertake an econometric analysis with two objectives:

- Whether JEEViKA members are more likely to adopt such practices than non-members,
- What are the other determinants of adopting the practices studied, and
- Whether there is any bandwagon effect.[2]

We have estimated the following regression model:

$$Y_{ij} = \beta_0 + \beta_1 JEEViKA_{ij} + \beta_2 X_{ij} + z_{ij} u_j + \varepsilon_{ij} \qquad [4.1]$$

Where

Y^{ij} is a binary variable indicating whether the ith respondent residing in the jth village has adopted the best practice or not.

$JEEViKA_{ij}$ is a dummy taking the value of 1 if the ith respondent in j^{th} village is a JEEViKA member and 0 otherwise.

X_{ij} are control variables (individual and household level characteristics of the ith respondent in j^{th} village).

The control variables are: age, education, standard of living index scores, socio-religious identity, number of living children, household size, whether respondent works, and whether her husband is a migrant. The error terms are explained subsequently.

It should be noted that a large number of JEEViKA members do not attend meetings at all, or do so irregularly. It implies that, although they are part of the treatment group, they do not actually receive the treatment. So we are finding out average intent-to-treat (AIT), not average treatment effect (ATE). The distinction between the two is that while ATE is "the average gain in outcomes of participants relative to nonparticipants, as if nonparticipating households were also treated" (Khandker et al., 2010), AIT is obtained if there is contamination between treatment and control groups – with all members of treatment group not receiving the treatment, while some members of the control group may receive the treatment.

As a robustness check, we will also estimate the local treatment effect (LTE), by dropping those JEEViKA members who did not receive the treatment (i.e., attend meetings regularly) and re-estimating (equation [4.1]). This is the impact of the programme on the subset of the sample that takes the treatment if and only if they were assigned to the treatment (Imbens & Angrist, 1994). Thus, the local average treatment effect (LATE) is only the ATE among the compliers.

The dependent variable (probability of adopting a practice) is binary. We have used a mixed-effects probit regression. It is a probit regression containing both fixed effects and random effects. In a two-level model, for a series of M independent clusters (say villages), and conditional on a set of fixed effects x_{ij} and a set of random effects u_j,

$$\text{Prob}(y_{ij} = 1 | x_{ij}, u_j) = H(x_{ij}\beta + z_{ij}u_j) \qquad [4.2]$$

For j = 1, ... , M clusters, with cluster j consisting of I = 1, ... ,n_j observations. The responses are the binary-valued y_{ij}, such that y_{ij} = 1 or 0. The 1 × p row vector x_{ij} are the covariates for the fixed effects, and are similar to the covariates of a standard probit regression model, with regression coefficients, β. They are often referred to as fixed effects. These variables are: whether the respondent is a JEEViKA member (the main study variable), age, education, standard of living index scores, socio-religious identity, number of living children, household size, whether the respondent works, and whether her husband is a migrant.

The 1 × q vector z_{ij} are the covariates corresponding to the random effects and can be used to represent both random intercepts and random coefficients. For example, in a random-intercept model, z_{ij} is simply the scalar 1. The random effects u are M realisations from a multivariate normal distribution with mean 0 and a q × q variance matrix Σ. The random effects are not directly estimated as model parameters but are instead summarized according to the unique elements of Σ, known as variance components. Finally, because this is probit regression, $H(\cdot)$ is the standard normal cumulative distribution function, which maps the linear predictor to the probability of success (y_{ij} = 1) with $H(v) = \Phi(v)$. The model may also be stated in terms of a latent linear response, where only $y_{ij} = I\ (y_{ij}^* > 0)$ is observed for the latent $y_{ij}^* = x_{ij}\beta + z_{ij}\ u_j + \varepsilon_{ij}$. The errors ε_{ij} are distributed as a standard normal with mean zero and variance one, and are independent of u_j.

As part of the post-estimation analysis, we have also estimated the intra-cluster coefficients (ICC), also referred to as the variance proportion coefficient. In multi-level models, random effects are useful for modelling intra-cluster correlation, reflecting the idea that observations in the same cluster are correlated because they share common cluster-level random effects. In multi-stage sampling surveys, the random assignment occurs at different stages, with multiple units observed within each cluster. A key parameter in these experiments is the intra-cluster correlation, which measures the proportion of the overall variance in the outcome explained by within-group variance.

The ICC at level 2 is defined, for a two-stage model, as:

$$ICC = \frac{\text{Level 2 residual variance}}{(\text{Level 2 residual variance} + \text{Level 1 residual variance})} \quad \text{for a continuous model.} \quad [4.3]$$

In the case of a binary dependent variable model, the level 1 residual variance is constant (at 3.29 for a logit model and 1 for a probit model). So, for a probit model, ICC at level 2 becomes

$$ICC = \frac{\text{Level 2 residual variance}}{\text{Level 2 residual variance} + 1} \quad [4.4]$$

This is interpreted as the amount of remaining variance in the likelihood to adopt a practice that is attributable to cluster variation. In our model, we can estimate ICC for village, block, and district levels as follows:

$$VPC_{Village} = \frac{(\text{Residual variance at village level} + \text{Residual variance at block level} + \text{Residual variance at district level})}{(1 + \text{Residual variance at village level} + \text{Residual variance at block level} + \text{Residual variance at district level})} \quad [4.5]$$

$$VPC_{Block} = \frac{(\text{Residual variance at block level} + \text{Residual variance at district level})}{(1 + \text{Residual variance at village level} + \text{Residual variance at block level} + \text{Residual variance at district level})} \quad [4.6]$$

$$\text{VPC}_{\text{District}} = \frac{\text{Residual variance at district level}}{(1+\text{Residual variance at village level}+}$$

Residual variance at block level +

Residual variance at district level)

[4.7]

When the VPC is close to 0, units in a cluster behave no more similarly than units in all other clusters at the same level. When the intra-cluster correlation is high and close to 1, on the other hand, units within each cluster are identical, so we effectively only have M independent observations, where M is the number of clusters at that level.

4.3.3 Analysing diffusion of best practices

The econometric analysis of the determinants of decision to adopt the best practices is followed by a discussion of the diffusion of adoption decisions (i) within the village and (ii) from JEEViKA members to non-members.

The former is the bandwagon effect. It refers to the tendency of an individual to acquire a particular style, behaviour, or attitude because everyone else is doing it (Leibenstein, 1950). It is a phenomenon whereby the rate of uptake of beliefs, ideas, fads, and trends increases with respect to the proportion of others who have already done so. In this case, a respondent adopts the practice simply because she wants to conform to what other women (comprising both JEEViKA member or non-member) in the village are doing. In order to test for diffusion of best practices within each village we have estimated the following regression model:

$$Y_{ij} = \beta_0 + \beta_{\text{Bandwagon effect}} VBPR_j + \beta_2 X_j + z_{ij} u_j + \varepsilon_{ij} \qquad [4.8]$$

Where

Y_{ij} is a binary variable indicating whether the ith respondent residing in the jth village has adopted the best practice or not.
$VBPR_j$ is the adoption rate of the best practice in j^{th} village.
X_j are control variables (individual and household level characteristics of the ith respondent).

These variables are: whether the respondent is a JEEViKA member (the main study variable), age, education, standard of living index scores, socio-religious identity, number of living children, household size, whether the respondent works, and whether her husband is a migrant.

Another important effect is a spill-over from the Health and Nutrition Strategy implemented by JEEViKA. We had seen that encouraging exclusive breastfeeding till six months of the child and supplementary feeding thereafter were objectives of the Health and Nutrition Strategy; further, the coefficient of the JEEViKA dummy is positive and significant for both these outcomes, indicating a program effect. Although non-members were not given any treatment, it is possible that the adoption of such practices by JEEViKA members may have influenced non-members also. The existence of such a spill-over effect may be tested by replacing the village-level adoption rates used in the model used to test for the existence of a peer effect with the adoption rate of these two practices among JEEViKA members in each village, a JEEViKA dummy and an interaction term between the JEEViKA dummy and an interaction term between the two as explanatory variables. While the coefficient of the JEEViKA adoption rates indicates the spill-over effect from JEEViKA members to non-members, the coefficient of the interaction term captures the program effect. The multi-level probit model is of the form:

$$Yij = \beta_0 + \beta_1 JBPRj + \beta_{Program\ Effect} JEEViKAj + \beta_{Spill\ Over} JEEViKA*JBPRj + \beta_4 Xj + z_{ij}\ u_j + \varepsilon_{ij} \qquad [4.9]$$

Where

Yij is a binary variable indicating whether the ith respondent residing in the jth village has adopted the best practice or not.

JBPRj is the adoption rate of the best practice among JEEViKA members in j^{th} village.

JEEViKA is a binary variable indicating whether the jth respondent is a JEEViKA member.

JEEViKA*JBPRj is the interaction term between the adoption level among JEEViKA members and JEEViKA dummy.

Xj are control variables (individual and household level characteristics of the ith respondent, stated earlier).

Both equations [4.8] and [4.9] are estimated using a multi-level probit model. The model is estimated for all the MCH practices stated earlier in Section 4.2.

The obvious question that crops up next is whether the spill-over effect is greater than the peer effect. The question is not easy to answer. What we can do is compare the spill-over effect (after factoring out the peer effect) with the peer effect (after factoring out the spill-over effect). This is undertaken as follows:

1. *Estimating spill-over effect (after factoring out the bandwagon effect)*: We first regress the probability of adopting the practice on the mean adoption rate for village and other control variables; the residual of this regression is regressed on the mean adoption rate among JEEViKA members and INTENSITY. The coefficient of mean adoption rate among JEEViKA members ($\beta_{Spill\ over}$) gives the spill-over effect, after factoring out the village effect.

2. *Estimating bandwagon effect (after factoring out the spill-over effect)*: The first stage regression is now probability of adopting the practice on mean adoption rate among JEEViKA members, INTENSITY, and other control variables. In the second stage, the residual is regressed on the village mean. The bandwagon effect, after factoring out the spill-over effect, is given by the coefficient of the village mean ($\beta_{\text{Bandwagon effect}}$).

A comparison of the two coefficients indicates which effect is stronger.

4.4 Results

4.4.1 Adoption levels of best practices

Table 4.1 represents the best maternal and child healthcare practices that have been adopted by our research participants. The table shows the total percentage of the respondents and the share of JEEViKA members and non-JEEViKA members who have adopted such practices. It also provides the corresponding statistical test results.

In most cases, adoption rates are substantially above the average for rural Bihar as estimated in the penultimate National Family Health Survey (fourth wave), undertaken in 2015–16 (IIPS, 2016). The exceptions are adoption of modern contraception methods, and percentage of women protected against neonatal tetanus. Corresponding state-level data for proportion of women receiving post-partum advise on contraception method, and percentage of children receiving OPV0 at birth, or provided complementary feeding between the age of 7 and 35 months are not available.

Preliminary results of the recently concluded fifth round of National Family Health Survey (NFHS) (undertaken in 2019–21), however, reveal that adoption rates have increased substantially for all indicators except exclusive breastfeeding. Adoption rates as revealed in our survey and adoption rates reported from NFHS-5 survey are similar for birth protection against neonatal tetanus, institutional delivery, post-partum check-ups within 48 hours of delivery, and exclusive breastfeeding up to six months. Adoption rates of modern contraception are higher in the NFHS survey, while adoption rates of ANC check-ups in the first trimester, availing recommended four ANC check-ups, provision of IFA tablets/syrup, delivery assisted by a skilled health worker, and complementary feeding after six months of birth are reported to be higher in our survey.

We can observe that 90.53% of the total respondents have availed tTetanus toxoid injections, making it the most adopted practice. The percentage of respondents who have given OPV0 to their children is also quite high, at 88.18%. The least adopted practice is the use of modern contraception, since only 19.82% of the respondents have availed such methods.

The table shows that JEEViKA members are better off with regard to four indicators, that is, the use of modern contraception after marriage as well

Table 4.1 Adoption levels of best practices

Practice	JEEViKA Member	Non-Member	t test	Total	Bihar 2015–16	Bihar 2019–21
Use of modern contraception methods after marriage	22.02	17.62	-2.63***	19.82	22.0	44.4
First ANC visit in the first trimester of pregnancy	64.21	64.77	0.28	64.49	32.7	52.9
Availed at least four ANC check-ups	43.43	43.77	0.16	43.60	13.0	25.2
Birth protected against neonatal tetanus	89.79	91.28	1.21	90.53	89.1	89.5
100 IFA tablets/syrup for anaemia during pregnancy	75.67	75.98	0.17	75.82	9.4	18.0
Full ANC services	32.42	32.83	0.21	32.62	3.0	NA
Delivery in an institution	78.06	82.56	2.69***	80.31	62.6	76.2
Delivery assisted by skilled person	85.61	88.52	2.06**	87.07	71.1	79.0
Availed post-partum check-ups within 48 hours of delivery	62.08	61.39	-0.34	61.73	41.1	57.3
Advice on post-partum contraception method	60.48	54.00	-3.11***	57.24	NA	NA
Giving OPV0 to child	87.74	88.61	0.64	88.18	NA	NA
Breastfeeding child at least up to six months of birth	89.61	86.03	-2.6***	87.82	54.1	58.9
Complementary feeding after six months of birth	79.84	74.56	-2.99***	77.20	29.5[a]	39.0[a]

Sources: Estimates from survey data; International Institute of Population Sciences (IIPS), 2016; and International Institute of Population Studies (IIPS), 2021.
Note:
*, **, and *** indicate significance at 10, 5, and 1% level, respectively.
[a] Children aged 6–8 months receiving solid or semi-solid food and breastmilk.

as advice on post-partum use, breastfeeding children for at least six months after birth, and also complementary breastfeeding post-six months of birth. There is no significant difference between JEEViKA and non-JEEViKA members in availing ANC check-up during the first trimester of pregnancy and four such check-ups in total, taking tetanus toxoid injections, taking 100 IFA tablets or syrup to prevent anaemia, availing post-partum check-up within 48 hours of delivery, and giving OPV0 to children. Our analysis also reveals that institutional delivery and deliveries assisted by a skilled person are significantly lower among JEEViKA members.

4.4.2 Variations in outcomes over correlates

From Table A4.1, we can say that the youngest age group, that is, 17–20 years, is the highest adopter of MCH practices. The highest proportion of JEEViKA members belonging to this group have availed first ANC visit in the first trimester of pregnancy, tetanus toxoid injections, tablets or syrup for anaemia, have had institutional delivery assisted by a skilled person, and have administered OPV0 to their children. Among non-JEEViKA members, the highest percentage from this age group have availed first ANC check-up in the first trimester and four such check-ups in total, tetanus toxoid injections, and have delivered in an institution.

However, out of these, there is a significant variation across age only for three practices, that is, first ANC visit in the first trimester, delivery in an institution and by a skilled person, and giving OPV0 to children, all adopted the most by JEEViKA members. Almost half (46.45%) of JEEViKA members belonging to the age group 21–25 years have availed at least four ANC check-ups, and 90.76% have breastfeed their children at least up to six months. However, while the former varies significantly with age, the latter does not. The highest proportion of non-JEEViKA members belonging to this age group has been assisted by a skilled person during delivery and has breastfeed for at least six months. Again, the former has a significant variation across age while the latter does not. Use of modern contraceptive methods after marriage and receiving advice on contraception post-partum, availing post-partum check-ups after delivery, and complementary feeding after six months of birth are practices that have been adopted the most by JEEViKA members belonging to the age group 26–30 years. Only the first practice has a significant variation across age. The highest proportion of non-JEEViKA members from this group have availed at least four ANC check-ups, received advice on post-partum contraception, and have given OPV0 to their children. However, only the second practice has a significant variation in the case of this age group. The highest share of respondents belonging to the age group 31–50 years who have adopted some of the best health practices are non-JEEViKA members. The practices include the adoption of modern contraception after marriage, having medications for anaemia during pregnancy, availing post-partum check-ups within 48 hours of delivery, and complementary feeding after six months of birth. Among these, only the first practice has a significant variation across age.

Table A4.2 shows that JEEViKA members who have received 11–17 years of education are the highest adopter of all MCH practices, with the exception of administering tetanus toxoid injections, which have been adopted the most by JEEViKA members with 1–5 years of education. Non-members from the latter group are the highest adopters of modern contraceptive method after marriage, anaemia medication, and complementary feeding, while non-members who are illiterate are the highest share of respondents who have breastfeed their children at least up to six months of birth. The highest proportion of non-JEEViKA members having 11–17 years of education have availed first ANC check-up within the first trimester of pregnancy and at least four such check-ups, administered tetanus toxoid injections, delivered in an institution and with the assistance of a skilled person, availed post-partum check-up within 48 hours of delivery, received advice on post-partum contraception, and have given OPV0 to children. In case of both JEEViKA members and non-members, women who have received 11–17 years of education have been the highest adopters of full antenatal check-up services (defined earlier), while women who are illiterate have been the least adopters of these facilities, and this variation is significant for both members and non-members. Variations across educational attainment for both JEEViKA members and non-members are insignificant for the adoption of modern contraception after marriage, breastfeeding children for at least up to six months, and complementary feeding. For only JEEViKA members, variations across educational achievement are insignificant in the case of availing tetanus toxoid injections and IFA tablets or syrup for anaemia during pregnancy. Again, such variations are not significant for institutional delivery, receiving advice on post-partum contraception, and giving OPV0 to children, but only for non-JEEViKA members.

In Table A4.3, we can observe that with regard to the standard of living, the most affluent respondents are the highest adopters of MCH practices for both JEEViKA members and non-members. However, the highest proportion of JEEViKA members and non-members who have breastfeed their children up to six months belong to the lowest tercile. Non-members from households with less assets are also the highest share of respondents who have administered tetanus toxoid injections. For tetanus toxoid injections and complementary feeding, the variation is not significant across asset scores for JEEViKA members and non-members. For both JEEViKA members and non-members, women belonging to affluent households have availed full ANC services the most, whereas, women belonging to less affluent households are the lowest adopters of full ANC services, and the variation is significant for both the scenarios.

Table A4.4 shows that the highest adopter of MCH practices is the Hindu-SC & ST (scheduled caste and scheduled tribe) category for both members and non-members of JEEViKAs. However, non-JEEViKA members belonging to the Hindu general category are the highest share of participants who have administered tetanus toxoid injections, and Muslim JEEViKA members are the highest share of respondents who have breastfeed their children up to six months. Hindu women belonging to ST and SC categories are the highest adopters of full ANC services and Hindu forward caste women are the lowest adopters of such services, and this holds true for both JEEViKA members and non-members. The variation is also significant for both members and non-members. For tetanus toxoid injections and anaemia medications, the variations across socio-religious categories are not significant. For post-partum contraception advice and breastfeeding children at least up to six months of birth, the variations across socio-religious identities are not significant for JEEViKA members. For non-members, it is insignificant for complementary feeding.

4.4.3 Results of econometric analysis

Table 4.2 presents the summary of the multi-level probit models estimated for adoption rates of different MCH practices. The Wald χ^2 likelihood ratio is above the tabulated value in all cases, indicating that the multi-level version of the probit model should be preferred to the ordinary probit model. The intercept term varies across districts, but is – under the assumptions of the multi-level model – not correlated with explanatory variables. Within each district, there are also block-level random effects; similarly, within each block, random effects vary across villages. The extent of variation, however, is generally small. The χ^2 statistic is statistically significant in all cases; it implies that the null hypothesis ($\beta_i = 0$) cannot be accepted.

The coefficient of the JEEViKA dummy is insignificant in nine out of the 12 models. It implies that adoption rates do not vary between JEEViKA members and non-members. In only three cases – given advice on post-partum contraception, exclusive breastfeeding up to six months, and complementary feeding after six months – is the coefficient of the JEEViKA dummy significant. In each of these cases, the coefficient is positive; it implies that the probability of adopting these practices is higher among JEEViKA members vis-à-vis non-members.

A major problem with estimating the program effect is self-selection. JEEViKA members often have unobservable characteristics that make them more amenable to treatment. In such cases the assumption of $E(u|x) = 0$ is violated, leading to endogeneity. In this situation, however, as intent to treat (ITT) is insignificant in most cases, self-selection is not likely to be an issue. Hence, we have not estimated instrumental variable models.[3]

Table 4.2 Adoption of best practices: Summary results of multi-level probit models

Variables	Modern Contraception methods after marriage	Whether first ANC visit was in the first trimester	At least four ANC check-ups	Whether given tetanus toxoid Injection
JEEViKA member	0.06	0.11	0.08	-0.05
Control variables	Yes	Yes	Yes	Yes
Constant	-1.62***	0.63*	0.15	0.94**
Var(District)	0.04	0.16	0.21	0.04
Var(District>Block)	0.03	0.07*	0.02	0.01
Var(District>Block>Village)	0.02	0.05*	0.04*	0.05
Statistics				
N	2250	2250	2250	2250
χ²	55.87	98.17	112.11	33.79
Wald χ²	42.11***	205.75***	221.14***	26.13***
Interclass correlation				
District	0.04	0.12	0.17	0.04
Block | District	0.07	0.18	0.18	0.05
Village | Block | District	0.09	0.22	0.22	0.09

Variables	IFA tablets/syrup for anaemia	Institutional Delivery	Delivery assisted by skilled person	Availed post-partum check-up within 48hrs
JEEViKA member	-0.08	-0.06	-0.03	0.07***
Control variables	Yes	Yes	Yes	Yes
Constant	0.30	0.80*	1.13**	-0.19
Var(District)	0.17	0.12	0.16	0.04
Var(District>Block)	0.04	0.22*	0.09	0.05
Var(District>Block>Village)	0.10**	0.16***	0.04	0.05*

(Continued)

Table 4.2 (Continued)

Variables	Modern Contraception methods after marriage	Whether first ANC visit was in the first trimester	At least four ANC check-ups	Whether given tetanus toxoid Injection
Statistics				
N	2250	2250	2250	2250
χ^2	27.53	88.37	77.69	57.95
Wald χ^2	170.28***	257.56***	135.26***	98.94***
Interclass correlation				
District	0.13	0.08	0.12	0.04
Block | District	0.16	0.23	0.19	0.09
Village | Block | District	0.24	0.33	0.22	0.13

Variables	Whether given advice on post-partum contraception	Whether child was given OPVO	Breastfeeding up to six months of birth	Complementary feeding after six months
JEEViKA member	0.12*	0.08	0.25**	0.14*
Control variables	Yes	Yes	Yes	Yes
Constant	-0.16	1.57***	1.46***	0.38
Var(District)	0.16	0.30	0.11	0.01
Var(District>Block)	0.02	0.19	0.01	0.00
Var(District>Block>Village)	0.06**	0.16**	0.01	0.01
Statistics				
N	2250	2250	2250	2250
χ^2	48.10	46.75	54.47	46.29
Wald χ^2	183.90***	164.82***	49.15***	6.99*
Interclass correlation				
District	0.13	0.18	0.10	0.01
Block | District	0.14	0.29	0.10	0.01
Village | Block | District	0.19	0.39	0.12	0.02

Source: Estimated from primary survey.

Table 4.3 Predicted probability for adopting best practices: Variations across socio-religious groups

Practices	H-SC & ST	H-OBC	H-FC	Muslim
Contraception	0.21	0.20	0.20	0.11
	0.00	0.00	0.00	0.00
First ANC visit	0.75	0.65	0.60	0.76
	0.00	0.00	0.00	0.00
First ANC check-ups	0.58	0.44	0.37	0.50
	0.00	0.00	0.00	0.00
Availed tetanus toxoid (TT) injections	0.91	0.90	0.92	0.90
	0.00	0.00	0.00	0.00
100IFA tabs/syrup for anaemia	0.72	0.76	0.76	0.78
	0.00	0.00	0.00	0.00
Full ANC services	0.39	0.32	0.28	0.38
	0.00	0.00	0.00	0.00
Institutional delivery	0.91	0.82	0.78	0.81
	0.00	0.00	0.00	0.00
Delivery assisted by skilled person	0.92	0.89	0.84	0.90
	0.00	0.00	0.00	0.00
Post-partum check-ups	0.65	0.63	0.59	0.64
	0.00	0.00	0.00	0.00
Post-partum contraception	0.58	0.58	0.56	0.55
	0.00	0.00	0.00	0.00
OPVO	0.96	0.89	0.87	0.88
	0.00	0.00	0.00	0.00
Breast feeding	0.81	0.88	0.90	0.92
	0.00	0.00	0.00	0.00
Complementary feeding	0.82	0.77	0.75	0.85
	0.00	0.00	0.00	0.00

Source: Estimated from primary survey.

The analysis of the detailed results of the regression models (Table A4.1) also reveals that women with more than five years of education, and particularly those with above ten years of education, are less likely to adopt the MCH practices. The probability of uptake of these practices also decreases with the age of respondents. Working women are less likely to avail of ANC check-ups within three months, take IFA tablets or syrups, and start complementary feeding of their child after six months. Respondents from households with higher asset holdings are also less likely to use modern contraception methods, avail of ANC check-up within the first trimester, breastfeed their child, and provide complementary food to their children. The probability of availing ANC check-ups in the first trimester is lower among H-SC & ST respondents; OBC respondents are less likely to breastfeed their children, and Muslim women have a lower uptake of ANC check-ups in the first trimester and delivering in an institution. Women from larger families are less likely to use modern contraception methods, avail of ANC services in the first trimester, avail of at least four ANC check-ups, seek protection against neonatal tetanus, take IFA tablets and syrups, avail of assisted deliveries, breastfeed their children, and provide complete food to their children after six months.

In Table 4.2 we summarized the results of multi-level probit models. The results showed the absence of statistically significant differences in the probability of adoption of the MCH practices between JEEViKA members and non-members in most cases. What we also need to study is how the adoption rates vary across socio-religious groups and educational levels.

In Table 4.3 we have presented the marginal effects of socio-religious practices. Results show that Hindu forward castes (H-FC) women are less likely to go for ANC check-ups in their first trimester, complete the recommended four ANC check-ups, avail the full ANC services, deliver in institutions, avail of skilled assistance during deliveries, avail of post-partum services, or contraception advise, and provide their child with complementary food after six months, compared to women from Hindu-other backward castes (H-OBC) and marginalised groups (H-SC & ST). Only the probability of exclusively breastfeeding children below six months is high among H-FCs.

Adoption rates of MCH practices among Muslims are relatively lower than that of H-SC & ST; however, Muslim women are more likely to exclusively breastfeed their children, or provide them with complementary food after six months. This is consistent with earlier studies (GoI, 2005).

In Table 4.4 we report variations in predictive probabilities for adopting MCH practices across education levels. Results show that the adoption rate of availing first ANC check-up within the first trimester, availing of the recommended four ANC check-ups, availing of full ANC services, delivering in institutions, availing assistance of skilled health worker during delivery, availing post-partum services including contraception advice, and ensuring polio vaccine at birth for their children is likely to be higher among more educated women.

On the other hand, an inverse U-shaped relationship is observed between education levels and predicted likelihood of using modern contraception methods, availing protection against natal tetanus and supplementing breastfeeding of child with semi-solid and solid food after six months.

Variations in the predicted likelihood of adopting MCH practices across asset index scores show a positive trend for most practices, implying that women from affluent households are more likely to adopt such practices. The exceptions are the likelihood of exclusive breastfeeding till six months (marginal variations across asset index scores), availing protection from tetanus, and complementary feeding of children after six months (women from affluent families are less likely to adopt such practices) (Figure 4.1).

As mentioned before, quite a few JEEViKA members do not attend meetings, or do so irregularly. During the focus group discussion, JEEViKA members reported that "Sometime we have work so we don't attend regularly".

Table 4.4 Predicted probability for adopting best practices: Variations across education levels

Practices	No schooling	1–5 years	6–10 years	11–17 years
Contraception	0.17	0.21	0.21	0.20
	0.00	0.00	0.00	0.00
First ANC visit	0.60	0.65	0.67	0.76
	0.00	0.00	0.00	0.00
First ANC check-ups	0.41	0.40	0.44	0.53
	0.00	0.00	0.00	0.00
Availed TT injections	0.89	0.92	0.91	0.91
	0.00	0.00	0.00	0.00
100 IFA tabs/syrup for anaemia	0.74	0.77	0.76	0.77
	0.00	0.00	0.00	0.00
Full ANC services	0.30	0.30	0.32	0.41
	0.00	0.00	0.00	0.00
Institutional delivery	0.79	0.80	0.83	0.88
	0.00	0.00	0.00	0.00
Delivery assisted by skilled person	0.87	0.86	0.89	0.91
	0.00	0.00	0.00	0.00
Post-partum check-ups	0.60	0.58	0.65	0.65
	0.00	0.00	0.00	0.00
Post-partum contraception	0.57	0.54	0.58	0.59
	0.00	0.00	0.00	0.00
Child given OPV0	0.87	0.88	0.90	0.92
	0.00	0.00	0.00	0.00
Breast feeding	0.87	0.90	0.88	0.90
	0.00	0.00	0.00	0.00
Complementary feeding	0.75	0.80	0.78	0.79
	0.00	0.00	0.00	0.00

Source: Estimated from primary survey.

Respondents also reported restrictions on their movement outside the home – "I don't generally move out from the house". In such cases, their mothers-in-law attended the meetings and deposited the monthly contributions to the JEEViKA common fund. About 31% of JEEViKA members reported that they had not attended any meetings in the last six months. About 4, 8, and 8% of the JEEViKA members reported that they had attended only one, two, and three meetings respectively in the six months prior to the survey. Thus, only 50% of respondents had attended more than three meetings in the last six months.

As half of the treatment group had not received treatment, or had received it partially, we dropped such respondents and re-estimated the multi-level models. We undertook this exercise only for those practices where a significant

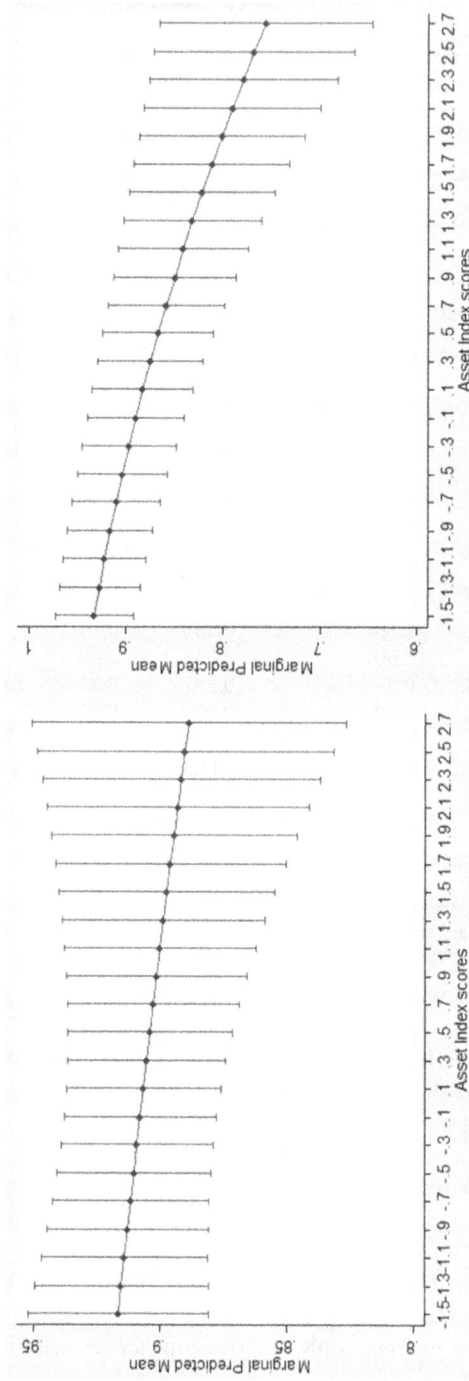

Figure 4.1 Predicted probability in select outcomes: Variations across asset index scores.

Source: Estimated from primary survey.

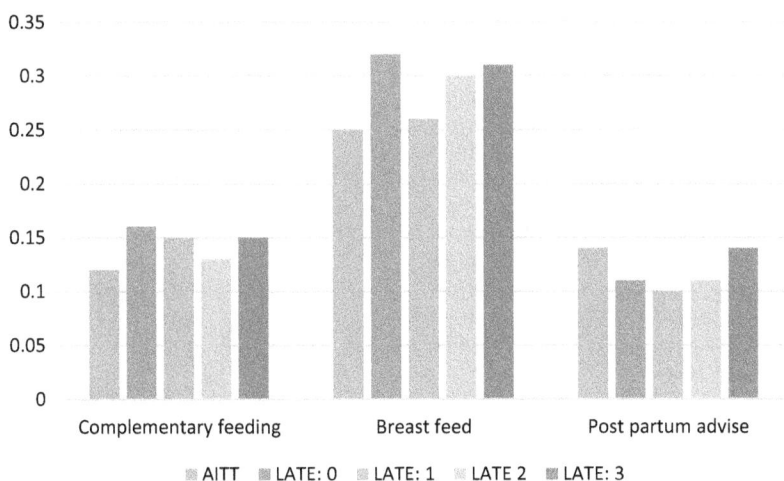

Figure 4.2 Comparison of AIT and LTE.

Source: Estimated from primary survey.

difference in adoption rates was observed between JEEViKA members and non-members. Four models were estimated dropping respondents as follows:

- who had not attended any meetings at all (LATE0),
- who had attended less than two meetings (LATE1),
- who had attended less than three meetings (LATE2), and
- who had attended less than four meetings (LATE3).

The LTE was compared with the AIT (Figure 4.2), and was found to be higher.

4.4.4 Diffusion of best practices: Bandwagon effects

Our analysis reveals relatively high rates of adoption in the case of most practices in the survey sites. Whether this reflects an overall improvement in Bihar after the last round of the NFHS or an increase in only our survey sites will be apparent after the next round of the District Level Household Survey (DLHS) or NFHS. What we have done is examined the possible role of peer effects in raising adoption rates of MCH practices.

One possible diffusion is within the villages. To test for the existence of a significant diffusion effect we have estimated [7] using a probit model. The summary of the results of the probit models for different MCH practices is given in Table 4.5. We can see that the coefficient is statistically significant at

Table 4.5 Bandwagon effect: Summary results of probit models

Variables	$B_{Bandwagon\ effects}$	N	Wald χ^2
Uses contraception	3.77***	2250	801.16 (0.00)
ANC visit	2.85***	2250	2475.57(0.00)
ANC check-up	2.73***	2250	3409.49 (0.00)
Availed tetanus injection	5.44***	2250	157.05 (0.00)
IFA tablets/syrup	1.56***	2250	42.84 (0.00)
Institutional delivery	3.44***	2250	868.40 (0.00)
Assisted delivery	4.35***	2250	520.53 (0.00)
Post-partum check-ups	2.74***	2250	2382.19 (0.00)
Post-partum advice	2.90***	2250	2591.73 (0.00)
Child given oral polio vaccine (OPV) at birth	4.31***	2250	382.84 (0.00)
Exclusive breastfeeding	4.79***	2250	457.51 (0.00)
Complementary feeding	3.32***	2250	696.29 (0.00)
Availed full ANC services	3.08***	2250	1668.51 (0.00)

Source: Estimated from primary survey.

1% level, and is positive for all outcomes. Apparently, therefore, a peer effect exists (Table A4.5).

4.4.5 Diffusion of best practices: Spill-over effects

The spill-over from the Health and Nutrition programme implemented by JEEViKA was revealed during the focus group discussions. The community mobilisers are not as active as Accredited Social Health Activists (ASHAs), but, every month, meetings are held to discuss maternal and child-related issues. All JEEViKA members do not attend, or do so irregularly; in some cases, such meetings are not held. However, in villages where such meetings are held regularly, they have played an important role in disseminating information among members: "Owing to JEEViKA we are also getting to know about dietary practices that should be followed. We learned about such practices and their benefits only after joining the JEEViKA group. So definitely the JEEViKA Health and Nutrition pogramme has played an important role in improving maternal health care seeking behaviour". During the focus group discussion, a non-member said, "Yes, we get to know something from them too, as they sometimes share the knowledge with us, so the meetings helped us too indirectly". This was confirmed by other participants also. Sometimes non-members are also invited to participate in the meetings to promote dietary practices: "Last month they have organized a programme and called some of us, there they have discussed about the diet that mothers and children should follow". Of course, spill-overs do not occur always; participants report "No one from JEEViKA told us anything ever" or "We never get anything specific from them". In some cases, non-members are too rigid and refuse to change their behaviour:

Q: So do you share your knowledge with people other than JEEViKA members?
P1: We try to make them understand but either they don't listen to us or they don't understand.
P3: We try but most of them don't listen to us and say they will do whatever they feel like.

However, in a revealing statement, a non-member lamented, "I want to know, but don't get to know anything, even I wanted to be a part of the group too, but that is also not happening ... no one is helping".

In order to test whether the adoption rate in the village affects the individual respondent's choices, we have re-estimated the multi-level probit models with two modifications:

a) We have dropped the dummy indicating whether the respondent is a JEEViKA member and
b) Incorporated the village adoption rates as an explanatory variable.

If the coefficient of the village mean is positive and statistically significant, it indicates a bandwagon effect. Coefficients are reported in Figure 4.3 for JEEViKA members and non-members.

We also include an interaction term with the JEEViKA dummy. Results indicate that the impact of the interaction term is significant and positively greater among JEEViKA members than that of non-members (Table 4.6). It implies that the program effect is greater than the spill-over effect – which is an expected result.

An examination of the marginal effects of the probit models shows how pervasive is the spill-over effect. The probit models are re-estimated, incorporating an interaction term between the adoption rate of the relevant practice among JEEViKA members and a variable INTENSITY. The latter is the number of JEEViKA meetings attended by the respondent if she is a JEEViKA member; it is zero for non-members.

The 95% predictive margins have been plotted against increasing values of the interaction term (Figure 4.4). It may be seen that the spill-over effect is positive even for non-members and those members who have not attended JEEViKA meetings in the last six months preceding the survey.

4.4.6 Spill-over versus bandwagon effect

The coefficient of the mean adoption rates among JEEViKA members is statistically insignificant (in case of exclusive breastfeeding), and 0.23 (in case of complementary feeding) (see Table 4.7). In contrast, the mean adoption rate for the village is statistically significant from zero; its values are 0.89 and 1.25. In both cases, the coefficient for village mean is greater than the

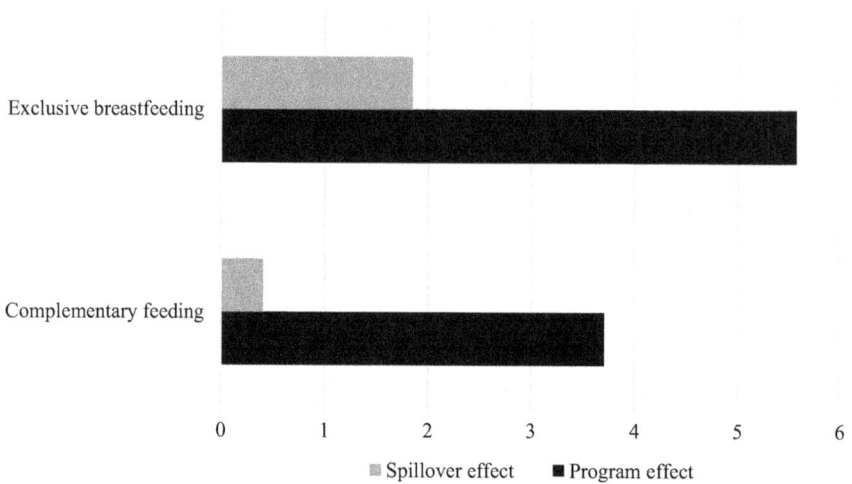

Figure 4.3 Comparison of spill-over and program effect.

Source: Estimated from primary survey.

Table 4.6 Spill-over effects vis-à-vis programme effects: Summary results for child health outcomes

Statistics	Exclusive breastfeeding		Complementary feeding	
	β	t	β	T
βSpill over	3.41	9.95	1.84	8.58
βProgramme effects	0.35	3.60	0.17	2.40
Control variables	Yes		Yes	
LR χ²	186.35		126.30	
Pseudo R²	0.11		0.05	
N	2250		2250	

Source: Estimated from primary survey

JEEViKA mean. The result implies that the bandwagon effect (after factoring out the spill-over effect) exceeds the spill-over effect (after factoring out the village effect).

4.5 Discussion and conclusion

Our analysis reveals high levels of adoption rates of recommended MCH practices in general in the survey sites, compared to state-level figures reported in the last wave of the NFHS survey. JEEViKA's Health, Nutrition and Sanitation program has played a major role underlying the change with

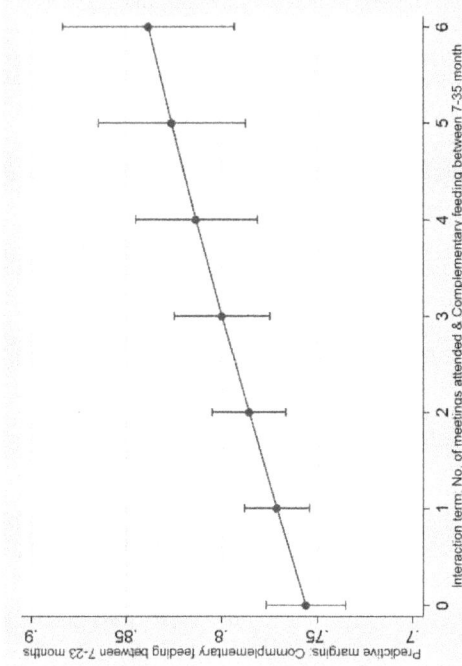

(a) Exclusive breastfeeding till 6 months

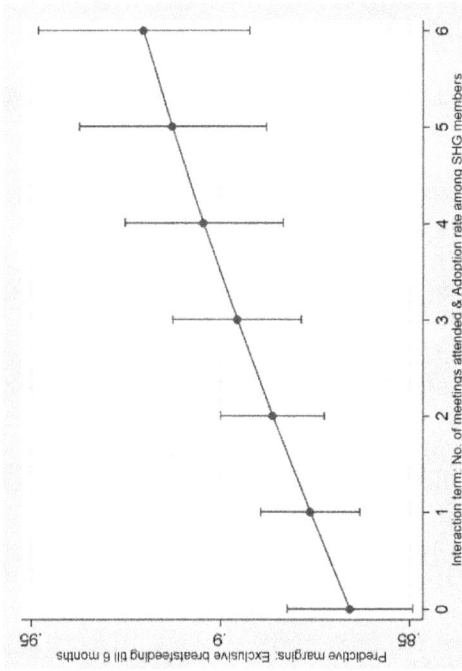

(b) Complementary feeding between 7-35 months

Figure 4.4 Predicted probability of child health outcomes: Variations across meetings attended and adoption levels among SHG members.

Source: Estimated from primary survey.

Table 4.7 Spill over vis-à-vis bandwagon effects for child health outcomes

	Coefficient	S.E.	t	R^2	F
Spill-over effects					
Breastfeeding	0.06	0.07	0.89	0.00	1.86
Complementary feeding	0.23	0.04	5.99	0.00	21.76
Diffusion effects					
Breastfeeding	0.89	0.12	7.45	0.01	55.45
Complementary feeding	1.25	0.10	12.77	0.02	162.97

Source: Estimated from primary survey

respect to two practices – exclusive breastfeeding of children below six months and supplementary feeding of children after six months. Moreover, socially backward groups (SCs and STs) have a higher predicted probability of adopting most of the practices that we have studied. In contrast, forward castes display resistance to adopt such practices. Female education plays a positive role in encouraging such practices, while affluent households are also more likely to adopt MCH practices.

The econometric analysis reveals that high (low) adoption rates of the MCH practices studied in the village positively affect the predicted probability of respondents adopting such practices. This indicates the existence of peer effects. We have also shown that the impact of such effects is greater than spill-over effects from the Health and Nutrition Scheme (HNS) of JEEViKA. Whether this comprises an exogenous peer effect is not certain at this point and needs to be examined carefully (Manski, 1993). This issue is examined comprehensively in the next chapter.

The high adoption levels of best practices in Bihar are in line with the improvement in MCH outcomes noted in Bihar after the inception of the National Health Mission (Ghosh et al., 2019; Walia et al., 2020). It is a welcome sign, given Bihar's historically poor health indicators. The results of this chapter, however, apparently do not validate the findings of earlier studies reporting better outcomes for SHG members (Saha et al., 2013; Saha et al., 2015; Mozumdar et al., 2018; Saggurti et al., 2018; Hazra et al., 2020; Mehta et al., 2020). The main reason for this is that the HNS did not focus on fertility control, and on improving utilisation of ANC services, PNC services, and immunisation. The HNS intervention was directed to improve dietary practices, and if we examine dietary practices of children, the results reveal that the HNS was successful in Bihar. This is consistent with results reported in evaluations of the pilot scheme (The World Bank, 2016; Gupta et al., 2019).

In contrast to existing studies reporting low adoption of MCH practices recommended by policymakers, planners, and NGOs among socially disadvantaged sections of the population (Singh et al., 2012; Patel et al., 2018; Bango & Ghosh, 2022; Pakrashi et al., 2022), we find that prevalence levels of such practices are higher among women belonging to SC and ST households. A possible reason for the contradictory findings is that the existing studies have mostly relied on NFHS data at the all-India level for their analysis. In Bihar, during previous visits to rural villages in Bihar (between 2015 and 2021), the authors had observed that the advantaged general caste households were socially conservative and were not receptive to ASHAs; they were less likely to change MCH practices than the SC/ST households. This observation was also supported by the discussion with officials of the State Health Department. In Chapter 5, when we examine the identity of motivators and variations across social classes, the validity of this explanation will be assessed.

Notes

1 Full ANC services are defined as taking an ANC check-up in the first trimester of pregnancy, availing of at least four ANC check-ups, taking 100 IFA tablets (or syrup), and providing natal protection from tetanus.
2 The bandwagon effect is the tendency of an individual to acquire a particular style, behavior, or attitude because everyone else is doing it (Leibenstein, 1950). It is a phenomenon whereby the rate of uptake of beliefs, ideas, fads, and trends increases with respect to the proportion of others who have already done so.
3 We ran Two Stage Least Square models, taking household size as Instrument, for post-partum advice ($\chi^2 = 0.55$; probability = 0.4573) and exclusive breastfeeding ($\chi^2 = 1.56$; probability = 0.2123) Hausman tests indicate that the null hypothesis of exogeneity cannot be rejected. In case of complementary feeding, the same result was obtained, taking whether respondent works as instrument ($\chi^2 = 2.27$; probability = 0.1323). Thus, in the three instances where the AIT was statistically significant there is no evidence to reject the assumption of exogeneity.

References

Bango, M., & Ghosh, S. (2022). Social and regional disparities in utilization of maternal and child healthcare services in India: A study of the post-national health mission period. *Frontiers in Pediatrics*, *10*. http://doi.org/10.3389/fped.2022.895033

Ghosh, S., Husain, Z., & S Ghosh, Z. H. (2019). Has the national health mission improved utilisation of maternal healthcare services in Bihar? *Economic & Political Weekly*, *54*(31), 44–51.

Government of India. (2005). *Millennium Development Goals (MDGs): India country report*. Government of India.

Gupta, S.Kumar, N., Menon, P., Pandey, S. and Raghunathan, K. (2019). *Engaging women's groups to improve nutrition: Findings from an evaluation of the Jeevika multisectoral convergence pilot in Saharsa, Bihar*. Washington D.C.: The World Bank.

Hazra, A. et al. (2020). Effects of health behaviour change intervention through women's self-help groups on maternal and newborn health practices and related inequalities in rural india: A quasi-experimental study. *EClinicalMedicine*, *18*, 100198. http://doi.org/10.1016/j.eclinm.2019.10.011

Imbens, G. W., & Angrist, J. D. (1994). Identification and estimation of local average treatment effects. *Econometrica, 62*(2), 467. http://doi.org/10.2307/2951620

International Institute of Population Studies (IIPS). (2021). *National family health survey: 2019–216, State fact sheet: Bihar*. Mumbai: IIPS.

International Institute of Population Studies (IIPS) and International Institute of Population Sciences (IIPS). (2016). *National Family Health Survey: 2015–16, State Fact Sheet: Bihar*. http://rchiips.org/nfhs/pdf/nfhs4/br_factsheet.pdf.

JEEViKA. (2019). *Proposal on JEEViKA as National Resource Organization (NRO) for integration Food, Nutrition, Health and WASH (FNHW) interventions*. Government of Bihar.

Khandker, S. R., Koolwal, G. B., & Hussain, A. S. (2010). *Handbook on impact evaluation: Quantitative methods and practices*. The World Bank.

Leibenstein, H. (1950). Bandwagon, snob, and Veblen effects in the theory of consumers' demand. *The Quarterly Journal of Economics, 64*(2), 183. http://doi.org/10.2307/1882692

Manski, C. F. (1993). Identification of endogenous social effects: The reflection problem. *The Review of Economic Studies, 60*(3), 531. http://doi.org/10.2307/2298123

Mehta, K. M. et al. (2020). Health layering of self-help groups: Impacts on reproductive, maternal, newborn and child health and nutrition in Bihar, India. *Journal of global health, 10*(2), 021007. http://doi.org/10.7189/jogh.10.021007

Mozumdar, A. et al. (2018). Increasing knowledge of home based maternal and newborn care using self-help groups: Evidence from rural Uttar Pradesh, India. *Sexual & Reproductive Healthcare, 18*, 1–9. http://doi.org/10.1016/j.srhc.2018.08.003

Pakrashi, D., Maiti, S. N., & Saha, S. (2022). Caste, awareness and inequality in access to maternal and child health programs: evidence From India. *Social Indicators Research, 163*(3), 1301–1321. http://doi.org/10.1007/s11205-022-02939-0

Patel, P., Das, M., & Das, U. (2018). The perceptions, health-seeking behaviours and access of Scheduled Caste women to maternal health services in Bihar, India. *Reproductive Health Matters, 26*(54), 114–125. http://doi.org/10.1080/09688080.2018.1533361

Prost, A. et al. (2013). Women's groups practising participatory learning and action to improve maternal and newborn health in low-resource settings: A systematic review and meta-analysis. *The Lancet, 381*(9879), 1736–1746. http://doi.org/10.1016/S0140-6736(13)60685-6

Rosato, M. et al. (2008). Community participation: Lessons for maternal, newborn, and child health. *The Lancet, 372*(9642), 962–971. http://doi.org/10.1016/S0140-6736(08)61406-3

Saggurti, N. et al. (2018). Effect of health intervention integration within women's self-help groups on collectivization and healthy practices around reproductive, maternal, neonatal and child health in rural India. *PLoS One, 13*(8), e0202562. http://doi.org/10.1371/journal.pone.0202562

Saha, S., Annear, P. L., & Pathak, S. et al. (2013). The effect of Self-Help Groups on access to maternal health services: Evidence from rural India. *International Journal for Equity in Health, 12*(1), 36. http://doi.org/10.1186/1475-9276-12-36

Saha, S., Kermode, M., & Annear, P. L. (2015). Effect of combining a health program with a microfinance-based self-help group on health behaviors and outcomes. *Public Health, 129*(11), 1510–1518. http://doi.org/10.1016/j.puhe.2015.07.010

Singh, P. K. et al. (2012). Determinants of maternity care services utilization among married adolescents in rural India. *PLoS One*, 7(2), e31666. http://doi.org/10.1371/journal.pone.0031666

The World Bank. (2016). *Livelihoods and nutrition: A women's empowerment and convergence initiative.* New Delhi. http://documents1.worldbank.org/curated/pt/109401572440521978/pdf/Livelihoods-and-Nutrition-A-Women-s-Empowerment-and-Convergence-Initiative-JEEViKA.pdf

Walia, M. et al. (2020). Effect of sharing health messages on antenatal care behavior among women involved in microfinance-based self-help groups in Bihar India. *Global Health Research and Policy*, 5(1), 3. http://doi.org/10.1186/s41256-020-0132-0

Wallerstein, N. (1992). Powerlessness, empowerment, and health: Implications for health promotion programs. *American Journal of Health Promotion*, 6(3), 197–205. http://doi.org/10.4278/0890-1171-6.3.197

Appendix

Table A4.1 Variation in adoption levels of best practices across the age of respondent

Age group	JEEViKA	Non-member
Use of modern contraception methods after marriage		
17–20 years	10	8.33
21–25 years	20.62	16.89
26–30 years	25.51	23.63
31–50 years	18.75	25.93
x^2	9.18(0.03)	21.46(0.00)
First ANC visit in the first trimester of pregnancy		
17–20 years	80	65.63
21–25 years	67.3	65.53
26–30 years	64.37	64.73
31–50 years	50.63	53.7
x^2	20.03(0.00)	3.11(0.37)
Availed at least four ANC check-ups		
17–20 years	42	44.79
21–25 years	46.45	43.69
26–30 years	45.14	44.52
31–50 years	30.63	37.04
x^2	12.87(0.01)	1.14(0.77)
Tetanus toxoid injections		
17–20 years	94	94.27
21–25 years	87.68	90.27
26–30 years	90.08	91.9
31–50 years	93.12	92.59
x^2	5.01(0.20)	3.03(0.39)
100 IFA tablets/syrup for anaemia during pregnancy		
17–20 years	80	78.65
21–25 years	73.7	73.21
26–30 years	77.33	78.42
31–50 years	74.38	83.33
x^2	2.28(0.52)	5.77(0.12)
Delivery in an institution		
17–20 years	94	84.37
21–25 years	79.86	82.76
26–30 years	78.34	81.16
31–50 years	67.5	81.48
x^2	18.66(0.00)	0.89(0.83)

(Continued)

Table A4.1 (Continued)

Age group	JEEViKA	Non-member
Delivery assisted by skilled person		
17–20 years	90	87.5
21–25 years	86.73	89.42
26–30 years	87.45	87.67
31–50 years	75.62	87.04
χ^2	15.52(0.00)	0.99(0.80)
Availed post-partum check-ups within 48 hours of delivery		
17–20 years	56	64.58
21–25 years	61.37	60.07
26–30 years	64.37	61.3
31–50 years	58.75	64.81
χ^2	2.73(0.43)	1.53(0.68)
Advice on post-partum contraception method		
17–20 years	58	47.4
21–25 years	58.77	52.9
26–30 years	63.97	59.59
31–50 years	55	59.26
χ^2	5.17(0.16)	7.93(0.05)
Giving OPV0 to child		
17–20 years	94	88.54
21–25 years	91.4	88.23
26–30 years	86.23	90.07
31–50 years	79.37	85.19
χ^2	20.21(0.00)	1.33(0.69)
Breast feeding child at least up to six months of birth		
17–20 years	90	81.25
21–25 years	90.76	88.74
26–30 years	90.49	86.3
31–50 years	83.75	72.22
χ^2	6.91(0.09)	15.81(0.00)
Complementary feeding after six months of birth		
17–20 years	70	69.79
21–25 years	79.15	74.57
26–30 years	81.38	76.71
31–50 years	80	79.63
χ^2	3.860(0.28)	3.75(0.29)

Source: Estimated from primary survey

Table A4.2 Variation in adoption levels of best practices across the education level of respondents

Education of respondents	JEEViKA	Non-member
Use of modern contraception methods after marriage		
No schooling	21.11	14.09
1–5 years of education	23.02	22.02
6–10 years of education	21.71	18.71
11–17 years of education	24.75	18.01
Chi-square	0.83 (0.84)	5.72 (0.12)
First ANC visit in the first trimester of pregnancy		
No schooling	54.8	55.8
1–5 years of education	62.7	61.9
6–10 years of education	73.03	68.59
11–17 years of education	85.15	77.64
Chi-square	47.88 (0.00)	27.82 (0.00)
Availed at least four ANC check-ups		
No schooling	37.1	37.57
1–5 years of education	37.7	34.52
6–10 years of education	51.32	46.19
11–17 years of education	63.37	60.87
Chi-square	35.05 (0.00)	31.65 (0.00)
Tetanus toxoid injections		
No schooling	88.49	87.85
1–5 years of education	91.67	93.45
6–10 years of education	90.79	92.15
11–17 years of education	88.12	94.41
Chi-square	2.48 (0.48)	8.75 (0.04)
100 IFA tablets/syrup for anaemia during pregnancy		
No schooling	74.63	70.99
1–5 years of education	72.62	80.95
6–10 years of education	76.97	77.37
11–17 years of education	84.16	78.26
Chi-square	5.78 (0.12)	8.12 (0.04)
Availed full ANC services		
No schooling	27.51	27.9
1–5 years of education	28.17	26.79
6–10 years of education	38.16	33.49
11–17 years of education	48.51	48.45
Chi-square	23.76 (0.00)	24.66 (0.00)

(Continued)

Table A4.2 (Continued)

Education of respondents	JEEViKA	Non-member
Delivery in an institution		
No schooling	72.49	76.8
1–5 years of education	71.03	82.74
6–10 years of education	88.16	84.06
11–17 years of education	91.09	91.3
Chi-square	43.87 (0.00)	17.59 (0.00)
Delivery assisted by skilled person		
No schooling	83.16	86.46
1–5 years of education	80.16	85.71
6–10 years of education	90.79	89.61
11–17 years of education	95.05	93.17
Chi-square	22.30 (0.00)	6.74 (0.08)
Availed post-partum check-ups within 48 hours of delivery		
No schooling	60.55	55.8
1–5 years of education	51.98	58.33
6–10 years of education	68.75	64.2
11–17 years of education	74.26	69.57
Chi-square	23.48 (0.00)	11.42 (0.01)
Advice on post-partum contraception method		
No schooling	58.42	54.14
1–5 years of education	53.57	52.38
6–10 years of education	66.78	51.96
11–17 years of education	68.32	60.87
Chi-square	13.50 (0.00)	3.96 (0.27)
Giving OPV0 to child		
No schooling	84.43	86.19
1–5 years of education	83.33	87.5
6–10 years of education	93.42	89.61
11–17 years of education	97.03	92.55
Chi-square	26.54 (0.00)	5.21 (0.16)
Breast feeding child at least up to six months of birth		
No schooling	87.85	88.67
1–5 years of education	90.87	87.5
6–10 years of education	90.46	84.99
11–17 years of education	92.08	81.37
Chi-square	2.90 (0.45)	5.71 (0.13)

(Continued)

Table A4.2 (Continued)

Education of respondents	JEEViKA	Non-member
Complementary feeding after six months of birth		
No schooling	77.83	72.1
1–5 years of education	83.33	77.98
6–10 years of education	77.96	75.29
11–17 years of education	86.14	74.53
Chi-square	6.25 (0.10)	2.31 (0.51)

Source: Estimated from primary survey.

Table A4.3 Variation in adoption levels of best practices across the standard of living index of respondents

Standard of living tercile class	JEEViKA	Non-member
Use of modern contraception methods after marriage		
Low	19.09	14.81
Medium	19.74	15.79
High	27.47	22.08
Chi-square	9.34 (0.01)	8.15 (0.02)
First ANC visit in the first trimester of pregnancy		
Low	56.99	57.14
Medium	61.54	65.37
High	74.45	71.69
Chi-square	26.26 (0.00)	17.77 (0.00)
Availed at least four ANC check-ups		
Low	33.87	32.01
Medium	42.31	44.32
High	54.4	54.81
Chi-square	31.85 (0.00)	40.33 (0.00)
Tetanus toxoid injections		
Low	88.98	92.33
Medium	89.49	89.2
High	90.93	92.21
Chi-square	0.83 (0.66)	2.91 (0.25)
100 IFA tablets/syrup for anaemia during pregnancy		
Low	70.43	69.31
Medium	75.64	75.9
High	81.04	82.6
Chi-square	11.26 (0.00)	18.45 (0.00)

(Continued)

Table A4.3 (Continued)

Standard of living tercile class	JEEViKA	Non-member
Availed full ANC services		
Low	23.92	21.69
Medium	31.54	35.73
High	42.03	41.04
Chi-square	27.75 (0.00)	34.41 (0.00)
Delivery in an institution		
Low	66.94	76.46
Medium	81.28	82.83
High	85.99	88.31
Chi-square	42.61 (0.00)	18.65 (0.00)
Delivery assisted by skilled person		
Low	79.03	83.33
Medium	86.92	88.92
High	90.93	93.25
Chi-square	21.99 (0.00)	18.53 (0.00)
Availed post-partum check-ups within 48 h of delivery		
Low	52.42	52.65
Medium	63.33	63.16
High	70.6	68.31
Chi-square	26.24 (0.00)	20.45 (0.00)
Advice on post-partum contraception method		
Low	51.08	46.56
Medium	64.62	52.91
High	65.66	62.34
Chi-square	20.64 (0.00)	19.37 (0.00)
Giving OPV0 to child		
Low	83.06	85.71
Medium	87.95	87.26
High	92.31	92.73
Chi-square	14.64 (.00)	10.26 (0.01)
Breast feeding child at least up to six months of birth		
Low	94.35	90.21
Medium	87.69	88.37
High	86.81	79.74
Chi-square	13.59 (0.00)	19.81 (0.00)

(Continued)

Table A4.3 (Continued)

Standard of living tercile class	JEEViKA	Non-member
Complementary feeding after six months of birth		
Low	78.23	74.07
Medium	72.97	73.41
High	82.42	76.1
Chi-square	2.29 (0.32)	0.78 (0.68)

Source: Estimated from primary survey.

Table A4.4 Variation in adoption levels of best practices across socio-religious groups

Socio-religious category	JEEViKA	Non-member
Use of modern contraception methods after marriage		
Hindu-SC & ST	30.36	26.19
Hindu OBC	21.3	18.66
Hindu-Gen	24.27	15.55
Muslims	12.77	9.41
Chi-square	8.24 (0.04)	9.63 (0.02)
First ANC visit in the first trimester of pregnancy		
Hindu-SC & ST	82.14	85.71
Hindu OBC	65.06	65.07
Hindu-Gen	56.53	56.4
Muslims	78.72	74.12
Chi-square	26.26 (0.00)	29.49 (0.00)
Availed at least four ANC check-ups		
Hindu-SC & ST	67.86	71.43
Hindu OBC	45.76	44.82
Hindu-Gen	35.2	32.01
Muslims	46.81	54.12
Chi-square	25.70 (0.00)	48.51 (0.00)
Tetanus toxoid injections		
Hindu-SC & ST	94.64	92.86
Hindu OBC	89.18	89.47
Hindu-Gen	90.4	94.21
Muslims	88.3	91.76
Chi-square	2.06 (0.58)	6.39 (0.09)
100 IFA tablets/syrup for anaemia during pregnancy		
Hindu-SC & ST	80.36	82.14
Hindu OBC	75.37	75.12

(Continued)

Table A4.4 (Continued)

Socio-religious category	JEEViKA	Non-member
Hindu-Gen	76.27	75.3
Muslims	72.34	78.82
Chi-square	1.33 (0.73)	2.46 (0.48)

Availed full ANC services

Hindu-SC&ST	53.57	53.57
Hindu OBC	33.44	32.85
Hindu-Gen	26.67	25
Muslims	36.17	42.35
Chi-square	17.99 (0.00)	29.00 (0.00)

Delivery in an institution

Hindu-SC & ST	92.86	97.62
Hindu OBC	79.87	84.37
Hindu-Gen	72.27	75
Muslims	80.85	83.53
Chi-square	16.08 (0.00)	27.73 (0.00)

Delivery assisted by skilled person

Hindu-SC & ST	94.64	95.24
Hindu OBC	88.19	90.59
Hindu-Gen	79.73	82.01
Muslims	87.23	91.76
Chi-square	17.66 (0.00)	20.93 (0.00)

Availed post-partum check-ups within 48 h of delivery

Hindu-SC & ST	78.57	69.05
Hindu OBC	64.39	64.43
Hindu-Gen	56.27	53.05
Muslims	60.64	63.53
Chi-square	13.30 (0.00)	14.32 (0.00)
Advice on post-partum contraception method		
Hindu-SC & ST	69.64	69.05
Hindu OBC	60.57	54.7
Hindu-Gen	60	50.61
Muslims	56.38	47.06
Chi-square	2.6652 (0.45)	10.95 (0.01)

Giving OPV0 to child

Hindu-SC & ST	98.21	97.62
Hindu OBC	88.69	89.79
Hindu-Gen	85.33	83.23
Muslims	85.11	91.76
Chi-square	8.84 (0.02)	17.87 (0.00)

(Continued)

Table A4.4 (Continued)

Socio-religious category	JEEViKA	Non-member
Breast feeding child at least up to six months of birth	14.64 (.00)	10.26 (.01)
Hindu-SC & ST	83.93	66.67
Hindu OBC	89.68	86.28
Hindu-Gen	89.33	88.11
Muslims	93.62	95.29
Chi-square	3.60 (0.31)	33.49 (0.00)

Complementary feeding after six months of birth		
Hindu-SC & ST	89.29	82.14
Hindu OBC	78.37	74.48
Hindu-Gen	78.67	71.65
Muslims	88.3	78.82
Chi-square	8.41 (0.04)	4.83 (0.19)

Source: Estimated from primary survey.

Table A4.5 Adoption levels of MCH practices: Results of multi-level regression

Variables	Cont.	ANC3m	ANC	TTI	IFA	ID	AD	PPC	PPACM	OPVO	BF	CF
Are you SHG member												
Non-member	-0.06	-0.13	-0.30 **	-0.42 ***	-0.27 **	-0.16 *	-0.30***	-0.21	-0.03	-0.28 **	-0.11	-0.21 ***
Years of education												
1–5 years of education	0.01	-0.17	-0.36 *	-0.10	-0.01	-0.06	-0.11	-0.49 **	0.23	-0.15	-0.13	0.08
6–10 years of education	-0.20	-0.18	-0.33	-0.33**	-0.40 ***	-0.25 **	-0.38 ***	-0.39**	-0.15	-0.48 ***	-0.35 ***	-0.10
11–17 years of education	-0.54 **	-0.45 ***	-0.63 ***	-0.50 ***	-0.40 **	-0.41 ***	-0.50 ***	-0.36	-0.58 ***	-0.51 ***	-0.27 **	-0.07
Socio-religious communities												
H-SC & ST	-0.20	-0.69 ***	-0.41	-0.25	-0.01	-0.19	0.09	-0.07	-0.37	-0.20	0.09	-0.23
H-OBC	0.10	-0.11	-0.07	0.07	0.13	-0.11	-0.01	-0.12	-0.21	-0.07	0.05	-0.17 **
Muslim	0.19	-0.35*	-0.37	-0.16	-0.15	-0.37 **	-0.20	0.18	0.05	0.14	-0.04	-0.10
Are you engaged in any work that brings income												
Yes	0.35	-0.24 *	-0.06	-0.13	-0.26 *	-0.08	0.01	0.16	-0.08	-0.17	-0.09	-0.33 ***
Age	-0.01	-0.02	-0.01	-0.01	-0.01	0.02 *	0.01	0.01	-0.01	0.02	0.00	0.03 **
Household size	-0.05*	-0.03*	-0.05	-0.04 **	-0.05	-0.02	-0.04 ***	-0.03	0.01	-0.02	-0.03 **	-0.02 *
Asset	-0.34 ***	-0.13 **	-0.01	-0.03	0.00	-0.05	-0.04	-0.13	-0.11	-0.03	-0.14 ***	-0.19 ***

(Continued)

Table A4.5 (Continued)

Variables	Cont.	ANC3m	ANC	TTI	IFA	ID	AD	PPC	PPACM	OPVO	BF	CF
If your partner is a migrant												
Non-migrant	0.33 **	0.02	0.03	-0.31 ***	-0.21	0.01	0.05	0.10	-0.06	-0.05	0.01	0.10
Total no of living children	0.02	0.15***	0.15 **	0.22 ***	0.10 *	0.01	-0.02	-0.11 *	-0.02	0.03	0.05	0.03
Constant	1.59 **	1.99 ***	2.25 ***	2.20 ***	2.47 ***	1.17 ***	1.94 ***	2.45 ***	2.11 ***	1.92 ***	1.61 ***	0.72 **
District	0.02	0.28	0.17	0.40	0.18	0.27	0.17	0.17	0.19	0.23	0.30	0.28
Block	0.00	0.00	0.03	0.02	0.00	0.09	0.09	0.03	0.06	0.01	0.08	0.11
Village	0.07	0.07	0.12	0.12	0.04	0.02	0.07	0.03	0.12	0.00	0.02	0.00
N	446	1451	981	2037	1706	1807	1959	1389	1288	1984	1976	1737
χ^2	1.62 (0.44)	97.42 ***	31.76 ***	171.63 ***	48.02 ***	116.49 ***	101.28 ***	37.17 ***	50.72 ***	69.04 ***	214.52 ***	185.72 ***
Wald χ^2	33.85***	65.11 ***	30.16 ***	60.78 ***	33.45 ***	31.94 ***	33.39 ***	22.72 **	31.61 ***	30.65 ***	39.75 ***	59.09 ***
Intra-class coefficients												
District	0.02	0.21	0.13	0.26	0.15	0.20	0.13	0.14	0.14	0.18	0.22	0.20
Block | District	0.02	0.21	0.15	0.30	0.15	0.26	0.19	0.17 (	0.19	0.19	0.28	0.28
Village | Block | District	0.09	0.26	0.24	0.35	0.18	0.27	0.24	0.19	0.27	0.19	0.30	0.28

Source: Estimated from primary survey.

Note: Cont: Uses modern contraception method; ANC3M: ANC check-up within three months; ANC: Availed recommended ANC check-ups; TTI: Availed tetanus toxoid injection; IFA: Availed IFA tablets/syrups; ID: Delivered in institution; AD: Delivery was assisted by skilled persons; PPC: Availed post-partum check-up; PPACM: Provided post-partum contraception advice; OPVO: Child given OPV at birth; BF: Exclusively breastfed child till six months; CF: Started complementary feeding after six months.

Chapter 5

Leveraging information diffusion

Peer effects versus individual counselling by ASHAS

5.1 Peer effects: An introduction

Chapter 4 revealed a high level of adoption level of maternal and child health (MCH) outcomes in the survey districts vis-à-vis levels reported in the National Family Health Survey undertaken in 2015–16. In this chapter we examine whether peer effects have played a role in increasing adoption levels.

Peer effects refer to the influence of friends, neighbours, and others in the social circle of an agent on the behaviour of an agent (Bramoullé et al., 2020). It refers to the tendency of an individual to behave in ways that resembles the behaviour of the group of which he/she is a member. In other words, "Peer effects refer to externalities in which the actions or characteristics of a reference group affect an individual's behaviour or outcomes" (Ryan, 2017). Such effects can be positive (Diani & McAdam, 2003; Katz & Lazarsfeld, 2005; Lim, 2010) or negative (Ennett & Bauman, 1993; Maxwell, 2002; Christakis & Fowler, 2007, 2008; Trogdon et al., 2008; Halliday & Kwak, 2009). There is no consensus on who forms such reference groups. Peer members are generally considered to be similarly aged reference groups with whom respondents regularly interact (Sacerdote, 2001; Ryan, 2017). However, depending on the context, peers can also refer to friends, roommates, classmates, colleagues, neighbours, health workers, and others.

In recent years, there has been considerable research on peer effects, and their impact on social and economic outcomes (An, 2011; Ryan, 2017). Researchers have shown the impact of peer effects on widening inequality (Finneran & Kelly, 2003; Calvó-Armengol & Jackson, 2004, 2007), social spreading of obesity (Christakis & Fowler, 2007; Trogdon et al., 2008; Halliday & Kwak, 2009; Carrell et al., 2011), autism (Liu et al., 2010), cigarette smoking (Ennett & Bauman, 1993; Maxwell, 2002; Christakis & Fowler, 2008), sexually transmitted diseases (Bearman, Moody and Stovel, 2004), flow of mass communication (Katz & Lazarsfeld, 2005), mobilisation of social movements and civic participation (Diani & McAdam, 2003; Lim, 2010), and so on.

DOI: 10.4324/9781003499251-5

The role of peer effects in promoting preventive health care behaviour is also established in the literature (Fletcher, 2014). A study of the Progressa scheme in Mexico reported that social interactions increased preventive care usage both among eligible and non-eligible households with respect to various types of prevention (Bouckaert, 2014). Similar findings have been obtained in other studies of peer effects (Webel et al., 2010; Houle et al., 2017). A study undertaken in the Philippines found the existence of significant peer effects from microfinance institutions (Hoffmann, 2019); similar findings have been reported for rural areas of Malawi (Lewycka et al., 2013) and India (Brooks et al., 2020).

5.2 Objectives and hypotheses

In this chapter we have examined the motivating factors that have led to behavioural change and adoption of best MCH practices in Bihar. The role of peer factors has been examined in three steps, each of which examines a specific hypothesis:

a) Step 1 (Hypothesis H1): In line with recent literature we have examined whether peer effects have facilitated the adoption of MCH practices.
b) Step 2 (Hypothesis H2): The adoption of MCH practices may also be the result of a confounding factor. The use of female grass-roots activists, referred to as Accredited Social Health Activists (ASHAs), in the National Rural Health Mission is one such confounding factor. ASHAs have been reported to have played a major role as a motivator in inducing behavioural practice (Kohli et al., 2015; Agarwal et al., 2019). The second hypothesis is that the ASHAs may have played a role in behavioural change among both JEEViKA members and non-members. If this hypothesis (H2) is accepted, then any peer effect observed when testing the first hypothesis (H1) is questionable. The reason is the peer effect observed initially may be explained by the presence of a confounding variable (ASHAs in this context).
c) Step 3 (Hypothesis H3): The analysis of this chapter, therefore, closes with an investigation of whether peer effects observed when testing H1 are still significant if we incorporate the role of ASHAs.

The methodology used to examine the three hypotheses has been discussed in the next section (Section 5.3). It is followed by the presentation and analysis of the results (Section 5.4). The "Results" section starts by testing the existence of possible peer effects (H1). It is followed by an investigation of the agents motivating the observed behavioural change. We first examine the comparative role of different motivators and their variations across socioeconomic correlates; the discussion is followed by the analysis of the main motivator and its variations across correlates. A regression model is also estimated to identify the characteristics of respondents motivated by ASHAs. In the final step we examine H3, namely, whether the peer effects observed when testing H1 is observed even after incorporating the motivating role of ASHAs. The chapter concludes with a discussion of the implications of the results.

5.3 Materials and method

5.3.1 Data

The analysis was undertaken using the data collected from the primary survey of six districts in Bihar – namely, Begusarai, Katiahar, Muzzafarpur, Nalanda, Purva Champaran, and Saharsa. The details of the sampling methodology are given in Chapter 2, Section 2.2. The study was administered in 120 villages spread over 24 blocks in the six districts. It was undertaken between January and March 2020. It covered 2250 women, selected using a stratified multi-stage sampling method, aged between 15 and 49 years who had at least one living child aged less than 36 months.

5.3.2 Estimating peer effects

The existence of peer effects may be tested using either static (one-period) or dynamic (multi-period) models. In the case of static models, the linear difference-in-difference (DID) approach is the most commonly used method to identify peer effects (Manski, 1993; Bramoullé et al., 2009; Graham & Hahn, 2009). The model assumes that the respondent i's outcome (Y_i) is determined by not only his or her own characteristics (X_i) but also by the respective mean values of the characteristics and outcomes of his or her peer group (X_j and Y_j, respectively). The structure of this model may be explained using a two-subject community. The outcomes of the two actors (i and j) are modelled by the following equations:

$$Y_i = \alpha_1 X_i + \alpha_2 X_j + \beta Y_j + e_i \qquad [5.1]$$

$$Y_j = \alpha_1 X_j + \alpha_2 X_i + \beta Y_i + e_j \qquad [5.2]$$

Manski (1993) argues that the DID model overlooks the fact that the propensity of individuals to behave in some way varies with the exogenous characteristics of the group. Referred to as the "reflection problem" by Manski (Manski, 1993), it leads to simultaneity in operational terms. It may be seen by combining the two equations to get the following reduced-form equation:

$$Y_i = \frac{\alpha_1 + \beta \alpha_2}{1-\beta^2} X_i + \frac{\alpha_2 + \beta \alpha_1}{1-\beta^2} X_j + (\beta e_j + e_i) \qquad [5.3]$$

There are only two exogenous variables but three parameters (α_1, α_2, and β) to be estimated, so that the above equations are under-identified, and cannot be estimated without making further assumptions.

In the case of binary outcome models, however, there is a trivial solution to the reflection problem (An, 2011). If the behaviour or outcome being studied is binary in nature, a logit or probit is adopted to model peer effects (Van den Bulte & Lilien, 2001; Brock & Durlauf, 2001a; Brock & Durlauf, 2001b; Krauth, 2006; Sorensen, 2006). The non-linear relationship between the explanatory variables and outcomes resolves the simultaneity problem (Brock & Durlauf, 2001a), so that the peer effect can be estimated easily. In our case, the outcome is a binary adoption (whether they have adopted maternal and child health (MCH) practices, or not). So we have estimated a non-linear probit model, thereby resolving the simultaneity problem. The likelihood function for a probit model is:

$$\text{Ln } L = \sum_i w_i \ln(_1X_i +_2 X_j + Y_j) + \sum_{ji} w_i \ln \left\{ 1 - \left(_1X_i +_2 X_j + Y_j\right) \right\}$$

$$= \sum_i w_i \ln(_1X_i +_2 X_j + Y_j) + \sum_{ji} w_j \ln\left(_1X_j +_2 X_i + Y_i\right) \tag{5.4}$$

5.3.3 Model specification

The regression model assumes the form:

$$Y_{ij} = \beta_0 + \beta_1 \text{VBPR}_j + \beta_2 \text{VX}_j + \beta_3 X_{ij} \tag{5.5}$$

when

Y_{ij} is a binary variable indicating whether the ith respondent in the jth village had adopted the best practice or not

VBPR_j is the adoption rate of the best practice in the jth village

VX_j is the characteristics of the jth village

X_{ij} is the characteristics of the ith respondent residing in the jth village

The individual characteristics are: age, education, and socio-religious identity of the respondent, whether the respondent is a JEEViKA member, whether the respondent is engaged in any work, standard of living measured using asset index scores, household size, whether the husband is a migrant worker, and the number of living children.

The village characteristics are mean years of schooling, and religious and caste profile of respondents in j^{th} village.

A probit model was used to estimate [5.5]. The Wald test indicates that multi-level models are not relevant; so the probit models are estimated after clustering at the village level. This yields robust standard errors. A positive and significant value of β_1 indicates the presence of peer effects.

5.3.4 Are ASHAs a confounding factor?

There is, however, another challenge in using static models to estimate peer effects. It is the possible presence of omitted variables, which will lead to biased and inconsistent estimates. As Manski (1993) points out, individuals in the same reference group may tend to behave similarly because they face a common environment. For instance, peer groups may be exposed to the same environmental shocks, which may affect the outcomes, even if the peer group members do not interact with each other (Van den Bulte & Lilien, 2001). Health shocks in a neighbourhood, for instance, could make people simultaneously decide to undergo medical check-ups, even without having directly influenced each other in their decisions.

For instance, under the National Rural Health Mission, every village is supposed to have an Accredited Social Health Activist (ASHA) who will "act as the interface between the community and the public health system". Their role is to promote child immunisation, and provide referral and escort services for reproductive child health and other health delivery programs. The role of ASHAs, therefore, is one such possible shock. The Community Mobiliser associated with JEEViKAs provides similar services, and holds monthly meetings to motivate JEEViKA members to follow MCH practices. The peer effects generated by the spill over of the programme effects may lead to an exogenous peer effect[1] that is quite different from the endogenous peer effect.

During the survey, we asked three questions about the motivating force underlying the adoption of the MCH practices studied. We asked whether the respondent adopted a particular practice (say, using modern contraception methods); those respondents who adopted such practices were asked who motivated the adoption of the practice. They could identify ASHAs, health workers, JEEViKA post-holders, JEEViKA members, husband, relatives, neighbours, and media as possible motivators. The question was of a multiple-response variety, and multiple motivators could be chosen. This was followed by another question where the respondent had to identify the main motivator who influenced their choice. These questions were asked for each of the MCH practices. Finally, we asked respondents to identify the main influence underlying the adoption of MCH practices in general. Analysis of these responses indicates the dominant influence of ASHAs. It indicates that ASHAs may be a common factor underlying the choice of an MCH practice by the community.

A regression model is also estimated. The specification is:

$$Y_{ij} = \beta_0 + \beta_1 X_{ij} \qquad [5.6]$$

where

Y_{ijk} is a binary variable indicating whether the ith respondent residing in the jth village was motivated by an ASHA in adopting the kth MCH practice.

X_{ij} is a vector indicating the characteristics (age, education, and socio-religious identity of the respondent, whether the respondent is engaged in any work, standard of living measured using asset index scores, household size, whether the husband is a migrant worker, and number of living children) of the ith respondent residing in the jth village.

A multi-level probit model was used to estimate the models for each of the MCH practices stated in Section 4.2.

5.3.5 Testing for exogenous peer effects

To rule out peer effects endogenously generated by confounding factors like ASHAs, we estimate a regression model incorporating variables capturing the influence of ASHAs on the individual (whether ASHA is the main motivator and proportion of respondents in the village motivated by ASHA). Including these variables will enable us to test whether an endogenous peer effect exists, even after controlling for the common environmental factor. The specification of the probit regression model is:

$$Y_{ij} = \beta_0 + \beta_1 VBPR_j + \beta_2 VX_j + \beta_3 X_{ij} + \beta_4 PVMA_j + \beta_5 ASHA_{ij} \qquad [5.7]$$

where

Y_{ij} is a binary variable indicating whether the ith respondent in the jth village had adopted the best practice or not.
$VBPR_j$ is the adoption rate of the best practice in the jth village.
VX_j is the characteristics of the jth village stated in Section 5.3.2.
X_{ij} is the characteristics of the ith respondent residing in the jth village stated in Section 5.3.2.
$PVMA_j$ is the proportion of villagers in the jth village motivated by the ASHA.
$ASHA_{ij}$ is a binary variable indicating whether the ith respondent in the jth village is motivated by ASHA

During the estimation process, village-level clustering ensured robust standard errors. As in the earlier case (Section 5.32), a positive and significant value of β_1 indicates the presence of peer effects.

5.4 Results

5.4.1 Estimates of peer effects

The summary results of the probit models specified in Section 5.5 are reported in Table 5.1.

Results show that, in all cases, the coefficient of the village outcome is positive and statistically significant from zero at the 1% level. The highest coefficient value is observed for availing tetanus injection, followed by

Table 5.1 Peer effects on MCH outcomes

MCH practices	β	t	Prob.	R^2
Modern contraception methods after marriage	3.80	23.69	0.00	0.12
The first ante natal care (ANC) visit was in the first trimester	2.84	33.12	0.00	0.19
At least four ANC check-ups	2.71	42.48	0.00	0.19
Given tetanus toxoid injection	5.41	9.68	0.00	0.15
Given iron folic acid (IFA) tablets/syrup for anaemia	3.46	26.60	0.00	0.16
Institutional delivery	3.49	25.39	0.00	0.27
Delivery assisted by skilled person	4.29	19.23	0.00	0.21
Post-partum check-up within 48 hours	2.75	37.99	0.00	0.13
Post-partum contraception advice	2.90	39.75	0.00	0.15
Whether child was given OPV0	4.31	16.02	0.00	0.24
Exclusive breast feeding up to six months of birth	4.89	16.89	0.00	0.15
Complementary feeding after six months	3.37	22.84	0.00	0.08

Source: Estimated from primary survey.

assisted delivery. The coefficient is lowest for availing the recommended four ANC check-ups and post-partum contraception advise. This indicates the prima facie existence of a positive peer effect. However, we still have to rule out the possibility of confounding factors. This requires us to identify the agents or forces motivating the adoption of MCH practices.

5.4.2 Alternative motivators of MCH practices

In Figure 5.1 we have analysed the multiple response data on persons motivating the adoption of MCH practices (for detailed results refer to Appendix A5.1). The data reveals that in all cases, grass-roots health workers (of which ASHAs constitute the majority) are the main motivators. In case of complementary feeding of child after six months (45%), exclusive breastfeeding till six months (49%), and institutional delivery (49%), their role is relatively low – though more influential than other agents. In case of promoting ANC services and adopting modern contraceptive methods, however, grass-roots workers are identified as motivators in at least 90% of responses. This is consistent with the findings of existing studies. Global experience shows that women, even when briefly trained, can successfully increase the coverage of healthcare, particularly if they are locally recruited and made accountable to the local clients (Reichenbach, 2007). Another study found that the introduction of ASHAs has had a positive impact in increasing the proportion of women taking at least three antenatal check-ups, delivering in institutions, and improving child immunisation (Bajpai, Sachs, and Dholakia, 2010).

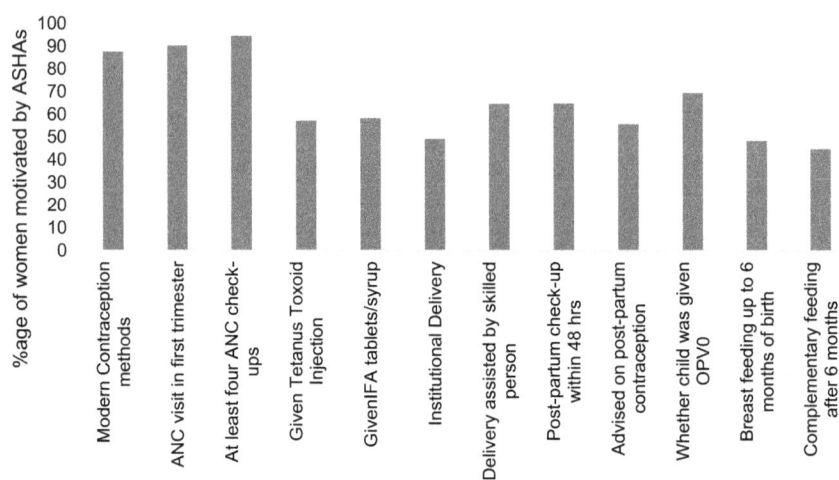

Figure 5.1 Role of ASHAs in motivating adoption of MCH practices.

Source: Estimated from primary survey.

Analysing data from India Human Development Survey 2012, Paul and Pandey (Paul & Pandey, 2020) found that the number of ANC contacts and exposure to ASHA workers both independently emerged as important determinants of institutional delivery. The study also argued that ASHA workers may have a crucial role in promoting antenatal care, thereby bridging the gap between ANC contacts and institutional delivery. A small-scale study carried out in Punjab found that the MCH services delivery definitely improved substantially after the inception of ASHA workers in rural communities (Panda et al., 2013). However, contrary to expectation, a study by Wagner et al. (Wagner et al., 2018a) found that between 2007 and 2008 and 2012 and 2013, an increase in ASHA placement in a village by 1% is likely to lower the unmet need for family planning and enhance full immunisation by 0.22%; however, no impact on institutional delivery was observed.

During the Focus group discussions, women reported that, over time, ASHAs had increased in numbers and had become proactive over time. Previously ASHAs were involved in immunisation drives. Now, however, "you can see her regularly roaming in the village". The reason why ASHAs were able to modify behaviour was that "ASHA comes home therefore when she tells something all the family members could learn and understand that. When she tells everyone listens to her and tries to understand and follow". Another participant observed that as "They not only talk to us, they also talk to our families, so it gets less difficult for us".

Analysis of the identity of other motivators also provides information about the rural society. For instance, husbands play an important role in the choice of modern contraception methods. This finding is similar to that of other studies in other developing countries (Blunch, 2008; Kaggwa et al., 2008; Myo-Myo-Mon & Liabsuetrakul, 2009; Samandari et al., 2010), including India (Sharma & Rani, 2009; Manna & Basu, 2011). Other family members play an important role in encouraging respondents to adopt contraceptives, avail antenatal care services, deliver in institutions, exclusively breastfeed children till six months, and supplement their diet after six months. During the interviews, in many cases, mothers-in-law intervened and claimed that they had a role. However, respondents spoke about the role of their *jethani* (sister-in-law) in encouraging the adoption of these practices. Although we had found a significant programme effect for exclusive breastfeeding and supplementary feeding in Chapter 4, only one out of seven respondents acknowledged the role of JEEViKA members and officers in the adoption of these two practices.

5.4.3 Variations in the identity of motivators across socio-economic correlates

This section analyses multiple response data on motivating persons of MCH practices across different socio-economic groups. Health workers have been the most important motivators with 43.64% of total responses for all practices, followed by family members and husband in some cases. While the role of husbands is important in the case of adoption of modern contraceptive methods (18.75% of responses), for all the other practices, husbands' role is relatively low. The role of other family members is relatively higher for certain practices, such as, it is more than 23% for the first ANC visit in the first trimester of pregnancy and four such visits in total, institutional delivery, breastfeeding, and complementary feeding. JEEViKA members and postholders also have some amount of influence, although it is quite low.

Table A5.2 shows responses by women who have been grouped into four categories with regard to their minimum years of education. Women with less education are with the highest share of responses (48.31%) in favour of ASHA workers as motivators for the use of modern contraception after marriage, and more educated women are more likely to acknowledge the role of family members as motivators (23.28%). Women with 6–10 years of education have given the highest share of responses (20.28%) stating husbands as important motivators for this practice.

For all antenatal care and post-partum healthcare practices, grass-roots health workers' influence is relatively higher among women with less education. This indicates that although ASHA is undoubtedly the most important motivator, its outreach is less in certain socio-economic groups. Women with more education are more likely to consider the role of family as important for these practices. The scenario is similar for husbands, with the exception of availing at least four ANC visits and giving polio vaccine to children, where their impact is higher among women with 1–5 years of education.

For breastfeeding children after six months of birth and complementary feeding post six months, illiterate women are more likely to observe ASHAs as their main motivators (52.35% and 47.14%). A majority of women who have received 6–10 years of education are influenced by their families after ASHAs (24.62% and 25.02% for exclusive breastfeeding and complementary feeding, respectively). More educated women are more likely to consider their husbands as important motivators of these two practices (11.30 % and 11.14%).

It is evident that for availing modern contraceptive methods, only the role of the media varies significantly with the education of respondents. Responses acknowledging grass-roots health workers as motivators vary significantly with the educational attainment of respondents in case of availing first ANC check-up within the first trimester of pregnancy and availing at least four such check-ups in total, and going for post-partum check-up within 48 hours of delivery. While variations of responses stating JEEViKA members as motivators across education are insignificant, that of JEEViKA post-holders is significant when it comes to availing a minimum of four ANC check-ups, delivering in an institution and with the assistance of a skilled person, receiving post-partum check-up within 48 hours of giving birth, and complementary feeding after six months of birth. The role of the family as a motivator varies significantly across minimum years of education of respondents in case of ensuring protection against natal Tetanus, institutional delivery, post-partum contraception advice, breastfeeding after six months of birth, and complementary feeding. Variations of the influence of husbands across education of their wives are insignificant except for visiting ANC check-up facilities within the first trimester of pregnancy and getting four such check-ups, delivering in an institution, receiving post-partum contraception advice, and exclusive breastfeeding.

Other than the adoption of modern contraception methods, the overall variations of motivators across education for all the other practices are significant.

In Table A5.3, we have analysed multiple responses of women across different household asset scores. For the adoption of modern contraception, responses recorded in favour of health workers are highest for women with a medium standard of living index (48.29%). For all the other practices, women from less affluent families are influenced by ASHAs the most, thereby again implying ASHA workers' outreach to underprivileged and marginalised sections of society. Women belonging to a higher class are more likely to respond that family is an important motivator (21.90%) for modern contraception use. This is followed by husbands, and respondents coming from affluent households have given the highest share of responses (20.87%) in this.

In the case of all antenatal care and post-partum health practices, women belonging to households with medium asset scores have given the highest share of responses acknowledging family members as motivators, except for advice on post-partum contraception (where the incidence is highest among women from higher classes). With the exception of taking IFA tablet or syrup for anaemia, institutional delivery, and OPV0 vaccine, the role of husband is relatively higher among women of affluent households.

For exclusive breastfeeding and complementary feeding, women from households with more asset are more likely to consider their family as an important motivator for these two practices (23.12% and 23.44%), followed by their husband (10.69% and 11.37%).

The variations across asset are insignificant for ASHAs with the exception of adoption of modern contraceptives and availing ANC services during the first trimester of pregnancy. In case of JEEViKA members, variations of their influence across classes are significant for administering tetanus toxoid injection, taking IFA tablet or syrup to prevent anaemia during pregnancy, giving birth in an institution, receiving advice on post-partum contraception, giving OPV0 to child, exclusive breastfeeding and supplementing diet, whereas for JEEViKA post-holders, the variation is significant only for the last two practices. The role of husbands as motivators varies significantly across the standard of living when it comes to visiting ANC facilities in the first trimester, undertaking institutional delivery, receiving advice on post-partum contraception, breastfeeding newborn child, and supplementing breastfeeding with semi-solid and solid food after six months. Again, the role of other family members varies significantly with asset score for institutional delivery, exclusive breastfeeding, and complementary feeding.

In the overall scenario, variations across the standard of living index are significant except for availing at least four ANC check-ups, taking anaemia medication, delivering with the assistance of a skilled person, and receiving post-partum check-up within 48 hours of delivery.

Table A5.4 represents multiple response data of women belonging to different socio-religious categories. For all practices, the influence of ASHA workers is highest among Hindu forward caste women, except for the use of modern contraception and advice on post-partum contraception, where their influence is highest among Muslim women. The role of family and husband is the most important when it comes to Hindu Scheduled Caste (SC) and Scheduled Tribe (ST) women and Muslim women. For the use of modern contraception, the role of family and husband as important motivators is the highest in the case of women from marginalised castes and tribes (27.63% for family and 26.32% for husband). Muslim women are more likely to consider family members as motivators when it comes to availing at least four ANC check-ups, taking anaemia medication, delivering in an institution and with the assistance of a skilled person, receiving post-partum advice on contraception, giving polio vaccine to a child, and complementary feeding. For the rest five practices, the role of family members is most important for Hindu lower caste and tribal women. The highest share of Muslim women has acknowledged the role of their husbands in anaemia medication, giving birth with the assistance of a skilled person, and ensuring the polio vaccine to children. In case of the other practices, the husbands' role is relatively higher among Hindu women from marginalised castes and tribes.

The influence of ASHA and other grass-roots level workers varies significantly across socio-religious category only for the first two practices, that is, the use of modern contraception methods, and availing first ANC check-up within the first trimester of pregnancy. The impact of JEEViKA members varies significantly across these categories in the case of the first ANC check-up in the first trimester, delivery assisted by a skilled person, and complementary feeding after six months of birth. For all the practices, the association between socio-religious identity and the role of family members as motivators is significant. Variations in the role of husbands across such identities are significant in the case of first ANC check-up in the first trimester, institutional delivery, and ensuring child protection from polio.

Overall, the variations across socio-religious category are significant in all cases except institutional delivery and advice on post-partum contraception. The absence of reliance of forward castes and affluent households on ASHAs was confirmed by the latter during the interaction. One ASHA reported that "upper caste people don't depend on ASHA"; it was claimed that "Most of them seek treatment from private facilities and doesn't bother to discuss anything with ASHA". As an ASHA worker complained, "they have money! Now what we will explain to them, they know it all". The main reason is that such households prefer to seek healthcare from private facilities:

> You know what happens to the upper caste they think that they have money so they will not take any government facilities, even we suggest them to do whatever they want to, but just to share the check-up dates.

As a result, ASHAs visit their homes as they have to maintain records, but interactions are minimal.

5.4.4 Who is motivating the adoption of MCH practices?

So far we have used the information elicited from respondents about the different actors who had motivated their adoption of the MCH practice studied in this paper. Respondents were allowed to identify several persons. The influence of these persons on the decision to adopt a practice may, however, vary. For instance, although two persons may identify their husband and

ASHA as influential persons, their relative influence may vary with ASHA being more influential for one person, and husband more influential for the other. So it is also necessary to study who exerted the *most* influence for each MCH practice. This section examines who is the main motivator behind each MCH practice, and the variations across socio-economic correlates. This analysis is undertaken for JEEViKA members and non-members separately.

Table A5.5 represents data on the main motivator for each healthcare practice, and it shows that in all cases, the majority of respondents have chosen health workers as the main motivators (Figure 5.2). ASHA and other health workers have been identified as main motivators in over 94% cases for IFA tablets or syrup to prevent anaemia, availing post-partum check-up within 48 hours of delivery, and ensuring the polio vaccine at birth for children. In comparison to other practices, the role of ASHA workers as main motivators is relatively low in case of supplementing breastfeeding of child with semi-solid and solid food after six months (79.97%) and adopting modern contraception methods (80.72%).

Our analysis shows that ASHAs have played a major role in changing the attitude and improving the uptake of MCH practices in the districts surveyed. A study of their age, education, and caste profile is important in understanding their success. ASHAs are aged, on an average, about 39 years. They have about ten years of schooling. About 97 of the ASHAs covered in the survey are Hindus. The majority belong to the OBC community (56%);

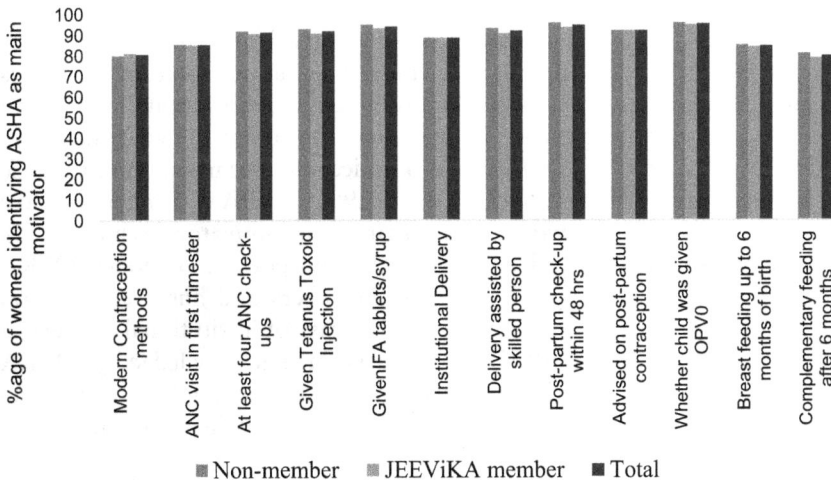

Figure 5.2 Percentage of women identifying ASHA as the main motivator.

Source: Estimated from primary survey.

a large proportion belong to the General (24%) and SC (19%) community. The higher level of education (mean year of schooling for respondents is only five years) and the fact that they belong to the numerically large OBC community enables them to approach target women easily. The fact that the ASHAs are middle-aged also facilitates them as there are less restrictions on their mobility.

Next to ASHAs, family members and husbands of our respondents, and JEEViKA workers and officers hold the second most acknowledged positions as main motivators for different MCH practices. Family and husband have an important role in motivating the adoption of several practices, the greatest influence being on the adoption of modern contraception (12.56%). In this, a higher proportion of women who are non-JEEViKA members have acknowledged family or husband's role as most important (15.15%) than women who have JEEViKA membership (10.48%). In the case of breastfeeding children up to six months of birth (8.55%) and complementary feeding after six months (10.54%), the total share of responses stating JEEViKA workers as main motivators is considerably higher, thus implying a significant program effect. For both these practices, therefore, a higher proportion of women who are JEEViKA members have considered JEEViKA workers as main motivators (10.31% for exclusive breastfeeding and 13.35% for complementary feeding) than women who do not have JEEViKA membership (6.72% in case of exclusive breastfeeding and 7.52% in case of complementary feeding). JEEViKA members also hold the second most common role as a main motivator for ensuring protection against natal tetanus and anaemia, administering OPV0 to children, availing post-partum check-up, and getting advice on post-partum contraception. Less than 2% of women have identified their family members or husbands as main motivators in taking medication to prevent anaemia during pregnancy, availing post-partum check-ups within 48 hours of delivery, and administering the polio vaccine to newborn child. A difference in responses among women who are JEEViKA members and those who are non-members is also noticeable. For instance, in the case of delivery assisted by a skilled person, 5.29% of JEEViKA members have observed that JEEViKA workers are their main motivators, while 2.81% non-members have responded so. A higher proportion of non-JEEViKA members (3.32%) have identified family members and husbands as main motivators for this practice. Similarly, in the case of institutional delivery, a lower proportion of non-JEEViKA members have acknowledged JEEViKA workers as their main motivators (2.82%), thereby making family members and husbands the main motivators for this practice when it comes to the total (6.64%).

Less than 1% of respondents have identified their friends, neighbours, or the media – who have been clubbed under the "Others" category – as main motivators of all the practices, except the adoption of modern contraception method after marriage, where the share is slightly higher (1.57%).

5.4.5 Variations in the identity of the main motivator across socio-economic correlates

In Table A5.6, we can observe that, illiterate women are more likely to state ASHAs as the main motivators for most practices, with the exception of the use of modern contraception after marriage and advice on post-partum contraception for JEEViKA members, and delivery assisted by a skilled person and complementary feeding for non-JEEViKA members. This indicates a relatively higher influence of grass-roots health workers among unprivileged socio-economic groups. With the exception of availing post-partum check-up within 48 hours of delivery, a higher share of responses in favour of family as main motivators has been given by more educated women who do not have JEEViKA membership. Again, for women with JEEViKA membership, a higher share of responses in favour of JEEViKA workers as main motivators is given by educated women, with the exception of exclusive feeding and complementary feeding. For half of the practices, a higher share of educated women who are non-JEEViKA members has acknowledged the role of JEEViKA workers as the main motivators. Women with 1–5 years of education who are JEEViKA members are more likely to consider family members as main motivators, except in the case of modern contraception use, first ANC visit in the first trimester of pregnancy, tetanus toxoid injection, and complementary feeding.

Variations of motivating persons for all respondents are significant across education for the first ANC visit in the first trimester of pregnancy, tetanus toxoid injections, institutional delivery, and advice on post-partum contraception. For only those respondents who are JEEViKA members, the variations are significant in case of availing at least four ANC check-ups, taking 100 IFA tablets or syrup for anaemia during pregnancy, giving birth with the assistance of a skilled person, availing post-partum check-up within 48 hours of delivery, and ensuring polio vaccine to a child. For non-JEEViKA members, it is significant only in the case of exclusive breastfeeding.

In Table A5.7, we can observe that, although ASHA workers are the main motivators for all practices and across all classes, their share is relatively lower in the case of affluent households, and this is true for both JEEViKA members and non-members. This again indicates that the outreach of ASHAs is lower in certain socio-economic groups. After grass-roots health workers, families come second for most MCH practices in the case of respondents who are non-JEEViKA members. The exceptions are post-partum check-ups within 48 hours of delivery, and giving polio vaccine to children, where JEEViKA workers have a greater role as motivators among non-JEEViKA members. For these two practices, the share of JEEViKA members as main motivators is higher in the case of women belonging to households with more assets. When it comes to respondents who are JEEViKA members, the role of JEEViKA workers as motivators is more important than family for most of the practices, with the exception of the first ANC visit in the first trimester of pregnancy. In this, women from affluent households are more likely to consider family members or JEEViKA workers as main motivators.

Motivators for all respondents vary significantly with asset only in case of adopting modern contraception after marriage, availing first ANC check-up in the first trimester of pregnancy, ensuring protection from natal Tetanus, and complementary feeding. For only JEEViKA members, the variation is significant only for availing at least four ANC check-ups, and for only non-members, it is significant only in case of receiving advice on post-partum contraception.

Table A5.8 shows that, for respondents who are non-JEEViKA members, next to ASHAs, family members come second as main motivators and are followed by JEEViKA workers for most of the practices. For respondents who are JEEViKA members, JEEViKA workers have the second highest share of responses as main motivators for most practices, followed by family. When it comes to non-JEEViKA members, for a majority of MCH practices, a higher share of Muslim women and Hindu women belonging to marginalised castes and tribes have acknowledged the role of ASHAs as main motivators, again implying ASHAs' greater outreach among deprived sections of society. When it comes to JEEViKA members, for half of the practices, forward caste Hindu women are more likely to consider ASHA workers as main motivators. A higher share of Muslim women who are JEEViKA members has chosen ASHAs as their main motivators for the use of modern contraception after marriage, availing post-partum check-up within 48 hours of delivery, and receiving advice on post-partum contraception methods. For taking anaemia medication and exclusive breastfeeding, a higher proportion of Hindu OBC women who are JEEViKA members have talked of ASHAs as main motivators, whereas, a higher share of JEEViKA members who are Hindu SC and ST women have said so for delivery assisted by a skilled person. In all the practices, for JEEViKA members, a higher share of Hindu SC and ST women have chosen family members as their main motivators.

The role of motivators for all respondents varies significantly across socioreligious categories only when it comes to the first ANC visit in the first trimester of pregnancy and availing of at least four such check-ups in total. For only JEEViKA members, the variation across such identities is significant only for receiving advice on post-partum contraception, and for only non-members, it is significant only in case of adopting modern contraception after marriage.

5.4.6 Econometric analysis

In Table 5.2 we present the results of multi-level probit models (Equation [5.6]) indicating whether the respondent was motivated by ASHA or some other person. Although inter-class correlation coefficients are low, the Wald χ^2 statistic indicates that multi-level models are more appropriate vis-à-vis probit models.

The influence of ASHA and other health workers is greater on JEEViKA members. In seven out of the 12 practices, the coefficient of JEEViKA is positive and significant. These practices are availing of the recommended four ANC check-ups, ensuring protection against Tetanus, taking IFA tablets or syrup, delivering in an institution, availing of assisted delivery, giving polio vaccine at birth to child, and complementary feeding of children aged between 7 and 35 months.

The influence of ASHAs declines among older respondents, but the coefficient is significantly negative only for institutional delivery, and complementary feeding after six months. More educated respondents, particularly those with at least 7–11 years of education, are less likely to be motivated by health workers. The influence of ASHAs is also less among respondents from affluent households (i.e. with higher asset scores). The coefficient for the asset is significant and negative for the adoption of contraception, availing ANC check-up in the first trimester, exclusive breastfeeding in the first six months, and complementary feeding thereafter till three years. Respondents who are engaged in income-earning activities are also less likely to be motivated by ASHAs; the coefficient is significantly different from zero for availing ANC check-up in the first trimester, taking 100 IFA tablets or syrup, and complementary feeding. If the husband is a migrant then respondents are less likely to be motivated by health workers; in case of ensuring protection against tetanus and taking IFA tablets, respondents with migrant workers are more likely to be motivated by ASHAs.

The influence of ASHAs vis-à-vis others is negligible across religion and caste groups. Larger households are less likely to be motivated by ASHAs. Respondents with more children are influenced by ASHAs in availing first ANC check-up in the first trimester, availing four ANC check-ups, seeking protection from Tetanus, taking IFA tablets, and obtaining post-partum contraception advice.

5.4.7 Endogenous peer effects

Our analysis reveals the presence of a common environmental factor underlying the improvement in MCH outcomes. The presence of an exogenous peer effect, however, does not rule out the presence of an endogenous peer effect – both may operate simultaneously. As a final step of our analysis, we have estimated (equation [5.7]). It enables us to test whether an endogenous peer effect exists, even after controlling for the common environmental factor, viz.

Table 5.2 Determinants of main motivator: Results of probit model

Variables	Use of contraception	ANC in trimester	Four ANC check-ups	Tetanus injection
Are you JEEViKA member				
Non-member	-0.06	-0.13	-0.30 **	-0.42***
Years of education				
1–5 years of education	0.01	-0.17	-0.36 *	-0.10
6–10 years of education	-0.20	-0.18	-0.33	-0.33**
11–17 years of education	-0.54 **	-0.45***	-0.63***	-0.50***
SRC				
H-SC & ST	-0.20	-0.69***	-0.41	-0.25
H-OBC	0.10	-0.11	-0.07	0.07
Muslim	0.19	-0.35*	-0.37	-0.16
Are you engaged in any work that brings income				
Yes	0.35	-0.24*	-0.06	-0.13
Age	-0.01	-0.02	-0.01	-0.01
Household size	-0.05*	-0.03*	-0.05**	-0.04**
Asset	-0.34 ***	-0.13**	-0.01	-0.03
If your partner is a migrant				
Non-migrant	0.33 **	0.02	0.03	-0.31 ***
Total no of living children	0.02	0.15***	0.15 **	0.22 ***
Constant	1.59 **	1.99***	2.20***	2.20***
District	0.02	0.28	0.17	0.40
Block	0.00	0.00	0.03	0.02
Village	0.07	0.07	0.12	0.12
N	446	1451	981	2037
χ^2	1.62 (0.44)	97.42***	31.76***	171.63***
Wald χ^2	33.85***	65.11***	30.16***	60.78***

	IFA tablet/syrup	Institutional delivery	Assisted delivery	Post-partum check-up
Intra class coefficient				
District	0.02	0.21	0.13	0.26
Block | District	0.02	0.21	0.15	0.30
Village | Block | District	0.09	0.26	0.24	0.35
Are you JEEViKA member				
Non-member	-0.27**	-0.16*	-0.30***	-0.21
Years of education				
1–5 years of education	-0.01	-0.06	-0.11	-0.49**
6–10 years of education	-0.40***	-0.25**	-0.38***	-0.39**
11–17 years of education	-0.40**	-0.41***	-0.50***	-0.36
Src				
H-SC & ST	-0.01	-0.19	0.09	-0.07
H-OBC	0.13	-0.11	-0.01	-0.12
Muslim	-0.15	-0.37**	-0.20	0.18
Are you engaged in any work that brings income				
Yes	-0.26*	-0.08	0.01	0.16
Age	-0.01	0.02*	0.01	0.01
Household size	-0.05 ***	-0.02	-0.04***	-0.03
Asset	0.00	-0.05	-0.04	-0.13
If your partner is a migrant				
Non-migrant	-0.21**	0.01	0.05	0.10
Total no of living children	0.10*	0.01	-0.02	-0.11 *
Constant	2.47***	1.17***	1.94***	2.45***
District	0.18	0.27	0.17	0.17
Block	0.00	0.09	0.09	0.03
Village	0.04	0.02	0.07	0.03

(Continued)

Table 5.2 (Continued)

Variables	Use of contraception	ANC in trimester	Four ANC check-ups	Tetanus injection
N	1706	1807	1959	1389
χ²	48.02***	116.49***	101.28***	37.17***
Wald χ²	33.45***	31.94 ***	33.39***	22.72**
Intra class coefficient				
District	0.15	0.20	0.13	0.14
Block | District	0.15	0.26	0.19	0.17
Village | Block | District	0.18	0.27	0.24	0.19

	Post-partum contraception advice	Child given OPVO	Exclusive breast feed	Complementary feeding
Are you JEEViKA member				
Non-member	-0.03	-0.28**	-0.11	-0.21***
Years of education				
1–5 years of education	0.23	-0.15	-0.13	0.08
6–10 years of education	-0.15	-0.48***	-0.35***	-0.10
11–17 years of education	-0.58***	-0.51***	-0.27**	-0.07
SRC				
H-SC & ST	-0.37	-0.20	0.09	-0.23
H-OBC	-0.21	-0.07	0.05	-0.17**
Muslim	0.05	0.14	-0.04	-0.10
Are you engaged in any work that brings income				
Yes	-0.08	-0.17	-0.09	-0.33***
Age	-0.01	0.02	0.00	0.03**
Household size	0.01	-0.02	-0.03**	-0.02*
Asset	-0.11	-0.03	-0.14***	-0.19***

If your partner is a migrant

Non-migrant	-0.06	-0.05	0.01	0.10
Total no of living children	-0.02	0.03	0.05	0.03
Constant	2.11***	1.92***	1.61***	0.72**
District	0.19	0.23	0.30	0.28
Block	0.06	0.01	0.08	0.11
Village	0.12	0.00	0.02	0.00
N	1288	1984	1976	1737
χ^2	50.72***	69.04***	214.52***	185.72***
Wald χ^2	31.61***	30.65***	39.75***	59.09***
Intra class coefficient				
District	0.14	0.18	0.22	0.20
Block | District	0.19	0.19	0.28	0.28
Village | Block | District	0.27	0.19	0.30	0.28

Source: Estimated from primary survey.
Note: The outcome variable was health worker (0) versus others (1).

motivating role played by ASHAs. Summary results are reported in Table 5.3. The coefficient of the village mean continues to be statistically significant in all cases. Results imply, therefore, that endogenous peer effects may exist.

The marginal effects of the peer effect (estimated at the mean value) for both equations [5.5] and [5.7] are reported in Figure 5.3. There is no difference between the two marginal effects, confirming H3, viz. presence of a positive peer effect for all the MCH practices analysed in this chapter.

5.5 Discussion and conclusion

To sum up, our analysis indicates the presence of positive peer effects. Although we found an exogenous peer effect in our study, with behaviour of actors influencing each other, there is also evidence of information diffusion from the grass-roots health workers, particularly the ASHAs, to women of reproductive age. ASHAs have played a major role in motivating women and their families to adopt MCH practices considered by policymakers to be desirable. They are observed to be especially active among less affluent and socially marginalised households and have created networks for information dissemination within the community. The features of such networks, and how such characteristics shape information flows are examined in the next chapter.

The findings of this chapter are, therefore, consistent with that of existing studies reporting peer effects on health care behaviour (Fowler & Christakis, 2008; Webel et al., 2010; Godlonton & Thornton, 2012; Lewycka et al., 2013; Bouckaert, 2014; Houle et al., 2017; Chatterjee et al., 2018; Hoffmann, 2019; Pruckner et al., 2020). This has important implications for policymaking. The existence of endogenous peer effects indicates the operation of a "social multiplier" for interventions (Fletcher, 2014) – if the health of one individual is increased, the effect of the intervention may be multiplied through peers and lead to sustained improvements in health outcomes (Chatterjee et al., 2018). The presence of endogenous peer effects in rural Bihar implies that the potential benefits of intervention will increase without a corresponding increase in the costs. The multiplicative impact of peer effects indicates the comparative efficacy of targeted (e.g., based on influential individuals within networks) over broad-based policy intervention strategies. Two important issues that emerge in this context are (1) identification of the catalytic agent or institution to effect behavioural change, and (2) whom to target during the behavioural change and awareness-generating campaigns.

The findings of this chapter validate findings from literature about the potentially game-changing role that may be played by grass-roots health workers, particularly in resource-poor settings (Thomas et al., 2021). Their ability to deliver MCH services by promoting healthcare seeking behaviour minimises delays in seeking health acre and improves MCH outcomes (Panday et al., 2017). Despite contextual variations in the technical quality of their knowledge (Okuga et al., 2015; Burnett-Zieman et al., 2021), such health

Table 5.3 Endogenous peer effects: Summary results from regression models

MCH practices	β	T	Prob.	R^2
Modern contraception methods after marriage	2.86	27.15	0.00	0.19
First ANC visit was in the first trimester	3.81	23.51	0.00	0.12
At least four ANC check-ups	2.65	37.23	0.00	0.19
Given tetanus toxoid injection	5.44	9.83	0.00	0.16
Given IFA tablets/syrup for anaemia	3.43	22.34	0.00	0.17
Institutional delivery	3.52	22.28	0.00	0.27
Delivery assisted by skilled person	4.31	17.04	0.00	0.21
Post-partum check-up within 48 hours	2.74	36.31	0.00	0.13
Post-partum contraception advice	2.90	37.69	0.00	0.15
Whether child was given OPV0	4.41	16.39	0.00	0.25
Exclusive breast feeding up to six months of birth	4.91	16.99	0.00	0.16
Complementary feeding after six months	3.35	23.23	0.00	0.08

Source: Estimated from primary survey.

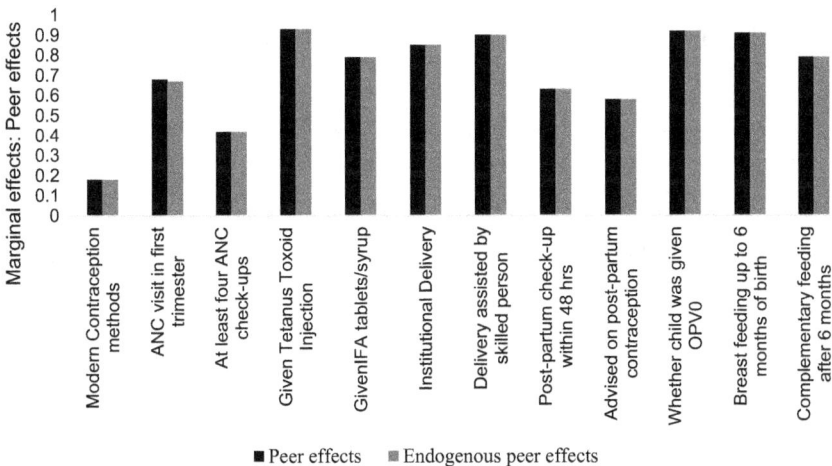

Figure 5.3 Predicted peer effects: Variations across best practices.

Source: Estimated from primary survey.

workers have notable advantages that make their outreach activities highly effective in transforming health outcomes in rural areas. For instance, they have been reported to have better contact with residents in their service area (Okuga et al., 2015; Bonifácio et al., 2019), are more proficient in identifying pregnant women through local networks (Okuga et al., 2015), and offer advice in culturally consistent terms enhancing likelihood of accomplishing behavioural change (Andrews et al., 2004).

Our findings are also consistent with the Indian experience regarding ASHAs. Some studies reported inadequate training and knowledge (Godhi et al., 2021) leading to poor delivery of services, particularly in the initial stages of the National Health Mission (Shrivastava & Shrivastava, 2012; Chaurasiya et al., 2020). However, most studies have reported improved MCH outcomes due to the activity of the ASHAs. Specifically, the probability of ANC utilization was higher, breast feeding was initiated earlier, and one-year mortality was lower among women who received ANC from an ASHA (Nadella et al., 2021). ASHAs have also been reported to have played a role in promoting demand for family planning and increasing institutional delivery and full immunisation coverage (Wagner et al., 2018b). However, ASHAs have not increased the likelihood of completing all ANC services along the continuum (Agarwal et al., 2019). Thus, ASHAs provide a highly cost-effective intervention strategy to increase health awareness and promote behavioural change (Nadella et al., 2021).

In contrast, JEEViKA's Health and Nutrition Strategy does not seem to have been so effective as a catalytic agent in enhancing awareness and inducing behavioural change. This is also consistent with a recent study that argues that the low participation of target women in SHG activities has constrained the effectiveness of SHGs in improving MCH outcomes among members (Husain & Dutta, 2022). It is a concerning feature, reflecting the focus of policymakers on visible targets like membership, rather than emphasising less intangible but more important activities like attendance in meetings and active participation.

Given that ASHAs have been identified to be more critical in encouraging rural women to adopt best MCH practices the associated question is whom should the ASHAs target. While the obvious answer seems to be a direct targeting of women in the reproductive age, we will see in the next chapter the actual dissipation process of information from the ASHAs to the target population is somewhat different.

Note

1 Exogenous peer effects refers to "the spillover effects of some exogenous policy intervention on subjects who are not originally targeted by the intervention but are connected to the original target population of the intervention" An, 515).

References

Agarwal, S., & Curtis, S. et al. (2019). Are community health workers effective in retaining women in the maternity care continuum? Evidence from India. *BMJ Global Health*, 4(4), e001557. http://doi.org/10.1136/bmjgh-2019-001557

Agarwal, S., Curtis, S. L. et al. (2019). The impact of India's accredited social health activist (ASHA) program on the utilization of maternity services: A nationally representative longitudinal modelling study. *Human Resources for Health*, *17*(1), 68. http://doi.org/10.1186/s12960-019-0402-4

An, W. (Edward) (2011). Models and methods to identify peer effects. In J. Scott & P. J. Carrington (Eds.), *The SAGE handbook of social network analysis2* (pp. 514–532). Sage Publications Inc.

Andrews, J. O. et al. (2004). Use of community health workers in research with ethnic minority women. *Journal of Nursing Scholarship*, *36*(4), 358–365. http://doi.org /10.1111/j.1547-5069.2004.04064.x

Bajpai, N., Sachs, J. D., & Dholakia, R. H. (2010). *Improving access and efficiency in public health services: Mid-term evaluation of India's national rural health mission*. Sage.

Bearman, P. S., Moody, J., & Stovel, K. (2004). Chains of affection: The structure of adolescent romantic and sexual networks. *American Journal of Sociology*, *110*(1), 44–91. http://doi.org/10.1086/386272

Blunch, N.-H. (2008). *Human capital, religion and Contraceptive use in Ghana*. http://www.csae.ox.ac.uk/conferences/2008-EdiA/papers/184-Blunch.pdf

Bonifácio, L. P., Marques, J. M. A., & Vieira, E. M. (2019). Assessment of the knowledge of Brazilian community health workers regarding prenatal care. *Primary Health Care Research & Development*, *20*, e21. http://doi.org/10.1017 /S1463423618000725

Bouckaert, N. (2014). Neighborhood peer effects in the use of preventive health care. *SSRN Electronic Journal* [Preprint]. http://doi.org/10.2139/ssrn.2381880

Bramoullé, Y., Djebbari, H., & Fortin, B. (2009). Identification of peer effects through social networks. *Journal of Econometrics*, *150*(1), 41–55. http://doi.org/10.1016 /j.jeconom.2008.12.021

Bramoullé, Y., Djebbari, H., & Fortin, B. (2020). Peer effects in networks: A survey. *Annual Review of Economics*, *12*(1), 603–629. http://doi.org/10.1146/annurev -economics-020320-033926

Brock, W. A., & Durlauf, S. N. (2001a). Discrete choice with social interactions. *The Review of Economic Studies*, *68*(2), 235–260. http://doi.org/10.1111/1467-937X .00168

Brock, W. A., & Durlauf, S. N. (2001b). Interactions-based models. In J. J. Heckman & E. Leamer (Eds.), *Handbook of econometrics volume V* (pp. 3299–3371). Elsevier Science.

Brooks, S. K. et al. (2020). The psychological impact of quarantine and how to reduce it: Rapid review of the evidence. *The Lancet*, *395*(10227), 912–920. http://doi.org /10.1016/S0140-6736(20)30460-8

Van den Bulte, C., & Lilien, G. L. (2001). Medical innovation revisited: Social contagion versus marketing effort. *American Journal of Sociology*, *106*(5), 1409– 1435. http://doi.org/10.1086/320819

Burnett-Zieman, B. et al. (2021). Community-based postnatal care services for women and newborns in Kenya: An opportunity to improve quality and access? *Journal of Global Health*, *11*, 07006. http://doi.org/10.7189/jogh.11.07006

Calvó-Armengol, A., & Jackson, M. O. (2004). The effects of social networks on employment and inequality. *American Economic Review*, *94*(3), 426–454. http:// doi.org/10.1257/0002828041464542

Calvó-Armengol, A., & Jackson, M. O. (2007). Networks in labor markets: Wage and employment dynamics and inequality. *Journal of Economic Theory, 132*(1), 27–46. http://doi.org/10.1016/j.jet.2005.07.007

Carrell, S. E., Hoekstra, M., & West, J. E. (2011). Is poor fitness contagious? *Journal of Public Economics, 95*(7–8), 657–663. http://doi.org/10.1016/j.jpubeco.2010.12.005

Chatterjee, C. et al. (2018). Government health insurance and spatial peer effects: New evidence from India. *Social Science & Medicine, 196*, 131–141. http://doi.org/10.1016/j.socscimed.2017.11.021

Chaurasiya, S. et al. (2020). Assessment of the services of ASHA workers on antenatal and postnatal care in a district of western Uttar Pradesh, India. *Journal of Family Medicine and Primary Care, 9*(7), 3502. http://doi.org/10.4103/jfmpc.jfmpc_381_20

Christakis, N. A., & Fowler, J. H. (2007). The spread of obesity in a large social network over 32 years. *New England Journal of Medicine, 357*(4), 370–379. http://doi.org/10.1056/NEJMsa066082

Christakis, N. A., & Fowler, J. H. (2008). The collective dynamics of smoking in a large social network. *New England Journal of Medicine, 358*(21), 2249–2258. http://doi.org/10.1056/NEJMsa0706154

Diani, M., & McAdam, D. (Eds.). (2003). *Social movements and networks: Relational approaches to collective action.* Oxford University Press.

Ennett, S. T., & Bauman, K. E. (1993). Peer group structure and adolescent cigarette smoking: A social network analysis. *Journal of Health and Social Behavior, 34*(3), 226. http://doi.org/10.2307/2137204

Finneran, L., & Kelly, M. (2003). Social networks and inequality. *Journal of Urban Economics, 53*(2), 282–299. http://doi.org/10.1016/S0094-1190(02)00513-2

Fletcher, J. M. (2014). Peer effects in health behaviors. In A. J. Culyer (Ed.), *Encyclopedia of health economics* (1st ed., pp. 467–472). Elsevier. http://doi.org/10.1016/B978-0-12-375678-7.00311-4

Fowler, J. H., & Christakis, N. A. (2008). Estimating peer effects on health in social networks: A response to Cohen-Cole and Fletcher; and Trogdon, Nonnemaker, and Pais. *Journal of Health Economics, 27*(5), 1400–1405. http://doi.org/10.1016/j.jhealeco.2008.07.001

Godhi, B. S., Kaul, S., & Shanbhog, R. (2021). Knowledge, attitude, and practices of grassroot health workers about early childhood caries, *Public Health Nursing, 38*(5), 913–919. http://doi.org/10.1111/phn.12913

Godlonton, S., & Thornton, R. (2012). Peer effects in learning HIV results, *Journal of Development Economics, 97*(1), 118–129. http://doi.org/10.1016/j.jdeveco.2010.12.003

Graham, B. S., & Hahn, J. (2009). Identification and estimation of the linear-in-means model of social interactions. *Economics Letters, 88*(1), 1–6.

Halliday, T., & Kwak, S. (2009). Weight gain in adolescents and their peers. *Economics & Human Biology, 7*(2), 181–190. doi: 10.1016/j.ehb.2009.05.002.

Hoffmann, R. (2019). Evaluating an MFI community health worker program: How microfinance group networks influence intervention outreach and impact. *Journal of Global Health, 9*(1). http://doi.org/10.7189/jogh.09.010435

Houle, J. et al. (2017). Peer positive social control and men's health-promoting behaviors. *American Journal of Men's Health*, *11*(5), 1569–1579. http://doi.org /10.1177/1557988317711605

Husain, Z., & Dutta, M. (2022). Impact of Self Help Group membership on the adoption of child nutritional practices: Evidence from JEEViKA's health and nutrition strategy programme in Bihar, India. *Journal of International Development* [Preprint]. http://doi.org/10.1002/jid.3703

Kaggwa, E. B., Diop, N., & Storey, J. D. (2008). The role of individual and community normative factors: A multilevel analysis of contraceptive use among women in union in Mali. *International family planning perspectives*, *34*(2), 79–88. http://doi .org/10.1363/ifpp.34.079.08

Katz, E., & Lazarsfeld, P. F. (2005). *Personal influence the part played by people in the flow of mass communications*. Transaction.

Kohli, C. et al. (2015). Knowledge and practice of Accredited Social Health Activists for maternal healthcare delivery in Delhi. *Journal of Family Medicine and Primary Care*, *4*(3), 359. http://doi.org/10.4103/2249-4863.161317

Krauth, B. V (2006). Simulation-based estimation of peer effects. *Journal of Econometrics*, *133*(1), 243–271. http://doi.org/10.1016/j.jeconom.2005.03.015

Lewycka, S. et al. (2013). Effect of women's groups and volunteer peer counselling on rates of mortality, morbidity, and health behaviours in mothers and children in rural Malawi (MaiMwana): A factorial, cluster-randomised controlled trial. *The Lancet*, *381*(9879), 1721–1735. http://doi.org/10.1016/S0140 -6736(12)61959-X

Lim, C. (2010). Mobilizing on the margin: How does interpersonal recruitment affect citizen participation in politics? *Social Science Research*, *39*(2), 341–355. http:// doi.org/10.1016/j.ssresearch.2009.05.005

Liu, K., King, M., & Bearman, P. S. (2010). Social influence and the autism epidemic. *American Journal of Sociology*, *115*(5), 1387–1434. http://doi.org/10.1086 /651448

Manna, N., & Basu, G. (2011). Contraceptive methods in a rural area of West Bengal, India. *Sudanese Journal of Public Health*, *6*(4), 164–169.

Manski, C. F. (1993). Identification of endogenous social effects: The reflection problem. *The Review of Economic Studies*, *60*(3), 531. http://doi.org/10.2307 /2298123

Maxwell, K. A. (2002). Friends: The role of peer influence across adolescent risk behaviors. *Journal of Youth and Adolescence*, *31*(4), 267–277. http://doi.org/10 .1023/A:1015493316865

Myo-Myo-Mon & Liabsuetrakul, T. (2009). Factors influencing married youths' decisions on contraceptive use in a rural area of Myanmar. *The Southeast Asian journal of tropical medicine and public health*, *40*(5), 1057–1064.

Nadella, P., Subramanian, S. V., & Roman-Urrestarazu, A. (2021). The impact of community health workers on antenatal and infant health in India: A cross-sectional study. *SSM - Population Health*, *15*, 100872. http://doi.org/10.1016/j .ssmph.2021.100872

Okuga, M. et al. (2015). Engaging community health workers in maternal and newborn care in eastern Uganda. *Global Health Action*, *8*(1), 23968. http://doi .org/10.3402/gha.v8.23968

Panda, P. et al. (2013). Role of ASHA in improvement of maternal health status in northern India: An urban rural comparison. *Indian Journal of Community Health*, 25, 465–471.

Panday, S. et al. (2017). The contribution of female community health volunteers (FCHVs) to maternity care in Nepal: A qualitative study. *BMC Health Services Research*, 17(1), 623. http://doi.org/10.1186/s12913-017-2567-7

Paul, P. L., & Pandey, S. (2020). Factors influencing institutional delivery and the role of accredited social health activist (ASHA): A secondary analysis of India human development survey 2012. *BMC Pregnancy and Childbirth*, 20(1), 445. http://doi .org/10.1186/s12884-020-03127-z

Pruckner, G. J., Schober, T., & Zocher, K. (2020). The company you keep: Health behavior among work peers. *The European Journal of Health Economics*, 21(2), 251–259. http://doi.org/10.1007/s10198-019-01124-4

Reichenbach, L. (Ed.). (2007). *Exploring the gender dimensions of the global health workforce*. Global Equity Initiative Harvard University.

Ryan, C. (2017). Measurement of peer effects. *Australian Economic Review*, 50(1), 121–129. http://doi.org/10.1111/1467-8462.12213

Sacerdote, B. (2001). Peer effects with random assignment: results for Dartmouth roommates. *The Quarterly Journal of Economics*, 116(2), 681–704. http://doi.org /10.1162/00335530151144131

Samandari, G., Speizer, I. S., & OConnell, K. (2010). The role of social support and parity in contraceptive use in Cambodia. *International perspectives on sexual and reproductive health*, 36(3), 122–131. http://doi.org/10.1363/ipsrh.36.122.10

Sharma, R. K., & Rani, M. (2009). contraceptive use among tribal women of Central India: Experiencesamong DLHS-RCH –II survey. *Research and Practice in Social Sciences*, 5(1), 44–66.

Shrivastava, S. R., & Shrivastava, P. S. (2012). Evaluation of trained Accredited Social Health Activist (ASHA) workers regarding their knowledge, attitude and practices about child health. *Rural and remote health*, 12(4), 2099. http://www .ncbi.nlm.nih.gov/pubmed/23198703

Sorensen, A. T. (2006). Social learning and health plan choice. *The RAND Journal of Economics*, 37(4), 929–945. http://doi.org/10.1111/j.1756-2171.2006.tb00064.x

Thomas, L. S., Buch, E., & Pillay, Y. (2021). An analysis of the services provided by community health workers within an urban district in South Africa: A key contribution towards universal access to care. *Human Resources for Health*, 19(1), 22. http://doi.org/10.1186/s12960-021-00565-4

Trogdon, J. G., Nonnemaker, J., & Pais, J. (2008). Peer effects in adolescent overweight. *Journal of Health Economics*, 27(5), 1388–1399. http://doi.org/10 .1016/j.jhealeco.2008.05.003

Wagner, A. L. et al. (2018a). Have community health workers increased the delivery of maternal and child healthcare in India? *Journal of Public Health*, 40(2), e164– e170. http://doi.org/10.1093/pubmed/fdx087

Wagner, A. L. et al. (2018b). Have community health workers increased the delivery of maternal and child healthcare in India? *Journal of Public Health*, 40(2), e164– e170. http://doi.org/10.1093/pubmed/fdx087

Webel, A. R. et al. (2010). A systematic review of the effectiveness of peer-based interventions on health-related behaviors in adults. *American Journal of Public Health*, 100(2), 247–253. http://doi.org/10.2105/AJPH.2008.149419

Appendix

Table A5.1 Motivators of MCH practices

Informant	Modern contraception methods after marriage	Whether the first ANC visit was in the first trimester	At least four ANC check-ups	Whether given a tetanus toxoid injection
Health worker	87.67	90.42	94.60	57.26
JEEViKA post-holder	4.71	4.96	4.49	2.66
JEEViKA member	15.47	12.20	10.19	7.91
Friend/neighbour	13.68	8.55	8.15	4.91
Media	1.57	0.69	1.02	0.29
Family	40.13	44.25	42.92	19.18
Husband	37.67	21.50	17.43	7.80
NA	0.00	0.00	0.00	0.00
DK	0.00	0.00	0.00	0.00
Responses	**896**	**2649**	**1754**	**3425**

Informant	IFA tablets/syrup for anaemia	Institutional delivery	Delivery assisted by skilled person	Availed post-partum check-up within 48hrs
Health worker	58.41	49.28	64.67	64.90
JEEViKA post-holder	3.33	2.45	2.57	2.33
JEEViKA member	7.81	7.74	4.46	5.10
Friend/neighbour	4.94	5.29	3.53	2.81
Media	0.35	0.40	0.27	0.29
Family	18.64	23.16	18.13	18.90
Husband	6.52	11.68	6.37	5.67
NA	0.00	0.00	0.00	0.00
DK	0.00	0.00	0.00	0.00
Responses	**2854**	**3476**	**2918**	**2100**

(Continued)

Table A5.1 (Continued)

Informant	Whether given advice on post-partum contraception	Whether child was given OPVO	Breastfeeding up to six months of birth	Complementary feeding after six months
Health worker	55.79	69.57	48.52	44.90
JEEViKA post-holder	3.22	2.55	4.87	4.68
JEEViKA member	8.18	4.18	8.42	9.54
Friend/neighbour	4.96	2.87	5.41	6.41
Media	0.67	0.35	0.83	0.80
Family	17.61	15.73	23.12	23.44
Husband	9.57	4.75	8.84	10.23
NA	0.00	0.00	0.00	0.00
DK	0.00	0.00	0.00	0.00
Responses	**2237**	**2823**	**3755**	**3481**

Source: Estimated from primary survey.

Table A5.2 Variations in the identification of motivators across the education level of respondents

Modern contraception methods	Years of education				Total	Chi²
	No schooling	1–5 years	6–10 years	11–17 years		
Health worker	42.06	48.31	45.20	37.07	43.64	4.92 (1.00)
JEEViKA post-holder	1.56	1.69	2.14	6.03	2.34	9.47 (0.20)
JEEViKA member	9.97	8.43	4.98	6.90	7.70	7.94 (0.33)
Friend/neighbour	9.03	5.62	5.69	5.17	6.81	6.14 (0.74)
Media	0.31	0.00	0.71	3.45	0.78	14.26 (0.02)
Family	18.69	18.54	21.00	23.28	19.98	3.34 (1.00)
Husband	18.38	17.42	20.28	18.10	18.75	1.32 (1.00)
NA	0.00	0.00	0.00	0.00	0.00	-
DK	0.00	0.00	0.00	0.00	0.00	-
Total	100.00	100.00	100.00	100.00	100.00	
N					446.00	
Pearson's Chi2	124.76 (0.09)					

First ANC visit in the first trimester	Years of education				Total	**Chi2**
	No schooling	1–5 years	6–10 years	11–17 years		
Health worker	52.61	49.15	50.05	42.62	49.53	21.21 (0.00)
JEEViKA post-holder	1.70	3.18	2.98	3.63	2.72	6.15 (0.73)
JEEViKA member	7.29	7.20	5.74	7.02	6.68	2.51 (1.00)
Friend/neighbour	5.95	4.87	4.04	3.39	4.68	4.66 (1.00)
Media	0.00	0.21	0.21	1.69	0.38	25.54 (0.00)
Family	23.09	22.25	24.97	27.12	24.24	10.26 (0.12)
Husband	9.36	13.14	12.01	14.53	11.78	12.83 (0.04)
NA	0.00	0.00	0.00	0.00	0.00	-

(Continued)

Table A5.2 (Continued)

First ANC visit in the first trimester	Years of education					
	No schooling	1–5 years	6–10 years	11–17 years	Total	Chi2
Total	100.00	100.00	100.00	100.00	100.00	
N	1451.00					
Pearson's Chi2	192.96 (0.01)					

Availed four ANC check-ups	Years of education					
	No schooling	1–5 years	6–10 years	11–17 years	Total	Chi²
Health worker	53.13	56.22	54.23	47.30	52.91	16.08 (0.01)
JEEViKA post-holder	2.43	2.41	1.47	4.76	2.51	11.92 (0.05)
JEEViKA member	6.08	3.61	5.54	6.98	5.70	5.70 (0.89)
Friend/neighbour	6.94	3.61	3.58	2.86	4.56	13.70 (0.02)
Media	0.00	0.00	0.49	2.22	0.57	22.38 (0.00)
Family	24.48	19.28	25.24	24.44	24.00	10.62 (0.10)
Husband	6.94	14.86	9.45	11.43	9.75	12.17 (0.05)
NA	0.00	0.00	0.00	0.00	0.00	-
DK	0.00	0.00	0.00	0.00	0.00	-
Total	100.00	100.00	100.00	100.00	100.00	
N	981.00					

Pearson Chi2   186.99 (0.00)

Tetanus toxoid injection	Years of education					
	No schooling	1–5 years	6–10 years	11–17 years	Total	Chi²
Health worker	58.35	59.27	57.40	51.11	57.26	6.39 (0.66)
JEEViKA post-holder	2.20	2.88	2.41	4.22	2.66	8.02 (0.32)
JEEViKA member	7.99	8.31	7.31	8.67	7.91	2.52 (1.00)

	No schooling	1–5 years	6–10 years	11–17 years	Total	Chi²
Friend/neighbour	6.36	4.95	4.19	2.67	4.91	10.46 (0.11)
Media	0.08	0.16	0.27	1.11	0.29	14.72 (0.01)
Family	18.34	15.65	21.03	21.78	19.18	19.57 (0.00)
Husband	6.68	8.79	7.04	10.44	7.80	11.81 (0.06)
NA	0.00	0.00	0.00	0.00	0.00	–
DK	0.00	0.00	0.00	0.00	0.00	–
Total	100.00	100.00	100.00	100.00	100.00	
N	2037.00					
Pearson's Chi2	222.66 (0.00)					

IF IFA tab/syrup taken for anaemia

	Years of education					
	No schooling	1–5 years	6–10 years	11–17 years	Total	Chi²
Health worker	57.63	61.21	59.27	54.64	58.41	4.68 (1.00)
JEEViKA post-holder	2.61	3.70	3.23	5.04	3.33	6.37 (0.66)
JEEViKA member	8.11	8.58	6.79	8.49	7.81	3.28 (1.00)
Friend/neighbour	6.08	4.87	4.31	3.45	4.94	6.03 (0.77)
Media	0.10	0.00	0.11	2.12	0.35	42.58 (0.00)
Family	19.11	14.81	20.15	18.83	18.64	9.98 (0.13)
Husband	6.37	6.82	6.14	7.43	6.52	1.68 (1.00)
NA	0.00	0.00	0.00	0.00	0.00	–
DK	0.00	0.00	0.00	0.00	0.00	–
Total	100.00	100.00	100.00	100.00	100.00	
N	1706.00					
Pearson's Chi2	199.10 (0.00)					

If respondent delivered in an institution

	Years of education					
	No schooling	1–5 years	6–10 years	11–17 years	Total	Chi²
Health worker	50.77	52.20	49.42	42.45	49.28	7.79 (0.35)
JEEViKA post-holder	1.79	2.29	2.31	4.40	2.45	15.63 (0.01)

(Continued)

Table A5.2 (Continued)

If respondent delivered in an institution	Years of education					
	No schooling	1–5 years	6–10 years	11–17 years	Total	Chi²
Friend/neighbour	6.29	5.29	4.55	4.78	5.29	3.90 (1.00)
Media	0.09	0.00	0.17	2.10	0.40	52.78 (0.00)
Family	22.62	20.63	24.30	24.47	23.16	17.16 (0.01)
Husband	10.54	11.64	11.74	14.15	11.68	12.48 (0.04)
NA	0.00	0.00	0.00	0.00	0.00	-
DK	0.00	0.00	0.00	0.00	0.00	-
Total	100.00	100.00	100.00	100.00	100.00	
N	1807.00					
Pearson's Chi2	258.26 (0.00)					

If delivery is assisted by skilled person	Years of education					
	No schooling	1–5 years	6–10 years	11–17 years	Total	Chi²
Health worker	64.80	68.31	65.50	57.99	64.47	2.16 (1.00)
JEEViKA post-holder	1.80	2.26	2.57	4.91	2.57	15.19 (0.01)
JEEViKA member	4.17	4.12	4.43	5.65	4.46	3.52 (1.00)
Friend/neighbour	4.65	2.88	2.78	3.19	3.53	7.05 (0.49)
Media	0.00	0.00	0.00	1.97	0.27	55.94 (0.00)
Family	18.41	15.84	18.74	18.67	18.13	6.03 (0.77)
Husband	6.17	6.58	5.98	7.62	6.37	3.28 (1.00)
NA	0.00	0.00	0.00	0.00	0.00	-
DK	0.00	0.00	0.00	0.00	0.00	-
Total	100.00	100.00	100.00	100.00	100.00	
N	1959.00					
Pearson's Chi2	180.51 (0.01)					

Post-partum check-up with 48 hours of delivery

	Years of education					
	No schooling	1–5 years	6–10 years	11–17 years	Total	Chi²
Health worker	64.48	71.15	66.07	57.32	64.90	17.18 (0.01)
JEEViKA post-holder	2.14	1.64	1.79	4.67	2.33	13.45 (0.03)
JEEViKA member	5.23	4.92	4.40	6.54	5.10	4.65 (1.00)
Friend/neighbour	3.49	1.64	2.34	3.43	2.81	5.77 (0.87)
Media	0.13	0.00	0.00	1.56	0.29	25.54 (0.00)
Family	18.77	15.74	19.92	19.94	18.90	9.78 (0.14)
Husband	5.76	4.92	5.49	6.54	5.67	3.01 (1.00)
NA	0.00	0.00	0.00	0.00	0.00	-
DK	0.00	0.00	0.00	0.00	0.00	-
Total	100.00	100.00	100.00	100.00	100.00	
N					1389.00	
Pearson's Chi2	169.69 (0.00)					

Advice on post-partum contraception method

	Years of education					
	No schooling	1–5 years	6–10 years	11–17 years	Total	Chi²
Health worker	57.87	58.02	57.28	45.53	55.79	3.46 (1.00)
JEEViKA post-holder	3.17	3.21	2.75	4.32	3.22	4.41 (1.00)
JEEViKA member	9.52	7.75	7.28	7.49	8.18	2.87 (1.00)
Friend/neighbour	5.20	5.08	4.40	5.48	4.96	2.33 (1.00)
Media	0.13	0.00	0.55	2.88	0.67	40.28 (0.00)
Family	16.24	15.24	18.96	20.46	17.61	16.89 (0.01)
Husband	7.87	10.70	8.79	13.83	9.57	22.84 (0.00)
NA	0.00	0.00	0.00	0.00	0.00	-
DK	0.00	0.00	0.00	0.00	0.00	-
Total	100.00	100.00	100.00	100.00	100.00	
N					1288.00	
Pearson Chi2	231.32 (0.00)					

(Continued)

Table A5.2 (Continued)

If child was given OPV0

	Years of education					
	No schooling	1–5 years	6–10 years	11–17 years	Total	Chi²
Health worker	70.19	72.60	69.14	65.07	69.57	4.88 (1.00)
JEEViKA post-holder	1.89	1.84	2.82	4.53	2.55	10.83 (0.1)
JEEViKA member	3.59	4.29	4.60	4.53	4.18	1.76 (1.00)
Friend/neighbour	3.19	2.66	2.72	2.67	2.87	0.60 (1.00)
Media	0.00	0.00	0.31	1.87	0.35	32.18 (0.00)
Family	16.45	12.68	16.63	15.47	15.73	6.32 (0.68)
Husband	4.69	5.93	3.77	5.87	4.75	4.98 (1.00)
NA	0.00	0.00	0.00	0.00	0.00	-
DK	0.00	0.00	0.00	0.00	0.00	-
Total	100.00	100.00	100.00	100.00	100.00	
N	1984.00					
Pearson's Chi2	150.02 (0.00)					

Breastfeeding up to six months

	Years of education					
	No schooling	1–5 years	6–10 years	11–17 years	Total	Chi²
Health worker	52.35	48.45	46.36	43.72	48.52	8.26 (0.29)
JEEViKA post-holder	4.02	5.79	5.12	5.23	4.87	6.13 (0.74)
JEEViKA member	8.19	10.45	7.83	7.53	8.42	4.94 (1.00)
Friend/neighbour	5.99	4.80	5.28	5.02	5.41	0.87 (1.00)
Media	0.15	0.56	0.64	3.56	0.83	61.61 (0.00)
Family	22.38	21.47	24.62	23.64	23.12	13.89 (0.02)
Husband	6.90	8.47	10.15	11.30	8.84	22.84 (0.00)
NA	0.00	0.00	0.00	0.00	0.00	-

DK	0.00	0.00	0.00	0.00	-
Total	100.00	100.00	100.00	100.00	100.00
N	1976.00				
Pearson's Chi2	264.46 (0.00)				

Complementary feeding after six months

	Years of education					
	No schooling	1–5 years	6–10 years	11–17 years	Total	Chi^2
Health worker	47.14	46.12	43.23	41.05	44.90	1.47 (1.00)
JEEViKA post-holder	3.48	7.15	4.66	4.37	4.68	13.07 (0.03)
JEEViKA member	9.53	10.05	8.80	10.70	9.54	3.38 (1.00)
Friend/neighbour	7.13	6.24	6.56	4.37	6.41	2.74 (1.00)
Media	0.33	0.15	0.78	3.06	0.80	42.11 (0.00)
Family	22.78	20.55	25.02	25.33	23.44	21.27 (0.00)
Husband	9.61	9.44	10.96	11.14	10.23	6.25 (0.70)
NA	0.00	0.00	0.00	0.00	0.00	-
DK	0.00	0.00	0.00	0.00	0.00	-
Total	100.00	100.00	100.00	100.00	100.00	
N	1737.00					
Pearson's Chi2	241.55 (0.01)					

Source: Estimated from primary survey.

Table A5.3 Variations in the identification of motivators across asset scores

Modern contraception methods	Standard of living index				
	Low	Medium	High	Total	Chi²
Health worker	46.06	48.29	38.79	43.64	20.13 (0.00)
JEEViKA post-holder	1.18	3.42	2.37	2.34	2.77 (1.00)
JEEViKA member	7.87	7.60	7.65	7.70	0.04 (1.00)
Friend/neighbour	6.69	6.46	7.12	6.81	0.25 (1.00)
Media	0.39	0.38	1.32	0.78	2.63 (1.00)
Family	16.93	20.15	21.90	19.98	3.82 (1.00)
Husband	20.87	13.69	20.84	18.75	9.55 (0.06)
NA	0.00	0.00	0.00	0.00	-
DK	0.00	0.00	0.00	0.00	-
Total	100.00	100.00	100.00	100.00	
N	446				
Pearson's Chi2	92.35 (0.04)				

First ANC visit in first trimester	Standard of living index				
	Low	Medium	Low	Total	Low
Health worker	54.17	49.44	46.29	49.53	14.40 (0.01)
JEEViKA post-holder	1.64	3.58	2.73	2.72	7.39 (0.17)
JEEViKA member	5.47	7.83	6.54	6.68	6.05 (0.34)
Friend/neighbour	5.47	3.80	4.88	4.68	1.80 (1.00)
Media	0.27	0.45	0.39	0.38	0.48 (1.00)
Family	22.44	25.17	24.71	24.24	8.75 (0.09)
Husband	10.53	9.73	14.45	11.78	16.06 (0.00)
NA	0.00	0.00	0.00	0.00	-
DK	0.00	0.00	0.00	0.00	-
Total	100.00	100.00	100.00	100.00	
N	1451				
Pearson's Chi2	133.09 (0.01)				

Availed four ANC check-ups	Standard of living index				
	Low	Medium	High	Total	Chi²
Health worker	53.55	52.15	53.16	52.91	6.44 (0.30)
JEEViKA post-holder	1.83	3.31	2.24	2.51	3.32 (1.00)
JEEViKA member	5.26	6.13	5.61	5.70	0.79 (1.00)
Friend/neighbour	4.81	5.30	3.79	4.56	2.60 (1.00)
Media	0.00	0.66	0.84	0.57	3.50 (1.00)
Family	24.49	24.50	23.28	24.00	1.84 (1.00)
Husband	10.07	7.95	11.08	9.75	2.63 (1.00)
NA	0.00	0.00	0.00	0.00	-
DK	0.00	0.00	0.00	0.00	-
Total	100.00	100.00	100.00	100.00	
N	981				
Pearson's Chi2	86.13 (0.40)				

(Continued)

Table A5.3 (Continued)

Tetanus toxoid injection	Standard of living index				
	Low	Medium	High	Total	Chi²
Health worker	60.64	54.69	56.64	57.26	7.73 (0.15)
JEEViKA post-holder	2.47	3.53	1.97	2.66	6.63 (0.25)
JEEViKA member	5.48	9.72	8.40	7.91	19.69 (0.00)
Friend/neighbour	5.30	5.07	4.37	4.91	0.93 (1.00)
Media	0.09	0.17	0.60	0.29	6.09 (0.33)
Family	17.63	20.29	19.54	19.18	7.58 (0.16)
Husband	8.40	6.53	8.48	7.80	3.03 (1.00)
NA	0.00	0.00	0.00	0.00	-
DK	0.00	0.00	0.00	0.00	-
Total	100.00	100.00	100.00	100.00	
N	2037				
Pearson Chi2	149.02 (0.00)				

IF IFA tab/syrup taken for anaemia	Standard of living index				
	Low	Medium	High	Total	Chi²
Health wker	59.98	56.33	59.44	58.41	0.15 (1.00)
JEEViKA post-holder	2.90	3.85	3.18	3.33	2.11 (1.00)
JEEViKA member	5.81	9.73	7.65	7.81	13.12 (0.01)
Friend/neighbour	6.27	4.36	4.37	4.94	4.21 (0.85)
Media	0.23	0.30	0.50	0.35	0.96 (1.00)
Family	17.77	19.86	18.19	18.64	4.29 (0.82)
Husband	7.43	5.57	6.66	6.52	1.82 (1.00)
NA	0.00	0.00	0.00	0.00	-
DK	0.00	0.00	0.00	0.00	-
Total	100.00	100.00	100.00	100.00	
N	1706				
Pearson's Chi2	81.45 (0.62)				

If respondent delivered in an institution	Standard of living index				
	Low	Medium	High	Total	Chi²
Health worker	55.90	46.76	47.06	49.28	0.47 (1.00)
JEEViKA post-holder	1.86	3.12	2.22	2.45	6.60 (0.26)
JEEViKA member	5.46	8.71	8.40	7.74	19.09 (0.00)
Friend/neighbour	4.91	6.00	4.89	5.29	4.72 (0.66)
Media	0.11	0.32	0.69	0.40	5.65 (0.42)
Family	21.40	24.06	23.53	23.16	20.81 (0.00)
Husband	10.37	11.03	13.22	11.68	13.22 (0.01)
NA	0.00	0.00	0.00	0.00	-
DK	0.00	0.00	0.00	0.00	-
Total	100.00	100.00	100.00	100.00	
N	1807				
Pearson's Chi2	134.82 (0.05)				

(Continued)

Table A5.3 (Continued)

If delivery is assisted by a skilled person	*Standard of living index*				
	Low	*Medium*	*High*	*Total*	*Chi²*
Health worker	65.47	64.31	64.31	64.67	0.35 (1.00)
JEEViKA post-holder	2.01	3.13	2.52	2.57	2.62 (1.00)
JEEViKA member	3.58	5.04	4.66	4.46	2.93 (1.00)
Friend/neighbour	4.02	3.43	3.20	3.53	0.85 (1.00)
Media	0.11	0.20	0.48	0.27	2.77 (1.00)
Family	17.65	18.55	18.14	18.13	0.61 (1.00)
Husband	7.15	5.34	6.69	6.37	2.58 (1.00)
NA	0.00	0.00	0.00	0.00	-
DK	0.00	0.00	0.00	0.00	-
Total	100.00	100.00	100.00	100.00	
N	1959				
Pearson Chi2	101.17 (0.20)				

Post-partum check-up with 48 hours of delivery	*Standard of living index*				
	Low	*Medium*	*High*	*Total*	*Chi²*
Health worker	66.38	63.41	65.21	64.90	0.97 (1.00)
JEEViKA post-holder	2.40	2.71	1.93	2.33	1.28 (1.00)
JEEViKA member	4.29	5.28	5.52	5.10	1.43 (1.00)
Friend/neighbour	2.92	3.66	1.93	2.81	4.79 (0.64)
Media	0.17	0.27	0.39	0.29	0.55 (1.00)
Family	17.67	19.92	18.87	18.90	2.48 (1.00)
Husband	6.17	4.74	6.16	5.67	1.33 (1.00)
NA	0.00	0.00	0.00	0.00	-
DK	0.00	0.00	0.00	0.00	-
Total	100.00	100.00	100.00	100.00	
N	1389				
Pearson's Chi2	85.06 (0.14)				

Advice on post-partum contraception method	*Standard of living index*				
	Low	*Medium*	*High*	*Total*	*Chi²*
Health worker	62.92	54.84	52.10	55.79	5.49 (0.45)
JEEViKA post-holder	2.32	4.15	2.95	3.22	5.81 (0.38)
JEEViKA member	5.88	9.69	8.29	8.18	12.17 (0.02)
Friend/neighbour	4.46	5.53	4.77	4.96	2.47 (1.00)
Media	0.00	0.50	1.25	0.67	9.91 (0.05)
Family	16.04	17.61	18.62	17.61	9.42 (0.06)
Husband	8.38	7.67	12.03	9.57	16.86 (0.00)
NA	0.00	0.00	0.00	0.00	-
DK	0.00	0.00	0.00	0.00	-
Total	100.00	100.00	100.00	100.00	
N	1288				
Pearson Chi2	127.98 (0.01)				

(Continued)

Table A5.3 (Continued)

If child was given OPV0	Standard of living index				
	Low	Medium	High	Total	Chi²
Health worker	71.89	67.50	69.54	69.57	1.33 (1.00)
JEEViKA post-holder	1.71	3.63	2.23	2.55	8.65 (0.09)
JEEViKA member	2.74	5.50	4.16	4.18	10.49 (0.04)
Friend/neighbour	2.63	3.12	2.84	2.87	0.71 (1.00)
Media	0.11	0.31	0.61	0.35	3.35 (1.00)
Family	15.54	16.10	15.53	15.73	0.85 (1.00)
Husband	5.37	3.84	5.08	4.75	2.02 (1.00)
NA	0.00	0.00	0.00	0.00	-
DK	0.00	0.00	0.00	0.00	-
Total	100.00	100.00	100.00	100.00	
N	1984				
Pearson's Chi2	91.51 (0.04)				

Breastfeeding up to six months	Standard of living index				
	Low	Medium	High	Total	Chi2
Health worker	55.96	44.86	45.58	48.52	3.35 (1.00)
JEEViKA post-holder	3.89	5.99	4.58	4.87	13.32 (0.01)
JEEViKA member	6.99	10.05	7.96	8.42	19.80 (0.00)
Friend/neighbour	5.61	5.54	5.06	5.41	1.43 (1.00)
Media	0.17	0.67	1.61	0.83	18.39 (0.00)
Family	20.38	24.17	24.52	23.12	41.75 (0.00)
Husband	6.99	8.72	10.69	8.84	22.59 (0.00)
NA	0.00	0.00	0.00	0.00	-
DK	0.00	0.00	0.00	0.00	-
Total	100.00	100.00	100.00	100.00	
N	1976				
Pearson's Chi2	196.62 (0.00)				

Complementary feeding after six months	Standard of living index				
	Low	Medium	High	Total	Chi²
Health worker	53.20	41.22	42.03	44.90	3.45 (1.00)
JEEViKA post-holder	3.96	5.85	4.08	4.68	12.40 (0.01)
JEEViKA member	6.90	11.07	10.09	9.54	30.07 (0.00)
Friend/neighbour	6.09	7.06	6.00	6.41	6.04 (0.34)
Media	0.41	0.56	1.36	0.80	9.43 (0.06)
Family	12.62	23.26	25.06	23.44	32.52 (0.00)
Husband	7.82	10.99	11.37	10.23	25.65 (0.00)
NA	0.00	0.00	0.00	0.00	-
DK	0.00	0.00	0.00	0.00	-
Total	100.00	100.00	100.00	100.00	
N	1737				
Pearson's Chi2	202.73 (0.00)				

Source: Estimated from primary survey.

Table A5.4 Variations in the identification of motivators across socio-religious category

Modern contraception methods	Socio-religious category					Chi²
	H-SC & ST	H-OBC	H-FC	Muslim	Total	
Health worker	35.53	42.36	47.19	52.78	43.64	14.08 (0.02)
JEEViKA post-holder	2.63	1.93	3.00	2.78	2.34	0.51 (1.00)
JEEViKA member	3.95	7.93	8.24	8.33	7.70	2.11 (1.00)
Friend/neighbour	2.63	7.74	6.74	2.78	6.81	5.27 (1.00)
Media	1.32	0.77	0.37	2.78	0.78	2.47 (1.00)
Family	27.63	21.28	16.10	13.89	19.98	13.01 (0.03)
Husband	26.32	17.99	18.35	16.67	18.75	4.19 (1.00)
NA	0.00	0.00	0.00	0.00	0.00	-
DK	0.00	0.00	0.00	0.00	0.00	-
Total	100.00	100.00	100.00	100.00	100.00	
N	446.00					
Pearson's Chi2	166.31 (0.00)					

First ANC visit in first trimester	Socio-religious category					Chi²
	H-SC & ST	H-OBC	H-FC	Muslim	Total	
Health worker	42.47	48.04	56.34	46.74	49.53	24.41 (0.00)
JEEViKA post-holder	1.37	2.79	3.32	1.92	2.72	2.40 (1.00)
JEEViKA member	5.48	8.10	4.23	5.75	6.68	17.50 (0.00)
Friend/neighbour	1.37	5.18	4.08	6.13	4.68	10.22 (0.12)
Media	0.46	0.53	0.15	0.00	0.38	3.24 (1.00)
Family	30.59	24.15	20.69	28.35	24.24	28.63 (0.00)
Husband	18.26	11.21	11.18	11.11	11.78	12.74 (0.04)
NA	0.00	0.00	0.00	0.00	0.00	-

	H-SC & ST	H-OBC	H-FC	Muslim	Total	Chi2
DK		0.00	0.00	0.00		-
Total		100.00	100.00	100.00	100.00	
N						
Pearson's Chi2		209.63 (0.00)				

1451.00

Availed four ANC check-ups

Socio-religious category

	H-SC & ST	H-OBC	H-FC	Muslim	Total	Chi2
Health worker	53.70	51.16	60.70	46.15	52.91	8.00 (0.32)
JEEViKA post-holder	1.23	2.61	2.67	2.75	2.51	1.83 (1.00)
JEEViKA member	5.56	6.27	4.28	5.49	5.70	4.62 (1.00)
Friend/neighbour	1.23	5.12	3.48	6.59	4.56	11.78 (0.06)
Media	1.23	0.68	0.00	0.55	0.57	3.78 (1.00)
Family	22.84	24.52	21.12	28.02	24.00	18.63 (0.00)
Husband	14.20	9.65	7.75	10.44	9.75	7.89 (0.34)
NA	0.00	0.00	0.00	0.00	0.00	-
DK	0.00	0.00	0.00	0.00	0.00	-
Total	100.00	100.00	100.00	100.00	100.00	
N	981.00					
Pearson's Chi2	155.53 (0.03)					

Tetanus toxoid injection

Socio-religious category

	H-SC & ST	H-OBC	H-FC	Muslim	Total	Chi2
Health worker	55.75	56.02	60.73	53.87	57.26	3.56 (1.00)
JEEViKA post-holder	0.88	2.24	3.37	4.23	2.66	8.39 (0.27)
JEEViKA member	7.52	8.32	7.51	7.04	7.91	1.82 (1.00)
Friend/neighbour	2.21	5.33	4.52	5.63	4.91	5.95 (0.80)
Media	0.88	0.32	0.10	0.35	0.29	4.51 (1.00)

(Continued)

Table A5.4 (Continued)

Tetanus toxoid injection	Socio-religious category					Chi2
	H-SC & ST	H-OBC	H-FC	Muslim	Total	
Family	22.57	20.10	16.27	21.13	19.18	18.07 (0.00)
Husband	10.18	7.68	7.51	7.75	7.80	2.97 (1.00)
NA	0.00	0.00	0.00	0.00	0.00	-
DK	0.00	0.00	0.00	0.00	0.00	-
Total	100.00	100.00	100.00	100.00	100.00	
N	2037.00					
Pearson's Chi2	196.48 (0.01)					

If IFA tab/syrup taken for anaemia	Socio-religious category					Chi^2
	H-SC & ST	H-OBC	H-FC	Muslim	Total	
Health worker	62.36	56.53	62.77	53.06	58.41	1.50 (1.00)
JEEViKA post-holder	2.25	2.94	4.22	3.67	3.33	2.65 (1.00)
JEEViKA member	6.74	8.18	7.35	7.76	7.81	3.01 (1.00)
Friend/neighbour	2.81	5.50	4.22	5.31	4.94	6.55 (0.61)
Media	1.69	0.31	0.00	0.82	0.35	13.22 (0.03)
Family	19.10	19.74	15.30	22.45	18.64	23.20 (0.00)
Husband	5.06	6.81	6.14	6.94	6.52	3.20 (1.00)
NA	0.00	0.00	0.00	0.00	0.00	-
DK	0.00	0.00	0.00	0.00	0.00	-
Total	100.00	100.00	100.00	100.00	100.00	
N	1706.00					
Pearson Chi2	152.21 (0.08)					

If respondent delivered in an institution

	Socio-religious category					Chi2
	H-SC & ST	H-OBC	H-FC	Muslim	Total	
Health worker	46.62	47.50	55.00	46.39	49.28	5.07 (1.00)
JEEViKA post-holder	1.50	2.43	2.44	3.44	2.45	2.61 (1.00)
JEEViKA member	7.14	8.17	7.33	6.53	7.74	4.05 (1.00)
Friend/neighbour	3.01	5.94	3.78	7.56	5.29	16.86 (0.01)
Media	1.13	0.40	0.22	0.34	0.40	4.77 (1.00)
Family	24.06	24.07	20.33	24.74	23.16	24.61 (0.00)
Husband	16.54	11.49	10.89	11.00	11.68	12.13 (0.05)
NA	0.00	0.00	0.00	0.00	0.00	–
DK	0.00	0.00	0.00	0.00	0.00	–
Total	100.00	100.00	100.00	100.00	100.00	
N	1807.00					
Pearson's Chi2	250.67 (0.00)					

If delivery is assisted by skilled person

	Socio-religious category					Chi2
	H-SC & ST	H-OBC	H-FC	Muslim	Total	
Health worker	70.81	62.02	71.95	56.51	64.67	2.92 (1.00)
JEEViKA post-holder	1.62	2.65	2.49	2.97	2.57	2.07 (1.00)
JEEViKA member	3.78	5.29	2.49	2.97	4.46	15.80 (0.01)
Friend/neighbour	1.62	3.88	2.75	4.83	3.53	9.07 (0.20)
Media	1.62	0.24	0.00	0.37	0.27	13.73 (0.02)
Family	13.51	19.58	14.94	21.19	18.13	30.58 (0.00)
Husband	7.03	6.35	5.37	8.92	6.37	9.23 (0.20)
NA	0.00	0.00	0.00	0.00	0.00	–

(Continued)

Table A5.4 (Continued)

If delivery is assisted by skilled person	Socio-religious category					Chi2
	H-SC & ST	H-OBC	H-FC	Muslim	Total	
DK	0.00	0.00	0.00	0.00	0.00	-
Total	100.00	100.00	100.00	100.00	100.00	
N	1959.00					
Pearson's Chi2	180.43 (0.01)					

Post-partum check-up with 48 hours of delivery	Socio-religious category					Chi2
	H-SC & ST	H-OBC	H-FC	Muslim	Total	
Health worker	69.23	61.34	73.17	62.64	64.90	0.85 (1.00)
JEEViKA post-holder	1.40	2.37	2.51	2.30	2.33	0.93 (1.00)
JEEViKA member	3.50	5.93	3.86	4.02	5.10	8.36 (0.30)
Friend/neighbour	0.00	3.48	1.74	3.45	2.81	11.71 (0.06)
Media	1.40	0.24	0.19	0.00	0.29	6.34 (0.70)
Family	17.48	20.55	14.29	21.84	18.90	26.22 (0.00)
Husband	6.99	6.09	4.25	5.75	5.67	5.60 (0.93)
NA	0.00	0.00	0.00	0.00	0.00	-
DK	0.00	0.00	0.00	0.00	0.00	-
Total	100.00	100.00	100.00	100.00	100.00	
N	1389.00					
Pearson's Chi2	126.99 (0.10)					

Advice on post-partum contraception method | Socio-religious category

	H-SC & ST	H-OBC	H-FC	Muslim	Total	Chi2
Health worker	48.92	53.73	60.61	61.74	55.79	4.44 (1.00)
JEEViKA post-holder	2.69	2.59	4.31	4.70	3.22	3.12 (1.00)
JEEViKA member	6.99	8.08	9.09	6.71	8.18	1.08 (1.00)
Friend/neighbour	2.69	6.27	2.71	6.04	4.96	17.20 (0.01)
Media	1.08	0.94	0.16	0.00	0.67	6.32 (0.68)
Family	23.66	18.90	14.19	13.42	17.61	28.94 (0.00)
Husband	13.98	9.49	8.93	7.38	9.57	10.42 (0.12)
NA	0.00	0.00	0.00	0.00	0.00	–
DK	0.00	0.00	0.00	0.00	0.00	–
Total	100.00	100.00	100.00	100.00	100.00	
N	1288.00					
Pearson Chi2	199.50 (0.00)					

If child was given OPV0 | Socio-religious category

	H-SC & ST	H-OBC	H-FC	Muslim	Total	Chi2
Health worker	75.57	66.00	78.24	62.95	69.57	7.19 (0.46)
JEEViKA post-holder	1.70	2.98	2.27	1.20	2.55	5.37 (1.00)
JEEViKA member	3.98	4.86	3.07	3.19	4.18	8.51 (0.26)
Friend/neighbour	1.14	3.40	2.00	3.19	2.87	9.40 (0.17)
Media	0.57	0.55	0.00	0.00	0.35	6.14 (0.73)
Family	11.93	17.18	11.62	21.12	15.73	43.02 (0.00)
Husband	5.11	5.04	2.80	8.37	4.75	21.61 (0.00)
NA	0.00	0.00	0.00	0.00	0.00	–

(Continued)

Table A5.4 (Continued)

If child was given OPV0	Socio-religious category					Chi2
	H-SC & ST	H-OBC	H-FC	Muslim	Total	
DK	0.00	0.00	0.00	0.00	0.00	-
Total	100.00	100.00	100.00	100.00	100.00	
N	1984.00					
Pearson Chi2	150.46 (0.00)					

Breastfeeding up to six months	Socio-religious category					Chi2
	H-SC & ST	H-OBC	H-FC	Muslim	Total	
Health worker	50	46.81	52.36	45.91	48.52	0.50 (1.00)
JEEViKA post-holder	4.17	4.34	5.90	5.26	4.87	2.36 (1.00)
JEEViKA member	5.73	8.82	8.26	7.89	8.42	4.49 (1.00)
Friend/neighbour	1.04	6.04	4.45	7.02	5.41	17.47 (0.00)
Media	1.04	0.94	0.54	0.88	0.83	2.19 (1.00)
Family	26.56	24.21	19.96	24.56	23.12	28.24 (0.00)
Husband	11.46	8.82	8.53	8.48	8.84	3.10 (1.00)
NA	0.00	0.00	0.00	0.00	0.00	-
DK	0.00	0.00	0.00	0.00	0.00	-
Total	100.00	100.00	100.00	100.00	100.00	
N	1976.00					
Pearson Chi2	218.78 (0.05)					

Complementary feeding after six months	Socio-religious category					Chi2
	H-SC & ST	H-OBC	H-FC	Muslim	Total	
Health worker	45.23	42.70	49.90	43.13	44.90	0.63 (1.00)
JEEViKA post-holder	2.90	4.37	5.52	5.43	4.68	2.67 (1.00)
JEEViKA member	8.30	10.63	8.33	7.35	9.54	13.42 (0.03)
Friend/neighbour	3.32	7.07	5.31	7.99	6.41	14.13 (0.02)
Media	0.83	1.07	0.21	0.96	0.80	7.56 (0.40)
Family	25.31	24.00	21.04	25.88	23.44	24.77 (0.00)
Husband	14.11	10.17	9.69	9.27	10.23	8.11 (0.31)
NA	0.00	0.00	0.00	0.00	0.00	-
DK	0.00	0.00	0.00	0.00	0.00	-
Total	100.00	100.00	100.00	100.00	100.00	
N	1737.00					
Pearson Chi2	272.07 (0.00)					

Source: Estimated from primary survey.

Table A5.5 Identification of the main motivator of different MCH practices

Motivator of practices	Non-member	JEEViKA member	Total
Adoption of modern contraception method after marriage			
Health worker	80.03	81.05	80.72
JEEViKA member	2.53	7.26	5.16
Husband/family	15.15	10.48	12.56
Others	2.02	1.21	1.57
First ANC visit in the first trimester of pregnancy			
Health worker	85.44	85.20	85.32
JEEViKA member	2.88	7.28	5.10
Husband/family	10.85	7.05	8.96
Others	0.82	0.41	0.62
Availed at least four ANC check-ups			
Health worker	91.87	90.59	91.23
JEEViKA member	1.63	5.11	3.36
Husband/family	6.50	4.29	5.40
Tetanus toxoid injections			
Health worker	92.88	90.80	91.85
JEEViKA member	2.73	6.33	4.52
Husband/family	4.00	2.57	3.29
Others	0.39	0.30	0.34
100 IFA tablets/syrup for anaemia during pregnancy			
Health worker	94.96	93.19	94.08
JEEViKA member	2.11	5.75	3.93
Husband/family	2.58	0.82	1.70
Others	0.35	0.23	0.29
Delivery in an institution			
Health worker	88.58	88.62	88.60
JEEViKA member	3.34	5.69	4.48
Husband/family	7.76	5.46	6.64
Others	0.32	0.23	0.28
Delivery assisted by skilled person			
Health worker	93.27	90.77	92.04
JEEViKA member	2.81	5.29	4.03
Husband/family	3.32	3.63	3.47
Others	0.60	0.31	0.46
Availed post-partum check-ups within 48 hours of delivery			
Health worker	95.94	93.71	94.82
JEEViKA member	2.32	4.43	3.38
Husband/family	1.59	1.86	1.73
Others	0.14		0.07

(Continued)

Table A5.5 (Continued)

Advice on post-partum contraception method			
Health worker	92.26	92.22	92.24
JEEViKA member	2.47	5.87	4.27
Husband/family	4.28	1.17	2.64
Others	0.99	0.73	0.85
Giving OPV0 to child			
Health worker	95.98	95.04	95.51
JEEViKA member	2.01	4.25	3.13
Husband/family	1.71	0.71	1.21
Others	0.30		0.15
Breastfeeding child at least up to six months of birth			
Health worker	85.11	84.14	84.62
JEEViKA member	6.72	10.31	8.55
Husband/family	7.45	5.05	6.22
Others	0.72	0.50	0.61
Complementary feeding after six months of birth			
Health worker	81.15	78.87	79.97
JEEViKA member	7.52	13.35	10.54
Husband/family	10.26	6.90	8.52
Others	1.07	0.89	0.98

Source: Estimated from primary survey.

Table A5.6 Identity of the main motivator of best practices: Variations across education level

Use of modern contraception method after marriage	JEEViKA member				Non-member			
	Health worker	SHG member	Family	Others	Health worker	SHG member	Family	Others
No Schooling	83.84	6.06	8.08	2.02	90.20	1.96	7.84	0.00
1–5 years of education	87.93	1.72	8.62	1.72	81.08	2.70	16.22	0.00
6–10 years of education	75.76	9.09	15.15	0.00	81.48	1.23	14.81	2.47
11–17 years of education	68.00	20.00	12.00	0.00	58.62	6.90	27.59	6.90
Chi-square	13.66 (0.13)				15.20 (0.09)			

First ANC visit in the first trimester of pregnancy	JEEViKA member				Non-member			
	Health worker	SHG member	Family	**Others**	Health worker	SHG member	Family	Others
No schooling	92.22	5.06	2.72	0.00	90.59	1.98	6.44	0.99
1–5 years of education	82.91	5.70	10.13	1.27	85.58	3.85	9.62	0.96
6–10 years of education	81.98	9.01	8.56	0.45	87.54	2.02	10.44	0.00
11–17 years of education	76.74	12.79	10.47	0.00	72.00	5.60	20.00	2.40
Chi-square	24.57 (0.00)				28.06 (0.00)			

Availed at least four ANC check-ups	JEEViKA member				Non-member			
	Health worker	SHG member	Family	**Others**	Health worker	SHG member	Family	Others
No schooling	96.55	3.45	0.00		95.59	1.47	2.94	
1–5 years of education	87.37	3.16	9.47		93.10	0.00	6.90	
6–10 years of education	89.74	4.49	5.77		91.00	2.00	7.00	
11–17 years of education	81.25	14.06	4.69		87.76	2.04	10.20	
Chi-square	27.44 (0.00)				6.46 (0.34)			

Tetanus toxoid injections

	Non-member				JEEViKA member			
	Health worker	SHG member	Family	Others	Health worker	SHG member	Family	Others
No schooling	95.91	1.26	1.89	0.94	94.46	4.34	0.72	0.48
1–5 years of education	93.63	3.82	2.55	0.00	90.48	5.19	3.90	0.43
6–10 years of education	90.98	3.76	5.01	0.25	88.77	7.97	3.26	0.00
11–17 years of education	90.79	1.97	7.24	0.00	80.90	13.48	5.62	0.00
Chi-square	18.92 (0.03)				25.66 (0.00)			

100 IFA tablets/syrup for anaemia during pregnancy

	Non-member				JEEViKA member			
	Health worker	SHG member	Family	Others	Health worker	SHG member	Family	Others
No schooling	96.50	0.78	1.95	0.78	96.00	3.71	0.00	0.29
1–5 years of education	94.85	3.68	1.47	0.00	95.63	2.73	1.64	0.00
6–10 years of education	93.13	2.99	3.58	0.30	90.17	8.12	1.28	0.43
11–17 years of education	96.83	0.79	2.38	0.00	84.71	14.12	1.18	0.00
Chi-square	10.89 (0.30)				25.49 (0.00)			

Delivery in an institution

	Non-member				JEEViKA member			
	Health worker	SHG member	Family	Others	Health worker	SHG member	Family	Others
No schooling	93.17	2.52	3.60	0.72	92.06	2.94	5.00	0.00
1–5 years of education	90.65	2.88	6.47	0.00	87.71	2.23	8.94	1.12
6–10 years of education	86.81	3.57	9.34	0.27	86.57	9.70	3.73	0.00
11–17 years of education	82.31	4.76	12.93	0.00	83.70	10.87	5.43	0.00
Chi-square	18.14 (0.03)				34.43 (0.00)			

(Continued)

Table A5.6 (Continued)

Delivery assisted by skilled person	Non-member				JEEViKA member			
	Health worker	SHG member	Family	Others	Health worker	SHG member	Family	Others
No schooling	94.89	1.28	2.56	1.28	94.36	3.85	1.54	0.26
1–5 years of education	96.53	2.08	1.39	0.00	88.61	2.97	7.92	0.50
6–10 years of education	91.49	4.12	4.12	0.26	89.13	7.61	3.26	0.00
11–17 years of education	91.33	3.33	4.67	0.67	85.42	9.38	4.17	1.04
Chi-square	13.61 (0.14)				28.35 (0.00)			

Availed post-partum check-ups within 48 hours of delivery	Non-member				JEEViKA member			
	Health worker	SHG member	Family	Others	Health worker	SHG member	Family	Others
No Schooling	98.02	0.99	0.99	0.00	95.42	3.87	0.70	
1–5 years of education	94.90	3.06	1.02	1.02	90.08	2.29	7.63	
6–10 years of education	94.96	2.52	2.52	0.00	93.78	5.74	0.48	
11–17 years of education	95.54	3.57	0.89	0.00	93.33	6.67	0.00	
Chi-square	11.25 (0.26)				32.54 (0.00)			

Advice on post-partum contraception method	Non-member				JEEViKA member			
	Health worker	SHG member	Family	Others	Health worker	SHG member	Family	Others
No schooling	96.43	1.02	2.55	0.00	92.34	5.84	0.73	1.09
1–5 years of education	93.18	4.55	2.27	0.00	95.56	2.22	2.22	0.00
6–10 years of education	92.89	2.22	4.00	0.89	92.61	5.42	1.48	0.49
11–17 years of education	81.63	4.08	10.20	4.08	84.06	14.49	0.00	1.45
Chi-square	28.45 (0.00)				17.34 (0.04)			

Giving OPV0 to child	Non-member				JEEViKA member			
	Health worker	SHG member	Family	Others	Health worker	SHG member	Family	Others
No Schooling	97.76	0.64	1.28	0.32	97.98	1.52	0.51	0.24
1–5 years of education	97.96	2.04	0.00	0.00	95.24	2.86	1.90	0.87
6–10 years of education	94.33	2.84	2.32	0.52	92.61	7.04	0.35	0.36
11–17 years of education	94.63	2.68	2.68	0.00	89.80	10.20	0.00	1.08
Chi-square	10.88 (0.28)				27.80 (0.00)			

Breastfeeding child at least up to six months of birth	Non-member				JEEViKA member			
	Health worker	SHG member	Family	Others	Health worker	SHG member	Family	Others
No schooling	90.97	2.80	5.30	0.93	87.14	9.22	3.40	0.24
1–5 years of education	85.03	10.20	4.76	0.00	82.10	9.61	7.42	0.87
6–10 years of education	82.34	8.42	8.42	0.82	80.36	12.36	6.91	0.36
11–17 years of education	78.63	7.63	12.98	0.76	87.10	10.75	1.08	1.08
Chi-square	24.58 (0.00)				14.32 (0.11)			

Complementary feeding child after six months of birth	Non-member				JEEViKA member			
	Health worker	SHG member	Family	Others	Health worker	SHG member	Family	Others
No schooling	83.14	4.60	11.49	0.77	82.74	11.78	4.66	0.82
1–5 years of education	87.02	7.63	5.34	0.00	78.10	12.86	8.57	0.48
6–10 years of education	80.37	8.28	10.12	1.23	73.42	15.61	10.13	0.84
11–17 years of education	72.50	11.67	13.33	2.50	79.31	14.94	3.45	2.30
Chi-square	16.34 (0.06)				14.35 (0.11)			

Source: Estimated from primary survey.

Table A5.7 Identity of the main motivator of best practices: Variations across asset score

Use of modern contraception method after marriage	Non-member				JEEViKA member			
	Health worker	SHG member	Family	Others	Health worker	SHG member	Family	Others
Low	87.50	3.57	8.93	0.00	92.96	4.23	1.41	1.41
Medium	89.47	1.75	7.02	1.75	89.61	6.49	3.90	0.00
High	69.41	2.35	24.71	3.53	66.00	10.00	22.00	2.00
Chi-square	13.75 (0.03)				29.62 (0.00)			

First ANC visit in the first trimester of pregnancy	Non-member				JEEViKA member			
	Health worker	SHG member	Family	Others	Health worker	SHG member	Family	**Others**
Low	88.43	2.31	8.33	0.93	91.51	3.77	4.25	0.47
Medium	88.98	3.39	6.78	0.85	87.08	8.75	3.75	0.42
High	80.07	2.90	16.30	0.72	78.60	8.86	12.18	0.37
Chi-square	14.45 (0.02)				23.85 (0.00)			

Availed at least four ANC check-ups by correlates

Correlate	Non-member				JEEViKA member			
	Health worker	SHG member	Family	Others	Health worker	SHG member	Family	**Others**
Low	91.74	3.31	4.96		92.86	3.97	3.17	
Medium	95.63	0.63	3.75		91.52	7.27	1.21	
High	89.10	1.42	9.48		88.38	4.04	7.58	
Chi-square	8.74 (0.07)				1145 (0.02)			

Tetanus toxoid Injections	Non-member				JEEViKA member			
	Health worker	SHG member	Family	Others	Health worker	SHG member	Family	Others
Low	94.84	2.58	1.72	0.86	93.96	3.63	1.51	0.91
Medium	90.37	3.11	6.21	0.31	89.40	8.60	2.01	0.00
High	93.24	2.54	4.23	0.00	89.12	6.56	4.23	0.00
Chi-square	12.55 (0.05)				18.83 (0.00)			

100 IFA tablets/syrup for anaemia during pregnancy	Non-member				JEEViKA member			
	Health worker	SHG member	Family	Others	Health worker	SHG member	Family	Others
Low	94.66	1.91	2.67	0.76	94.27	4.20	1.15	0.38
Medium	95.99	1.82	1.82	0.36	92.88	6.78	0.34	0.00
High	94.34	2.52	3.14	0.00	92.54	6.10	1.02	0.34
Chi-square	3.84 (0.70)				4.13 (0.66)			

Delivery in an institution	Non-member				JEEViKA member			
	Health worker	SHG member	Family	Others	Health worker	SHG member	Family	Others
Low	91.35	2.77	5.19	0.69	89.56	4.42	5.62	0.40
Medium	88.63	3.34	7.69	0.33	88.96	5.99	4.73	0.32
High	86.18	3.82	10.00	0.00	87.54	6.39	6.07	0.00
Chi-square	7.97 (0.24)				2.78 (0.83)			

(Continued)

Table A5.7 (Continued)

Delivery assisted by skilled person	Non-member				JEEViKA member			
	Health worker	SHG member	Family	Others	Health worker	SHG member	Family	Others
Low	93.97	3.17	1.90	0.95	91.50	4.42	3.74	0.34
Medium	94.08	2.18	3.43	0.31	91.15	6.78	1.77	0.29
High	91.92	3.06	4.46	0.56	89.73	4.53	5.44	0.33
Chi-square	5.21 (0.52)				8.51 (0.20)			

Availed post-partum check-ups within 48 hours of delivery	Non-member				JEEViKA member			
	Health worker	SHG member	Family	Others	Health worker	SHG member	Family	Others
Low	96.48	2.01	1.01	0.50	94.36	4.10	1.54	
Medium	97.81	1.32	0.88	0.00	94.33	4.86	0.81	
High	93.92	3.42	2.66	0.00	92.61	4.28	3.11	
Chi-square	8.17 (0.23)				3.96 (0.41)			

Advice on post-partum contraception method	Non-member				JEEViKA member			
	Health worker	SHG member	Family	Others	Health worker	SHG member	Family	Others
Low	93.75	2.84	3.41	0.00	94.21	3.16	2.11	0.53
Medium	95.81	1.57	2.09	0.52	92.86	6.75	0.00	0.40
High	88.33	2.92	6.67	2.08	89.96	7.11	1.67	1.26
Chi-square	12.32 (0.05)				9.82 (0.13)			

Giving OPV0 to child

	Non-member				JEEViKA member			
	Health worker	SHG member	Family	Others	Health worker	SHG member	Family	Others
Low	97.22	1.54	0.93	0.31	97.09	1.94	0.97	
Medium	94.92	2.22	2.54	0.32	93.88	5.83	0.29	
High	95.80	2.24	1.68	0.28	94.35	4.76	0.89	
Chi-square	3.05 (0.80)				7.60 (0.11)			

Breast feeding child at least up to six months of birth

	Non-member				JEEViKA member			
	Health worker	SHG member	Family	Others	Health worker	SHG member	Family	Others
Low	88.27	5.28	5.87	0.59	88.60	7.12	3.99	0.28
Medium	84.64	7.84	7.52	0.00	80.41	13.74	5.56	0.29
High	82.08	7.17	9.12	1.63	83.23	10.13	5.70	0.95
Chi-square	10.65 (0.10)				11.94 (0.06)			

Complementary feeding of child after six months of birth

	Non-member				JEEViKA member			
	Health worker	SHG member	Family	Others	Health worker	SHG member	Family	Others
Low	87.86	5.36	6.07	0.71	86.25	9.62	3.78	0.34
Medium	78.11	9.06	12.08	0.75	75.00	16.88	7.79	0.32
High	77.47	8.19	12.63	1.71	75.67	13.33	9.00	2.00
Chi-square	14.01 (0.03)				21.51 (0.00)			

Source: Estimated from primary survey.

Table A5.8 Identity of the main motivator of best practices: Variations across socio-religious category

Use of modern contraception method after marriage	Non-member				JEEViKA member			
	Health worker	SHG member	Family	Others	Health worker	SHG member	Family	Others
Hindu-SC & ST	59.09	0.00	40.91	0.00	64.71	5.88	29.41	0.00
Hindu OBC	84.62	1.71	11.97	1.71	79.69	8.59	9.38	2.34
Hindu-Gen	80.39	3.92	13.73	1.96	83.52	6.59	9.89	0.00
Muslims	75.00	12.50	0.00	12.50	100.00	0.00	0.00	0.00
Chi-square	22.5 (0.01)				12.54 (0.2)			

First ANC visit in the first trimester of pregnancy	Non-member				JEEViKA member			
	Health worker	SHG member	Family	Others	Health worker	SHG member	Family	Others
Hindu-SC & ST	68.06	2.78	29.17	0.00	69.57	8.70	21.74	0.00
Hindu OBC	87.50	3.43	8.09	0.98	84.14	8.95	6.39	0.51
Hindu-Gen	87.57	2.70	9.73	0.00	91.04	4.25	4.72	0.00
Muslims	85.71	0.00	11.11	3.17	83.78	6.76	8.11	1.35
Chi-square	36.92 (0.00)				25.33 (0.00)			

Availed at least four ANC check-ups	Non-member				JEEViKA member			
	Health worker	SHG member	Family	Others	Health worker	SHG member	Family	Others
Hindu-SC & ST	81.67	0.00	18.33		84.21	2.63	13.16	0.00
Hindu OBC	93.24	1.42	5.34		91.27	6.18	2.55	0.00
Hindu-Gen	92.38	3.81	3.81		93.94	2.27	3.79	0.00
Muslims	95.65	0.00	4.35		81.82	9.09	9.09	0.00
Chi-square	20.68 (0.00)				16.59 (0.01)			

Tetanus toxoid injections	Non-member				JEEViKA member			
	Health worker	SHG member	Family	Others	Health worker	SHG member	Family	Others
Hindu-SC & ST	93.59	0.00	6.41	0.00	86.79	7.55	5.66	0.00
Hindu OBC	92.87	3.21	3.92	0.00	90.30	6.72	2.80	0.19
Hindu-Gen	92.23	2.91	3.88	0.97	92.92	5.01	1.47	0.59
Muslims	94.87	1.28	2.56	1.28	87.95	8.43	3.61	0.00
Chi-square	11.60 (0.24)				7.72 (0.56)			

100 IFA tablets/syrup for anaemia during pregnancy	Non-member				JEEViKA member			
	Health worker	SHG member	Family	Others	Health worker	SHG member	Family	Others
Hindu-SC & ST	98.55	0.00	1.45	0.00	88.89	6.67	4.44	0.00
Hindu OBC	95.12	2.12	2.55	0.21	93.60	5.96	0.22	0.22
Hindu-Gen	94.33	2.43	2.43	0.81	93.36	5.59	0.70	0.35
Muslims	92.54	2.99	4.48	0.00	92.65	4.41	2.94	0.00
Chi-square	5.48 (0.79)				13.80 (0.13)			

Delivery in an institution	Non-member				JEEViKA member			
	Health worker	SHG member	Family	Others	Health worker	SHG member	Family	**Others**
Hindu-SC & ST	89.02	1.22	9.76	0.00	88.46	3.85	7.69	0.00
Hindu OBC	87.90	3.59	8.32	0.19	87.71	6.67	5.42	0.12
Hindu-Gen	89.43	3.66	6.10	0.84	91.88	2.95	5.17	0.00
Muslims	90.14	2.82	7.04	0.00	82.89	10.53	5.26	1.32
Chi-square	5.58 (0.78)				13.69 (0.13)			

(Continued)

Table A5.8 (Continued)

Delivery assisted by skilled person	Non-member				JEEViKA member			
	Health worker	SHG member	Family	Others	Health worker	SHG member	Family	Others
Hindu–SC & ST	97.50	0.00	2.50	0.00	92.45	1.89	5.66	0.00
Hindu OBC	92.43	3.17	3.87	0.53	90.57	5.66	3.40	0.38
Hindu–Gen	93.68	2.97	2.23	1.12	91.97	4.68	3.34	0.00
Muslims	93.59	2.56	3.85	0.00	86.59	7.32	4.88	1.22
Chi-square	6.64 (0.68)				6.81 (0.66)			

Availed post-partum check-ups within 48 hours of delivery	Non-member				JEEViKA member			
	Health worker	SHG member	Family	Others	Health worker	SHG member	Family	Others
Hindu–SC & ST	100.00	0.00	0.00	0.00	88.64	4.55	6.82	
Hindu OBC	94.80	2.72	2.23	0.25	93.54	4.65	1.81	
Hindu–Gen	97.13	2.30	0.57	0.00	94.31	5.21	0.47	
Muslims	96.30	1.85	1.85	0.00	96.49	0.00	3.51	
Chi-square	5.67 (0.77)				11.87 (0.06)			

Advice on post-partum contraception method	Non-member				JEEViKA member			
	Health worker	SHG member	Family	Others	Health worker	SHG member	Family	Others
Hindu–SC & ST	93.10	1.72	3.45	1.72	82.05	10.26	7.69	0.00
Hindu OBC	90.67	2.33	5.54	1.46	91.76	5.77	1.10	1.37
Hindu–Gen	94.58	2.41	3.01	0.00	93.78	5.78	0.44	0.00
Muslims	95.00	5.00	0.00	0.00	96.23	3.77	0.00	0.00
Chi-square	8.24 (0.51)				22.40 (0.01)			

Giving OPV0 to child

	Non-member				JEEViKA member			
	Health worker	SHG member	Family	Others	Health worker	SHG member	Family	Others
Hindu-SC & ST	97.56	0.00	2.44	0.00	92.73	3.64	3.64	0.00
Hindu OBC	95.38	2.49	1.95	0.18	94.00	5.44	0.56	0.37
Hindu-Gen	95.97	2.20	1.10	0.73	96.88	2.81	0.31	0.60
Muslims	98.72	0.00	1.28	0.00	96.25	2.50	1.25	1.14
Chi-square	7.59 (0.58)				12.03 (0.06)			

Breastfeeding child at least up to six months of birth

	Non-member				JEEViKA member			
	Health worker	SHG member	Family	Others	Health worker	SHG member	Family	Others
Hindu-SC & ST	91.07	0.00	8.93	0.00	82.98	8.51	8.51	0.00
Hindu OBC	82.81	8.13	8.13	0.92	85.34	9.65	4.64	0.37
Hindu-Gen	87.89	5.54	5.88	0.69	82.99	11.64	4.78	0.60
Muslims	86.42	6.17	7.41	0.00	81.82	10.23	6.82	1.14
Chi-square	9.61 (0.38)				4.25 (0.89)			

Complementary feeding child after six months of birth

	Non-member				JEEViKA member			
	Health worker	SHG member	Family	Others	Health worker	SHG member	Family	Others
Hindu-SC & ST	82.61	2.90	14.49	0.00	78.00	10.00	12.00	0.00
Hindu OBC	77.30	9.21	11.78	1.71	77.92	14.65	6.16	1.27
Hindu-Gen	86.38	5.96	7.23	0.43	81.02	11.53	7.46	0.00
Muslims	88.06	5.97	5.97	0.00	77.11	14.46	6.02	2.41
Chi-square	16.47 (0.06)				10.58 (0.30)			

Source: Estimated from primary survey.

Chapter 6

Obstacles to information networks

Results from social network analysis

6.1 Social network analysis: An introduction

Data from the last two rounds of the National Family Health Survey indicates that there has been substantial improvement in maternal and child health (MCH) outcomes since the inception of the National Rural Health Mission in 2005. This is also supported by our study, with both the quantitative analysis and focus group discussions conducted in November and December providing evidence of improved MCH outcomes. It appears that the grassroots health workers have played a crucial role in this transformation. The process of information dissemination may be studied using social networks (Rogers, 1962; Coleman et al., 1966). Social network analysis refers to the study of interpersonal relationships. It is formally defined as a collection of nodes (actors) linked by several relationships indicated by unidirectional or bidirectional ties.

Social network analysis has been used to study ties between job market applicants (Granovetter, 1983; Granoveter, 1994), heart patients (Fowler & Christakis, 2009), terrorists (Krebs, 2002), migrants (Garip, 2008; Munshi, 2011), cyberbullies (Barlett et al., 2018), telecommunication firms (Barnett, 2001), and so on. Social networks are increasingly being recognised as having an important influence on health and healthcare use, as they facilitate the exchange of information on healthcare-related issues (Mukong & Burns, 2020). Applications in the area of maternal and child health care-seeking behaviour, particularly in developing countries, are limited and comprise an under-researched area. A study of community health workers under the Manoshi scheme of BRAC in urban Bangladesh reports improvements in maternal and neonatal health best practices (Adams et al., 2015). The community health workers were observed to provide support, facilitate ideational change, connect mothers to resources, and strengthen or counter the influence of strong ties. Such networks may constitute of household family, non-household family, community, children's initial school, and health workers (Reyes et al., 2022). Another study of the role of social networks in the context of child health behaviour reports that such networks may connect the

DOI: 10.4324/9781003499251-6

child directly, or through their parents, to influential peers (Lois, 2022). The influence of networks may operate through mechanisms like social support, social contagion, and social control (Lois, 2022) to facilitate decision-making, increase information and awareness, and impart guidance (Mukong & Burns, 2020). The influence of social networks on social norms, behaviour, and practices helps to translate policy to delivery of services in developing countries (Ssegujja et al., 2022). These studies have, however, failed to study the nature of the social networks using analytic concepts developed in this field. Rather, they have either used econometric models to analyse quantitative data, or qualitative data to provide a descriptive analysis. This chapter, in contrast to existing studies, has used social network methods developed by theorists working in this field to examine the nature of networks among women in Bihar, analyse the diffusion of information within the community, and identify factors that facilitate or constrain such diffusion.

Social network analysis involves description and analysis of the structural features of the social relations existing between actors (Scott, 2017). The analysis will help us to trace the dissemination of information from Accredited Social Health Activists (ASHAs) and community mobilisers (CM) to women of reproductive age. It will enable us to assess the role of different actors and social relations in facilitating or obstructing such information flows and identify areas where social change may be attempted to accelerate information dissemination and reduce social resistance to such dissemination. The use of formal methods to study network data enables us to present the results of our analysis succinctly; it also helps us to identify features and patterns, and communicate such results effortlessly.

6.2 Objectives

This chapter examines the nature of the networks that dissipate information about maternal and child healthcare practices. These networks are the embodiment of the formal and informal structures existing at the grass-roots level. We examine the characteristics of the network structures, the role of individual actors, and the basis of interaction. It is followed by an analysis of the content from focus group discussions (FGDs) providing information on the role of family and external actors in facilitating information flow to target recipients. The dynamics of the family form an important part of this discussion.

In this chapter, we commence with a discussion of the key network terms and concepts used to analyse the data. In the first step the basic characteristics of the networks (viz. size and density) are described, followed by an analysis of the patterns of connections. The opportunities offered to actors and the constraints faced by them are analysed using centrality measures. A discussion of the hierarchical nature of the networks, their stability, and embedded relations follows. It leads to a discussion of the clusters within each network

– analysed using the concept of homophily. Section 6.3 is followed by a short description of the data used for analysis. Section 6.4 contains the results. It is followed by a discussion of the FGD contents relating to the flow of information and the barriers to the dissemination of the information.

6.3 Materials and method

Social network analysis has developed formal tools and concepts – based on the theory of graphs and matrices – that may be used to summarise the structural features of networks. Such summaries help us to appreciate the "texture of the social fabric" (Hanneman & Riddle, 2011, p. 340). In this section, we discuss the measures relevant to our analysis and describe the source of the data.

6.3.1 Data

The data used in the analysis of the networks was collected through a survey of 12 networks in the districts of Begusarai, Katiahar, Muzzafarpur, Nalanda, Purva Champaran, and Saharsa, in Bihar. A starting point was randomly selected using the recruitment criterion that the respondent had to be a woman aged 15–49 years, normally residing in the village and with at least one child aged <36 months. She was asked about the sources of information about maternal and child health care services. Using a snowballing method other sources of information were identified. In case a health worker or a person residing outside the village was named, the link was not followed. The details of the data collection method are described in Section 3.3.2.

The analysis was undertaken on eight out of the 12 networks; four networks were too sparse for their statistical analysis to reveal significant information. However, they were analysed later to reveal important information on the potential resistances to behavioural change through the diffusion of information.

In addition, focus group discussions (FGDs) were undertaken with eight members each. The same recruitment criterion was used to identify possible participants. After undertaking eight FGDs, saturation was observed. Section 2.3.1 presents further details about the method of undertaking FGDs.

6.3.2 Basic properties of network

Actors and connections, or ties, between the actors, define networks; hence, a convenient starting point is to look at the size of the network and how actors are connected. For instance, given the limited resources and capacities of individual agents for creating and maintaining ties, an important characteristic of network is its size. The size is measured by counting the number of nodes (actors in the network). Given n number of nodes, it is easy to see that there are potentially $n \times (n - 1)$ possible directed ties.[1] It implies that as more actors join the network, its complexity increases exponentially. All possible ties, however, may not actually materialise. The density of the network is the proportion of ties that have actually materialised (actual number of ties/potential number of ties). It provides information on the speed at which information diffuses among the nodes and the extent to which actors have high levels of social capital (facilitating social forces) and social constraints (social features obstructing flows within the network).

6.3.3 Patterns of connections

While size and density provide useful information on the range of possible interactions feasible in a social system, the actual pattern or texture of such interactions is more important. One way to capture the pattern of interactions between actors is through the concept of path. Path refers to a connection between two pairs of actors – it does not matter whether the two actors are directly connected, or whether others lie in between (indirect connection). If reachability is high, it implies that a signal will diffuse throughout the network whereever it originates. Even if pairs of actors are able to reach each other, however, the connection between the pair may not be strong. In such situations, the number of alternative paths through which A and B are connected is important; if there are multiple pathways between two actors, they have high connectivity (Burris, 2005). Connectivity measures the number of nodes that would have to be removed to ensure that A cannot reach B.

The concept of walks and distance is important to understand how actors are embedded in a social system. A walk is a sequence of actors and relations that begins with, say, an actor A and ends with (generally another) actor, say, B. The distance of the walk looks at the number of nodes between any two pair of actors, say A and B. If they are directly connected, then the distance is one; if A and B are connected through C and D (i.e., A → C → D → B) then the distance is three. The shortest distance between A and B is called the geodesic distance. The longest path is called eccentricity, with the largest eccentricity in the network being referred to as the diameter of the network. In small and less dense networks distances are short, permitting speedy diffusion of information.

6.3.4 Centrality measures for network

The embedded structure of the network has another important implication – it offers individual actors opportunities and also imposes constraints (Granovetter, 1982). Given that a node may face fewer constraints and enjoy more opportunities than others, the actor may be in a favourable structural position.

A macro measure of centrality based on connectedness has been proposed by Freeman (1978). He defines the out-degree network centralisation measure as a measure of inequality or variance in the ability to reach out to others for information.

The source of the relative (dis)advantage of an individual actor may be examined from three perspectives, using the concept of centrality:

a) *Degree-based approach to centrality*: This is closely associated with the notion of social capital and focuses on the number of ties that an agent possesses.

Considered to be the most intuitive form of centrality, degree central-ity measures the number of ties that an actor has. In the case of directed ties, it is important to distinguish between how many ties an individual receives (in-degree) and how many alter the ego seeks ties with (out-degree). Since our network is based on how many persons an actor seeks information from – rather than how many people the actor receives information from – the out-degree connectedness, in our context, focuses on how many alters an ego approaches for information. Actors with high out-degree connectedness indicate that the actor has high prestige. After normalising for group size, it is given by:

$$C_0(i) = \frac{1}{n-1} \sum_{j=1}^{n} x_{ij}$$

where x_{ij} is the value of the tie from actor j to actor I (value being either 0 or 1), and n is the number of nodes.

b) *Closeness-based approach to centrality*: On the other hand, if an actor can reach more alters easily and with less effort, he/she may be in a more advantageous position.

Normalised closeness is given by:

$$C_C = \frac{n-1}{\sum_{j=1}^{n} d_{ij}}$$

where d_{ij} is the distance connecting actor i to actor j.

A peripheral actor is dependent on others for obtaining information (Bavelas, 1950; Freeman, 1978). On the other hand, an actor close to many others is relatively independent and can reach out to others with-out relying on intermediaries. For instance, an actor can reach the target of information dissemination easily if they are close. Leavitt (1951) has also associated centrality with ease of accessing information.

c) *Betweenness-based approach to centrality*: Finally, an actor who bridges gaps between alters may be at a more advantage relative to others.

Despite their intuitive appeal, degree centrality is limited by their nar-row perspective – they focus on only the immediate neighbourhood of the network, rather than its entire structure. Betweenness builds upon eigenvector centrality, focussing on the entire network, but extends it to consider the placement of an actor. Betweenness counts how many times an actor is placed on the geodesic path between pairs of actors (Freeman, 1978; Freeman et al., 1991). The normalised betweenness measure is given by:

$$C_B = 2 \frac{\sum \delta_{ikj}/\delta_{ij}}{(n-1)(n-2)}, \ i \neq j \neq k$$

where δ_{ikj} is the number of geodesics linking actors i and j that pass through the node k, and δ_{ij} is the number of geodesics linking actors i and j.

Bonacich (1987) pointed out that the above centrality measures often varied in their conclusions. Further, they neither examined the wider network structure – focussing on the immediate neighbourhood – nor considered whether the ties comprised positive relations or negative relations. These issues, Bonacich argued, could be addressed by an alternative measure of centrality, β-centrality. This is given by:

$$C_\beta (i) = \sum_{j=1}^{n} A_{i,j} \left(\alpha + \beta C_\beta (j) \right)$$

where

α is a scaling parameter set to normalise the score,
β is a value selected by the analyst to reflect the amount of dependence of actor i's centrality on the centralities of the alters to whom actor i is tied directly,
$A_{i,j}$ is the adjacency matrix, and
Cβ(j) is the centrality of j (actor i's partners).

The value of β is chosen to assign weightage to the wider network structure, relative to the locality of actor i.

6.3.5 Embedded nature of networks

The texture of the social relations is also revealed through its hierarchical nature. This notion is based on the observation that actors may be embedded in clusters. The structure that emerges is said to be horizontally differentiated – with each cluster being ranked equally. Hierarchies, in which individuals or sub-populations are not only differentiated but also ranked, are extremely common in social life. Such differentiation is called vertical differentiation.

Krackhardt (1994) provided a definition of the meaning of hierarchy, based on the notion of a pure, "ideal-typical" hierarchy as an "out-tree" graph. An out-tree graph is a directed graph in which all points are connected, and all nodes, except one, have an in-degree of one. The exception is the "boss" or a superior node, who is placed at the top of the hierarchy. In our case, the ASHA is one such "boss". This means that all actors in the graph (except the ASHA or CM) have a single superior node. The simplest "hierarchy" is a directed line graph from A to B to C to D..., ending with ASHA. More complex hierarchies, however, exhibit wider, and varying out-degrees of points (spans of control).

This definition of the pure type of hierarchy was deconstructed into four individually necessary and jointly sufficient conditions by Krackhardt (1994), who developed four measures of the extent to which a given structure resembles the ideal-typical hierarchy:

1) *Connectedness*: To be a pure out-tree, a graph must be connected into a single component – all actors are embedded in the same structure. We can measure the extent to which this is not true by looking at the ratio of the number of pairs in the directed graph that are reachable relative to the number of ordered pairs. That is, what proportion of actors cannot be reached by other actors? Where a graph has multiple components – multiple un-connected sub-populations – the proportion not reachable can be high. If all the actors are connected in the same component, if there is a "unitary" structure, the graph is more hierarchical.

2) *Hierarchy*: To be a pure out-tree, there can be no reciprocated ties. Reciprocal relations between two actors imply equal status, and this denies pure hierarchy. We can assess the degree of deviation from pure hierarchy by counting the number of pairs that have reciprocated ties relative to the number of pairs where there is any tie; that is, what proportion of all tied pairs have reciprocated ties.

3) *Efficiency*: To be a pure out-tree each node must have an in-degree of one. That is, each actor (except the ultimate boss) has a single boss. This aspect of the idea type is termed "efficiency" because structures with multiple bosses have unnecessary redundant communication of orders from superiors to subordinates. The amount of deviation from this aspect of the pure out-tree can be measured by counting the difference between the actual number of links (minus 1, since the ultimate boss has no boss) and the maximum possible number of links. The bigger the difference, the greater the inefficiency. This dimension then measures the extent to which actors have a "single boss".

4) *Least upper bound (LUB)*: To be a pure out-tree, each pair of actors (except pairs formed between the ultimate boss and others) must have an actor that directs ties to both – that is, the command must be unified. The

deviation of a graph from this condition can be measured by counting the number of pairs of actors that do not have a common boss relative to the number of pairs that could (which depends on the number of actors and the span of control of the ultimate boss).

(Hanneman & Riddle, 2011, p. 230.

6.3.6 Fragmentation

Fragmentation is the proportion of pairs of nodes that cannot reach each other. Distance-weighted fragmentation is one minus the average recipro-cal distance between all pairs of nodes. Node-level fragmentations are these values that involve the specified node. Fragmentation centrality of a node is the difference in the total score with the node and the score with the node removed. The same process is used for distance-weighted fragmentation.

6.3.7 Sociograms

As mentioned before, networks comprise nodes (or agents) and the ties (or relationships) that link the nodes. The relationships may indicate the dissemi-nation of information, the flow of resources and assistance, etc. Analysing the relational data (i.e. numerical information about the links between nodes) provides information about the structure and pattern of interactions, and their implications for social actions. The numerical information is often ana-lysed using visual techniques. Analysing networks using mathematical graphs drawn in two or three- dimensional space reveal "patterns that are generally not apparent to human observers" (Scott, 2017, p. 2), particularly in the case of small and low-density networks. Such visual depictions enable research-ers to understand how actors are embedded in the global structure. Freeman (1996) suggests that coding such visual depictions using different colours, shapes, and sizes adds value to such maps, thereby expanding possibilities of discovering new patterns and facilitating communication of such struc-tural findings. As observed by Bertin (1983), visual depiction permits *differ-ent categories of numerical information to be communicated simultaneously*, whereas the information communicated through numbers, equations, and textual matter is absorbed *sequentially*. We concentrated on three attributes – caste, JEEViKA membership, and the nature of relationship. The coding of attributes is described in Table 6.1.

6.3.8 Homophily

A social situation where actors prefer to have social relations with other actors who are similar in respect to some attribute is referred to as homophily (Easley & Kleinberg, 2010; Prell, 2012). This phenomenon has been studied fairly extensively by researchers (Lazarsfeld & Merton, 1954; Blau, 1977;

Table 6.1 Coding patterns employed in network maps

Colour	Caste	Size	Relation	Shape	JEEViKA
Red	SC	Small	Kin	Circle	Member
Green	Other backward castes (OBCs)	Medium	Neighbour	Triangle	Non-member
Blue	General	Large	Health worker	NA	NA

Source: From primary survey.

McPherson et al., 2001). The notion that ties are not formed randomly, but shaped by "surrounding context" (Easley & Kleinberg, 2010, p. 78), underlies the concept of homophily. It may be attributed to two forces:

a)   Organisational settings determining ties between similar actors (Coleman et al., 1981; Feld, 1981, 1982); and,
b)   Self-selection, wherein actors are drawn to seek out and establish ties with 'similar' actors (Skvoretz, 1985, 1990).

Krackhardt and Stern (1988) have proposed a simple measure of homophily using an E-I (external-internal) index. It is given by:

$$\text{E-I Index} = \frac{T_E - T_I}{T_E + T_I}$$

where T_E is the number of external ties, and T_I is the number of internal ties. This is a raw measure and is adjusted by the maximum possible external and internal ties to get the Expected E-I index. It is also possible to adjust for group size and density to get the rescaled value of the Index. In this chapter we have examined caste- and kinship-based homophily.

6.4 Results

6.4.1 Size and density of the networks

The networks analysed are small networks among which network 3 is the largest with 12 nodes and 20 ties. The mean average degree across networks, as in Table 6.2, is 1.32 and ranges from 1 to 1.88. It implies that a single member of the network is barely connected with other members within each network. This apparent sparseness in the association may indicate how the severance of a single tie can act as an information barrier.

6.4.2 Connectivity of the networks

Table 6.3 shows how well the members of the networks are connected. The connectivity measure suggests that all the networks are unstable. Moreover, the compactness measure of all networks is less than 0.5 – with some reaching as low as 0.2, making the networks barely compact. In contrast, the average distance indicates that the network members are close to each other. A closely-knit small network will allow quick permeation of information, which is beneficial even when the networks are unstable.

The mean of all reciprocal distances is low, indicating a small-size network structure. The sum of geodesic distances, given by the Wiener Index, varies substantially across networks – ranging from 18 to 64.

In our network, we are primarily interested in the flow of information from the ASHA or community mobiliser (CM) to the ego, with other actors facilitating or obstructing such flows. So these concepts are not relevant in our context. We are interested in the reachability, connectivity, and geodesic distance between the ego and the ASHA or CM.

The network egos are connected to at least one ASHA or Anganwadi worker despite the low density, small network structure. The average geodesic distance across these networks is approximately 1.5, indicating a close, direct tie for egos with health workers. A geodesic distance of one indicates there is at least one direct tie between our network egos and health workers. The availability of multiple ties between the ego and health worker in these networks indicates the absence of reliance on a particular ASHA

Table 6.2 Size and density of the networks

Statistic	1	2	3	4	5	6	7	8
No. of nodes	10	9	12	10	8	8	7	9
No. of ties	15	10	20	11	15	8	9	9
Average degree	1.50	1.11	1.67	1.10	1.88	1.00	1.23	1.00
Density	0.17	0.14	0.15	0.12	0.27	0.14	0.214	0.13

Source: Estimated from primary survey.

Table 6.3 Connectivity and compactness of the networks

Statistic	1	2	3	4	5	6	7	8
Connectivity	0.23	0.236	0.288	0.267	0.411	0.268	0.31	0.222
Average distance	1.33	1.529	1.684	1.667	1.391	1.667	1.385	1.563
Compactness	0.20	0.183	0.21	0.189	0.336	0.196	0.28	0.169
Wiener index	28	26	64	40	32	25	18	25

Source: Estimated from primary survey.

or health worker. The exceptions are networks 5 and 6. Network 5's ego (Sundar) has two relations, one being a direct tie. The geodesic distance of three with the other tie essentially increases the reliance on the direct tie; her efficiency will determine the speed with which information flows to Sundar. On the other hand, the ego of network 6 has only one direct tie with an Anganwadi making her dependent on this health worker. If the latter does not undertake her duties effectively, this will affect the diffusion of information to the ego.

While speedy information dissemination is important, the information must also be credible for it to be acted upon. Credibility often depends upon how many sources provide the actor with the information (Frank, 1996). The number of alternative sources that ASHAs can use to relay information to the alter depends upon how many nodes lie on the multiple paths between the two. It is defined as flow and indicates the availability of alternative routes to transmitting information.

Most of our networks are in an advantageous position when it comes to passing the information from health workers to the target through varied channels to our network egos. All the networks, except networks 2, 4, 6, and 8, have at least one health worker with three or more channels to transmit critical information. It reduces reliance on a single health worker, who may or may not be performing her duties actively. There is also the additional advantage that the credibility of the information increases, as it is repeated by multiple sources (Frank, 1996). In particular, the egos of networks 1 and 2 with a total of 11 and 7 flows, respectively, are assured of receiving communication. Despite having a single flow, network 4's three health workers and their geodesic distances put the ego in a better position than that of network 6's.

6.4.3 Centrality of the networks

The normalised out-degree centrality measure for the network egos is substantially high ranging from 0.38 (network 4) to 0.56 (network 1) given the low number of ties in individual networks. The egos, therefore, have 30%–60% of one-hop relations within their respective networks.

Compared to the star network, which is the most unequal network structure, networks 1, 3, and 8 register a moderately high degree of unequal distribution to a tune of 43% (Table 6.4). Network 5 has a substantially low out-degree centrality of 18%. The individual network range of in-degree and out-degree centrality measure points to a positional advantage of some actors within the system in securing information, notably network 8.

While degree centrality focuses on a number of nodes directly tied with the actor, eigenvector centrality measures the number of direct ties weighted by the degree centrality of each of these nodes (Bonacich, 1987). It is given by the ith entry of the unit eigenvector e when e is the largest eigenvalue obtained

Table 6.4 Degree centrality of the networks

Statistic	1	2	3	4	5	6	7	8
Out-degree	0.43	0.27	0.43	0.36	0.18	0.33	0.33	0.42
In-degree	0.19	0.13	0.23	0.11	0.35	0.16	0.53	0.14
Eigenvector	0.50	0.43	0.41	0.52	0.31	0.56	0.55	0.44

Source: Estimated from primary survey.

by solving $Ae = \lambda e$ given A is the adjacency matrix. As Borgatti (1995)points out, an eigenvector is a more refined version of degree centrality, as it captures the possibility that an actor may have limited ties, but one such tie is with an alter who has a high degree of centrality.

The eigenvector centralisation index for each network attains almost 47% of the maximum possible degree of concentration. There is only a 0.6% variation within the indices, keeping the measure consistent for all networks. At the micro level, the egos are the most central actors each reflecting almost 50% of the global pattern within networks, except for networks 8, 6, and 7. The egos therefore enjoy a positional advantage in information exchange, even with a limited number of ties.

In networks studying information flows, betweenness helps to identify actors with high potential control over the diffusion of information (Cook et al., 1983). For instance, focus group discussions have revealed that mothers-in-law play an important role in acting as the conduit through which information flows to the respondent:

P2: *See now my mother-in-law is a member of JEEViKA, now she comes to attend the group meeting and she understands how to keep a child and she also suggests me the same with the child as it was advised in the group.*

P2: *I don't usually go anywhere from the house so I don't know … my mother-in-law goes … I don't go out, she goes, she attends* (JEEViKA meetings) *and she tells (me).*

Unless there are alternative channels, it becomes very easy for the mother-in-law to control the flow of information by withholding or distorting information, thereby preventing the behavioural change of the respondents.

Barring network 8, the Freeman betweenness centralisation index seems to be moderately high, given the low density of our networks (Table 6.5). This may be accredited to the number of interpersonal ties within actors of a network, which may also result in high brokerage for a few members within a network group. Within each network, however, we can expect the

Table 6.5 Betweenness of the networks

Statistic	1	2	3	4	5	6	7	8
Freeman	3.55	7.03	8.76	11.42	7.82	12.93	5.00	8.04
Flow	47.63	64.96	50.98	50.82	7.14	58.16	23.89	40.85

Source: Estimated from primary survey.

mother-in-law's betweenness score to be high. We observe this to be true for networks 3, 4, 7, and 8 as per Freeman's approach. For networks 3 and 6, the mother-in-law scores the highest. For the rest, alters take the lead.

Alternately, instead of focussing on which node is central, we can concentrate on identifying which *relations* are more central. Using Freeman's definition, a relation is between if it lies on the geodesic path between two actors. It will give the *flow* betweenness centrality measure.

The flow betweenness macro measures are larger than the Freeman measure but it does not alter the picture much other than a distinct although marginal dip for network 6 – from 7.8 to 7.1. Actor-level flow measure, on the other hand, takes into consideration all the possible pathways including the "inefficient ones" which can be used to relay information to the target audience. This changes the "influencing factor" of actors compared to Freeman's measure. For example, while Freeman assigned a value of zero to the ego of network 1, she received a flow score of 61, the highest among network 1 members. Rubi who was rather unimportant, when we considered the Freeman measure, became the most important under-flow centrality. For the rest of the networks, however, the intra-network actor ranking remains the same as was under the Freeman approach.

Compared to the individual integration averages, the network in-centrality measures reported in Table 6.6 indicate overall node closeness within networks. The scenario is different for networks 4 and 6 where the share of peripheral actors may be larger than nodes in close proximity, driving the gap between the measure and the average. Interestingly, the individual nodes of each network have a high reaching-out tendency. The difference between average radiality and out centrality is positive and quite high, specifically in network 1 (46.75) and network 4 (46.75).

Information channels often entail influencing. In such situations, the advantage lies in connections with those who are well-connected. High out-β centrality measures of the egos in Table 6.7 suggest that our respective network egos are well-connected to those who are central in their networks. Compared to their out-degree centrality measures, the Bonacich power index reflects the egos' wider influence outside their immediate neighbourhood. Intentionally, we focus on the health workers' in-β centrality measure β's to observe whether people in our networks seek them when needed. There is at

Table 6.6 Measures of closeness of the networks

Statistic	1	2	3	4	5	6	7	8
Integration: Average	20.741	19.444	23.864	20.741	35.714	20.833	26.984	18.056
Network in-centrality	22.22	15.62	21.07	9.88	46.26	8.84	46.3	17.19
Radiality: Average	20.741	19.444	23.864	20.741	35.714	20.833	26.984	18.056
Network: Out centrality	67.49	57.81	63.22	67.49	46.26	52.38	59.26	64.06

Source: Estimated from primary survey.

Table 6.7 Measures of Beta centrality[1] of the networks

Beta = 0.5	1	2	3	4	5	6	7	8
Ego[2]	2.43	2.32	2.57	2.65	1.67	2.03	2.12	2.34
Health Worker 1	1.87	1.42	1.90	0.46	1.92	1.59	2.33	0.65
Health Worker 2	0.91	1.71	2.14	1.21	1.56		0.61	1.79
Health Worker 3	0.91	0.99	1.01	1.21				0.98
Health Worker 4			0.65					

Source: Estimated from primary survey.
Notes:
1. The Bonacich centrality measures, corresponding to $\beta = 0.5$.
2. Measures are estimated for the ego based on her out-degree nodes; in the case of health workers, we use their in-degree nodes.

least one health worker in every network who is well-connected with other members. In most of our cases, these health workers are situated in the one-walk neighbourhood of the network egos. The only exceptions are networks 4 and 6, where far-located health workers enjoy an influential position.

6.4.4 Dimensions of hierarchy

The homogenous nature of the networks studied is clear from a comparison of the graph theoretic dimensions (GTD) measures (Table 6.8). Either values do not vary or do so marginally. The GTD measures indicate that the networks are connected, hierarchical, highly efficient, and have a unified command. It indicates the highly hierarchical nature of the information flow, originating from the health workers and filtering to the egos. While the absence of redundant links implies a high degree of "organisational efficiency", it has potential dangers as some agents may acquire considerable power to control information flow. This aspect of the networks is examined next.

Table 6.8 Krackhardt's graph theoretic dimensions (GTD) measure of the networks

Statistic	1	2	3	4	5	6	7	8
Connectedness	1.00	1.00	1.00	1.00	1.00	1.00	1.00	1.00
Hierarchy	1.00	1.00	1.00	1.00	1.00	1.00	1.00	1.00
Efficiency	0.83	0.93	0.84	0.94	0.62	0.95	0.80	0.96
LUB	1.00	1.00	1.00	1.00	1.00	1.00	1.00	1.00

Source: Estimated from primary survey.

Table 6.9 Fragmentation measures of the networks

Statistic	1	2	3	4	5	6	7	8
Fragmentation	0.767	0.764	0.712	0.733	0.589	0.732	0.690	0.778
Distance weighted fragmentation	0.802	0.817	0.790	0.811	0.664	0.804	0.742	0.831

Source: Estimated from primary survey.

6.4.5 Fragmentation

Our networks, on average, are highly fragmented with 50% or more node pairs unable to reach each other within their respective structure (Table 6.9). The proportions for most networks are closer to one which is not unexpected given the densities are low. The distance-weighted fragmentation measure, additionally, takes into account the reciprocal distances between any pair of nodes. Therefore, it imparts a sense of closeness between a pair of nodes. Considering the distances, the distance-weighted fragmentation measure boosts the previous measure. The ranking of the networks under the latter measure changes from that of the former. However, the overall scenario remains almost untouched. The latter measure also confirms that the networks have more peripheral actors than portrayed by the closeness measures.

6.4.6 Visual depiction of the networks

In this section we present the information flow between the actors using graphs. The direction of the arrow between (say) A to B indicates that A seeks information from B.

The data for the first network studied (Figure 6.1) was obtained from the village of Jhitkaiya, in the Mehsi block of Purba Champaran district. The respondent, Anu, was asked who provided her with information regarding antenatal care (ANC) services. It can be seen that Anu is provided the information from multiple people; of them, Sushinta is an ASHA worker, while Sangita is an Anganwadi worker. The geodesic distance with grassroots health workers is, therefore, just one. This places her in a position of

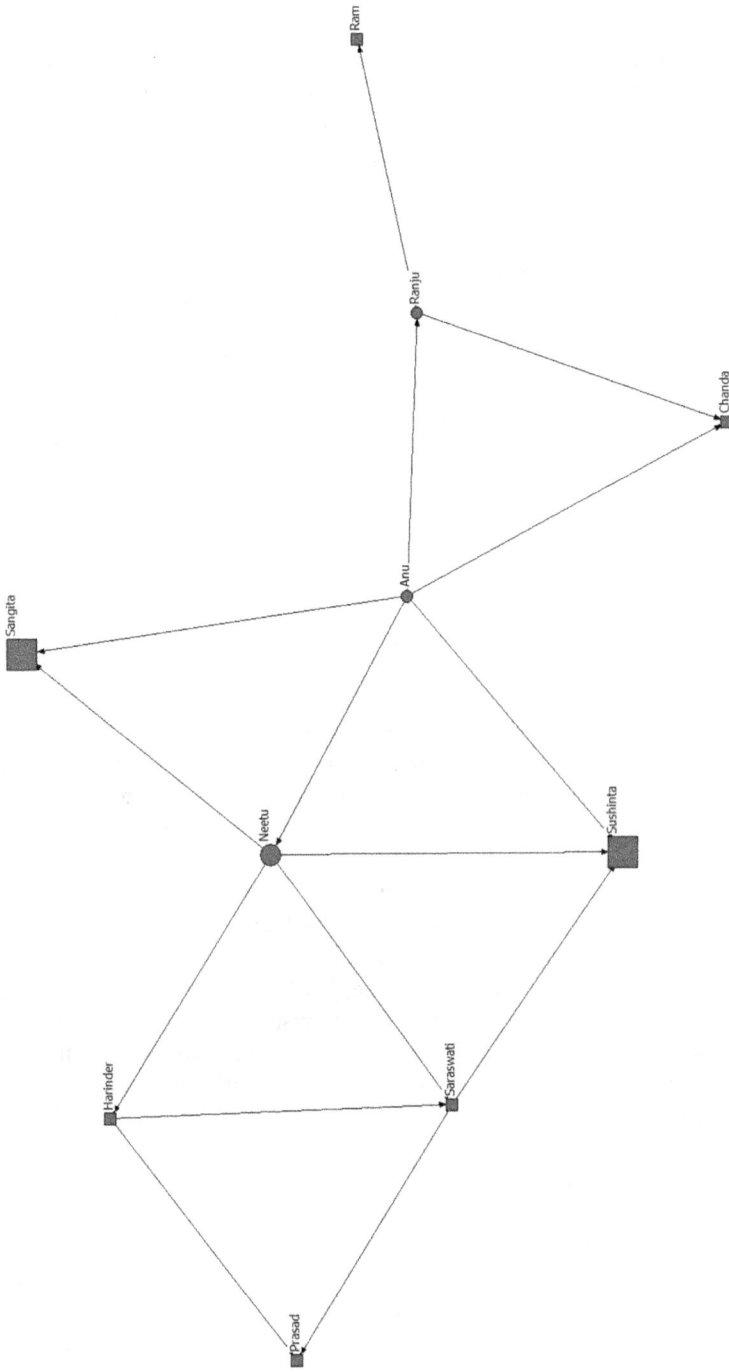

Figure 6.1 Sociogram of network 1.

strength. She does not have a mother-in-law, which prevents any potential blocks to her information flow. Her neighbour, Neetu, and Neetu's mother-in-law, Saraswati, are key players[2] who can fragment the network; but this will not affect Anu's access to information as she has direct links with Sangita and Sushinta. The network demonstrates strong caste-based homophily – with all respondents belonging to OBCs.

The second network studied (Figure 6.2) also relates to information on ANC services. The respondent, Pinki, is a resident of Bahuragopisingh village, Terariya block, Purba Champaran district. In this case, Pinki's geodesic distance from one of the two ASHAs, Lalsa Devi, is one. She also has two other channels of information, through which she receives information from the ASHA workers, Lalsa, Puja, and Soyel; these channels of diffusion, however, pass through two important members of her family – Shanti (her mother-in-law) and Raviranjan (her husband). They, along with Kamal (Raviranjan's elder brother), are key players whose removal would fragment the network. Shanti's role is not crucial; removing her would block information flow from only Puja, as Pinki would still be able to maintain links with Lalsa. Raviranjan's removal would result in the removal of contact with Soyel, as well as other (indirect) informants. Thus, the combination of husband and mother-in-law is able to control the information being received by Pinki. We find homophily in this network also, with links between only scheduled castes (SCs).

In Figure 6.3, we depict the information flow on institutional delivery to Neelam, an OBC woman residing in Kantapiraucha village, Gaighat block, in Muzaffarpur district. The network is denser relative to the other networks studied in this chapter. Neelam has considerable autonomy, which is manifested in her ability to access Bharti (ASHA), Manju (Anganwadi worker), and Ramrati (CM). The distance between Neelam and these four actors is only one. The position of strength is derived from Neelam's JEEViKA membership; it enabled her to come in contact with the four grass-roots health workers, who are also members of JEEViKA. It implies that, although links between JEEViKA members are not dense, JEEViKA enables actors to establish close links with influential persons. Consequently, the ability of the mother-in-law, Malti, to control the flow of information to Neelam is considerably undermined. The key players in this network, Suresh and Puja, are both at a distance from Neelam and so are not in a position to block her access to the ASHA.

The network depicted in Figure 6.4 is for Puja, a resident of Lachmannagar village, Gaighata block, in Muzaffarpur district. The residents of this area are mostly from the forward caste community. Although, there are two grass-roots health workers (Sushila and Saroj) and one doctor (Anit), the ego, Puja, does not have any direct link with health workers. In her case, both her mother-in-law (Rita) and *jethani* (Mani) play an important role as gatekeepers through which information diffuses to Puja. They are key players, whose

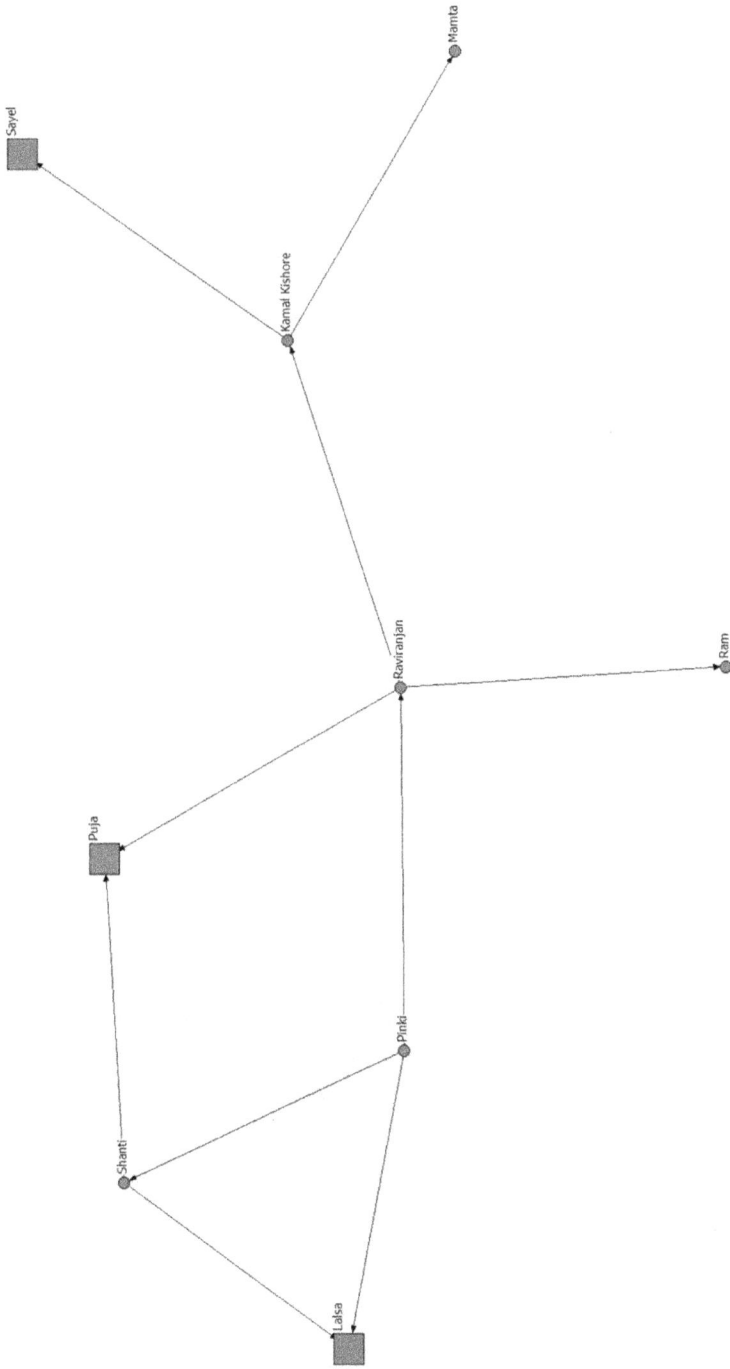

Figure 6.2 Sociogram of network 2.

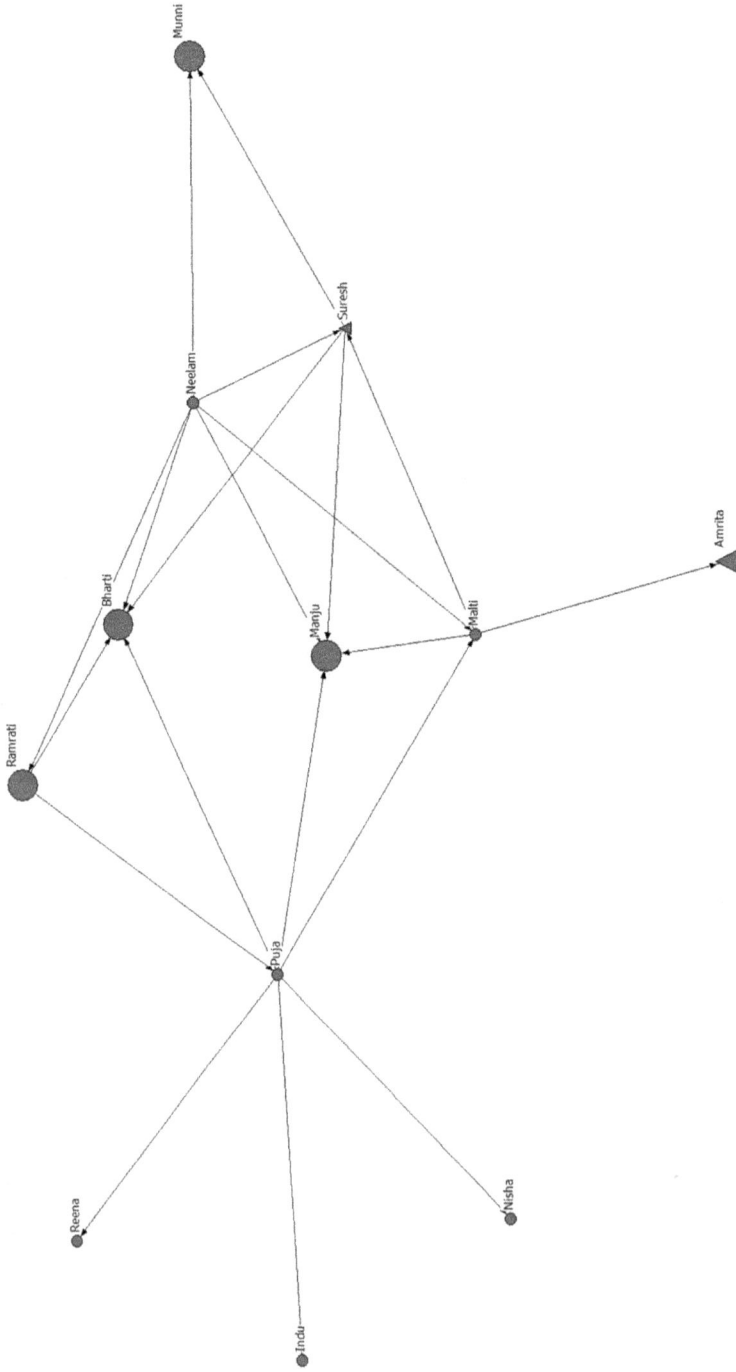

Figure 6.3 Sociogram of network 3.

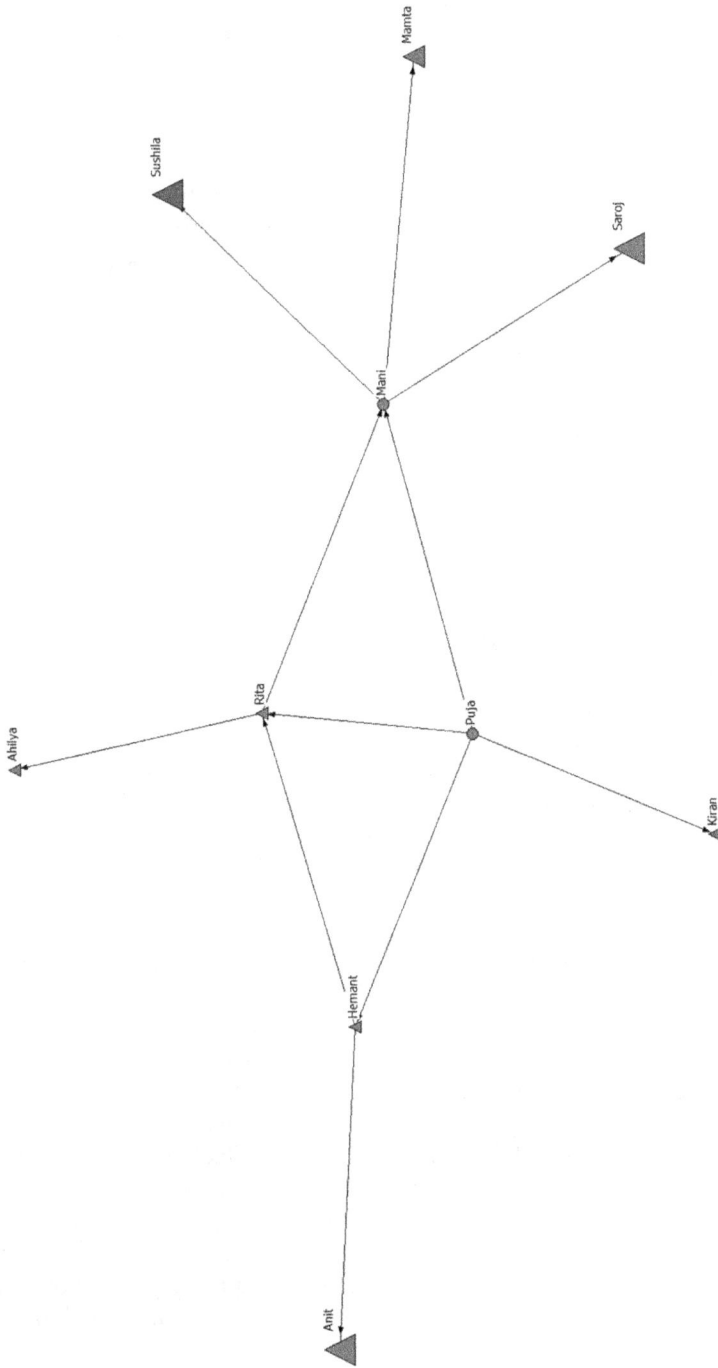

Figure 6.4 Sociogram of network 4.

removal would lead to a substantial breakdown in the network. Although Puja is a JEEViKA member, it does not help her to establish direct channels with any ASHA. This possibly reflects a Veblen effect (Veblen, 1989), as upper caste members have been reported to prefer private doctors over ASHAs:

> You know what happens to the upper caste, they think that they have money so they will not take any government facilities; even we suggest them to do whatever they want to, but just to share the check-up dates.

The next network (Figure 6.5) is for Sundar, an SC woman residing in Jamina village, Barauni block, Begusarai district. Sundar has three direct contacts, of whom one is Krishna, an ASHA. The other two alters are her husband (Shivlal) and her mother-in-law (Mamta). Through these two actors, Sundar is able to access other nodes. Most of these nodes are, however, family members (sisters-in-law), with only Rajeswari being a CM. Of the actors indirectly linked to Sundar, one of her sisters-in-law, Rubi, is a key player, along with Shivlal.

In Figure 6.6 we depict the ego network for Maya. Her residence is in the village of Sartha, in Chandi block of Nalanda district. Maya's contacts are through her mother (Renuka) and mother-in-law (Seema). As Seema resides in a different village, her control over Maya is minimal. In contrast, Maya's mother is better positioned to control the information flow to Maya; she is a key player. Although Maya also has a direct tie with Inku (an Anganwadi worker), the path to Preeti Kumari (Cluster Facilitator) is relatively long (geodesic distance is three). She does not have any path with ASHA.

Data for the network depicted in Figure 6.7 were obtained in the village of Binnawar, in Chandi block, Nalanda district. The ego was Ribha, an OBC woman. Ribha has three links with Indu, the village ASHA. Although one of them is direct, the other two are via her husband (Chotelal) and mother-in-law (Urmila). The mediation of these two family members in Ribha's interaction with the ASHA reflects their influential role in controlling the process of information diffusion, similar to that manifested in other networks.

The last network studied focusses on OBC women in the village of Tetrawan, Bihar Shariff block, Nalanda district. The ego is Sita. She is a JEEViKA member; her membership has enabled her to establish a route with a geodesic distance of one with Kusum (CM). Her geodesic distance to Pratima (Anganwadi worker) is also one. But her link to the ASHA (Sanju) is through Debi, her mother-in-law. In fact, Debi plays a crucial role in the information flow, as she is situated on paths between Sita and Sunita, Parmod, and Sunaina – as well as between Kusum and Sanju. Without Debi, Sita's network would get fragmented, and shrink substantially; Debi is, therefore, a key player in the network.

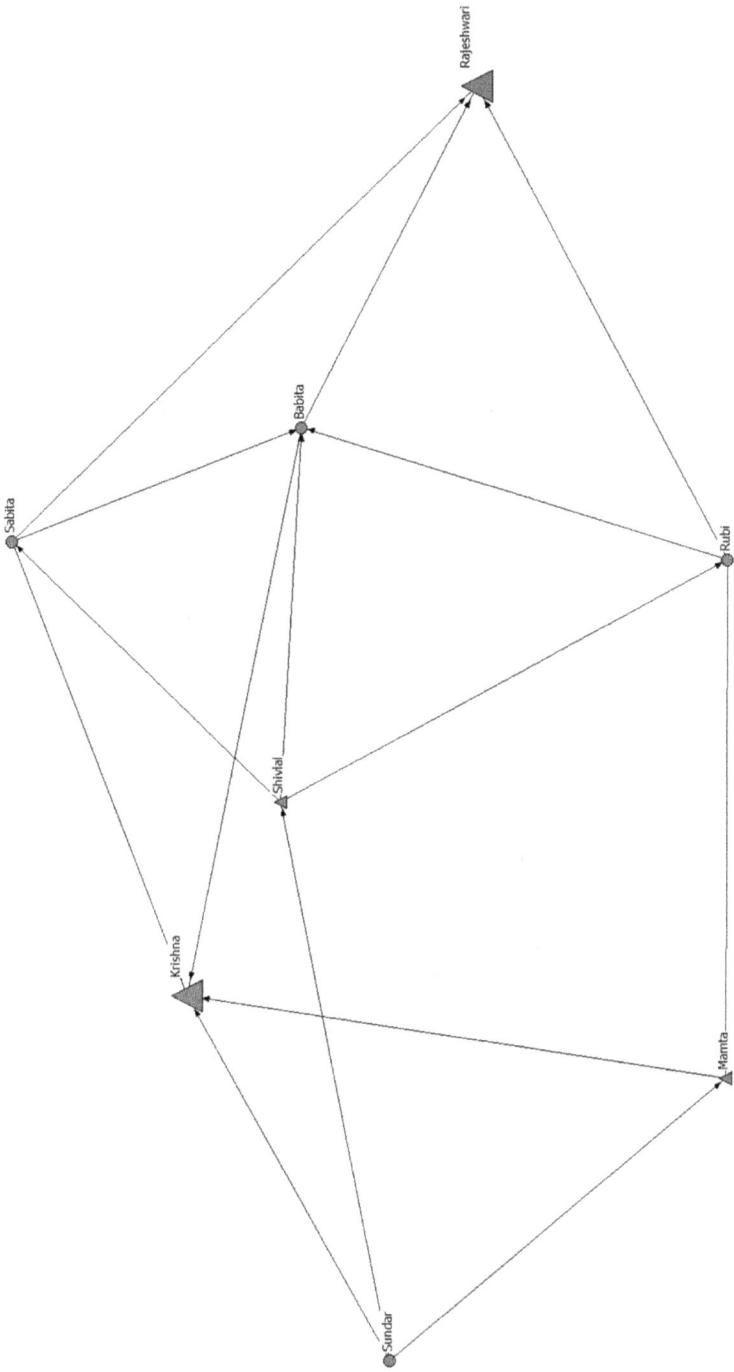

Figure 6.5 Sociogram of network 5.

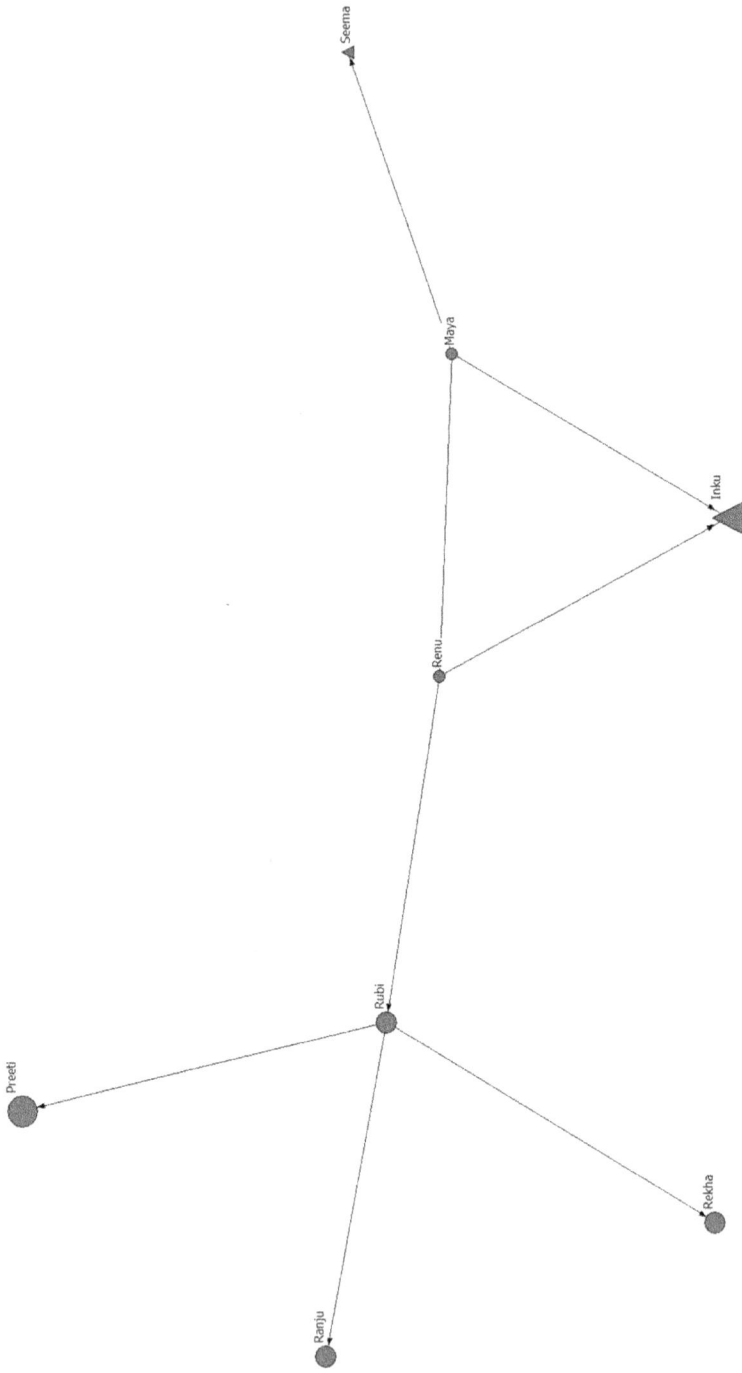

Figure 6.6 Sociogram of network 6.

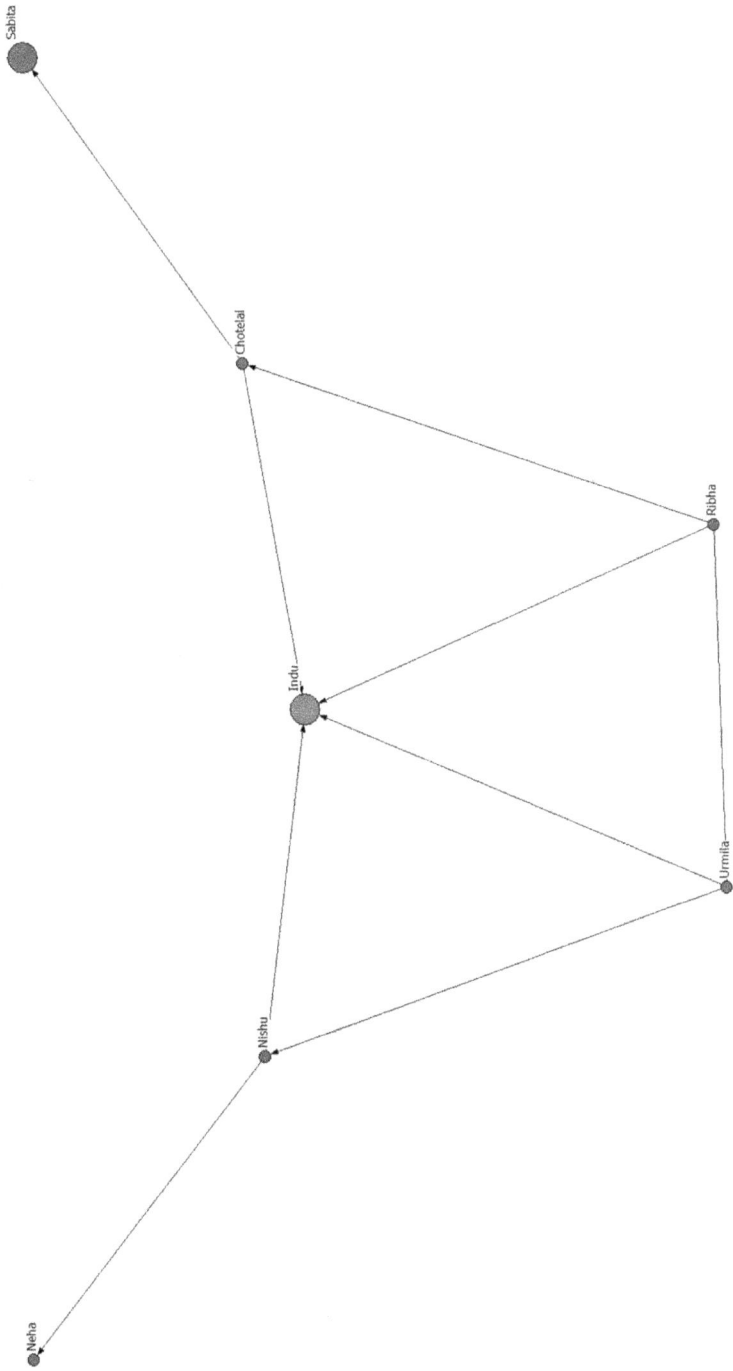

Figure 6.7 Sociogram of network 7.

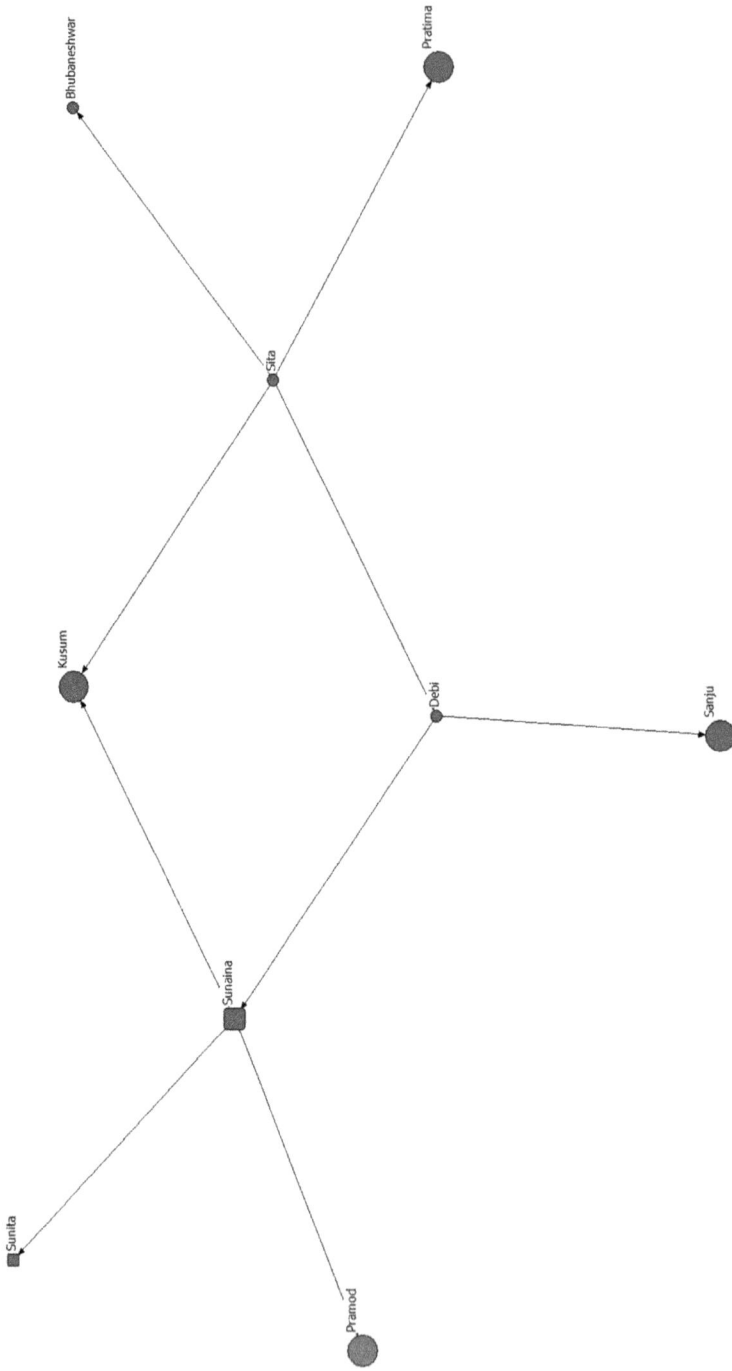

Figure 6.8 Sociogram of network 8.

Table 6.10 E–I Index (caste) of the networks

E–I Index Measures	1	2	3	4	5	6	7	8
E–I Index	-1.00	-1.00	-1.00	-0.27	-0.60	-1.00	-0.11	-0.78
Expected E–I	-1.00	-1.00	-1.00	-0.60	-0.50	-1.00	-0.43	-0.56
Rescaled E–I	-1.00	.	.	-0.11	.-0.14	.	-0.33	-0.75
Probability	1.00	1.00	1.00	0.30	1.00	1.00	0.146	1.00

Source: Estimated from primary survey.

An important feature of all the maps is the high proportion of links with members of the same caste. This feature is analysed in the next sub-section.

6.4.7 Caste-based homophily

Table 6.10 gives the values of the raw E–I index, and its adjusted values, when actors are grouped by caste. In some networks, however, the actors all belong to the same caste. In such cases, UCINET does not give the rescaled E–I index. Results reveal a strong element of caste-based homophily, with raw values ranging from -0.11 (network 7) to -1 (first three networks). Expected values (when available) are higher, with a minimum of -0.43 (network 7). These results indicate the tendency of respondents to self-select among establishing ties with the same caste members. Even though the E–I values are high, an important question is whether such results are genuine, or a result of the way in which networks are drawn, or sampling variability. The probability values given in the last row indicate that the observed deviation from randomness is statistically significant.

6.4.8 Kinship relations

We have also examined two possible forms of homophilic interactions – based on kinship and between JEEViKA members. Except for network 5, there does not seem to be any preference for interaction with JEEViKA members either (Table 6.11). A possible reason for this is that the mobility of most women of childbearing age is restricted, thereby hindering their interactions with other JEEViKA members. The only scope for interaction is the meetings; but, even in the case of meetings, in many cases, mothers-in-law deposit the weekly subscriptions, and attend the meetings on their behalf. During FGDs, JEEViKA members reported that "Sometimes we have work so we don't attend regularly"; in such cases "we send our mothers-in-law if (we) can't go ....", or "... send money through my mother-in-law to submit".

While kinship may often form an important basis of networks (Hamberger et al., 2011), in this case, prima facie it does not seem to be an important

Table 6.11 E–I Index (JEEViKA) of the networks

E–I Index Measures	1	2	3	4	5	6	7	8
E–I Index	-0.07	0.00	-0.80	-0.27	-0.07	0.00	-1.00	0.11
Expected E–I	-0.07	0.00	-0.39	-0.29	0.14	-0.14	-1.00	-0.05
Rescaled E–I	-0.07		-0.80	-0.27	-0.33			0.11

Source: Estimated from primary survey.

Table 6.12 E–I Index (kinship) of the networks

E–I Index measures	1	2	3	4	5	6	7	8
E–I Index	0.07	0.00	0.00	0.46	-0.20	-0.25	0.11	0.33
Expected E–I	0.02	0.00	0.18	0.20	-0.14	0.50	-0.05	0.33
Rescaled E–I	0.07			0.46	0.00	0.14	0.11	0.33
Dropping health workers and doctors								
E–I Index	-0.25	-1.00	-0.78	0.25	-1.00	0.33	-1.00	-0.60
Expected E–I	-0.04	-1.00	-0.50	0.05	-1.00	0.43	-1.00	-0.33
Rescaled E–I	0.00		-0.71	0.25	1.00	0.33		-0.60
Probability	0.43	1.00	1.00	0.38	1.00	0.78	1.00	1.00

Source: Estimated from primary survey.

basis for forming social ties (Table 6.12). However, if we exclude health workers and doctors, we will find that the resultant networks exhibit a high degree of kin-based homophily. Moreover, the majority of existing ties are with relatives belonging to the husband's family.

6.5 Evidence from FGDs

According to ASHA workers, mothers-in-law played a very important role in the utilisation of MCH services for pregnant women. The reason is that, in most households, the former is treated as the guardian. Young women had to obey them, and any opposition would create marital discord and result in oppression by other family members. As participants in FGDs revealed:

P8: *See, before taking any decision you need to consult with your guardians, right? So without asking your husband and discussing this with your guardians at home – like mother-in-law or father-in-law – how can you take such decisions?*

P3: *Yes, and mostly from our mother-in-law.*

P7: *See, our husband may be our overall guardian; but within our house, the guardian is our mother-in-law. So we have to ask her and discuss these things with her before finalising anything.*

The control of the mothers-in-law partly stems from the absence of the husband from the home:

> *They (husbands) are busy with their work and so they don't have that much information about what we do ... This is the matter of women and so women who are guardians, like my mother-in-law, take care of these matters.*

Seeking the husband's approval becomes a matter of routine: "*Mostly we tell them by phone and they approve*".

As mothers-in-laws are old and hold outdated beliefs, there is a scope for potential conflict between her values, and those held by younger women. One of the FGD participants remarked

> "*See, my mother-in-law is from an older generation ... She doesn't understand the need to limit fertility*".

P2: *This is not the concern of her, she would always want as much as kids, but then it's the parents who have to feed them.*

Most of the conflict arises over limiting fertility by adopting contraception methods, choice of delivery (i.e., home or health facility), and immunisation of children. In such situations, mothers-in-law feel threatened if the younger women establish connections outside the home, as they feel that it may lead the latter to adopt MCH practices that she disapproves of (Anukriti et al., 2020).

ASHA workers reported that, to minimise intra-household conflict, they generally involve the mother-in-law in their discussion during visits to the home of a pregnant women and try to convince the older women. Convincing the mothers-in-law, according to the ASHAs, is the "*key to behaviour change*". Participants of FGDs also acknowledged that, as ASHAs visit their home, "*when she tells something all the family members could learn and understand that. When she provides information everyone listens to her and also tries to understand and follow*". Respondents also admitted that the approach followed by ASHAs makes adopting new practices "*less difficult for us*".

The positive "brokerage" role played by the mother-in-law is facilitated by three factors. The first factor is an overall increase in awareness in the villages:

In the past no one was aware about the MCH practices that should be followed. ... Now people are getting to know about such practices and understand that a lot has changed; it leads them to modify their behaviour from what they did in the past.

Secondly, behaviour change is facilitated by the young age of the mother-in-law. While it is true that mothers-in-law are older, the term "old" is a misnomer, as women marry early in rural Bihar, and generally complete their fertility period by the age of 25. So a mother-in-law would be about 45 years. The age gap with the daughters-in-laws, therefore, is not very large.

Thirdly, in some cases, it is the mother-in-law who joins the JEEViKA. In such cases, she is the target of the motivating campaigns, and passes on the knowledge to her daughters-in-law:

My mother-in-law is a member of JEEViKA, and she regularly attends the group meetings. She understands what dietary practices should be followed to keep a child healthy, and she passes on the information imparted in group meetings to me to so that I can feed my child as advised in the group meetings.

This situation, however, has the potential danger since the mother-in-law becomes the gatekeeper through which information must flow to her daughter-in-law. Even if the woman is a JEEViKA member, she is often unable to attend the meetings as she has to look after her child and undertake other household chores. There are also restrictions on their movement. In such circumstances, if the JEEViKA member is *"not able to attend the JEEViKA meetings, my mother-in-law attends them ... If someone is unable to go to the meetings, then what else can she do?"* The mother-in-law acquires the ability to manipulate the information received by the younger women and govern the latter's reproductive and fertility choices, and healthcare-seeking behaviour:

I have only one son and a daughter and she is afraid that something might happen to them. That is why she wants me to not go for ligation. I have to listen to her on this. I have no other option ... we can't deny our elders...

Q: Who mainly decides about opting for institutional delivery or home delivery?

P3: My mother-in-law says that it will increase the expense and so you should deliver at home.

In some cases, particularly as younger women are more educated and aware, the situation can plant the seed for a potential conflict:

*P2: My mother-in-law belongs to an older generation; she maintains tradi-
tional outdated beliefs and tells me to have as many children as possible.
She doesn't understand the benefits of family planning. ... She will always
want as many kids as possible. But it's the parents who have to feed them.*
*P7: My mother-in-law also keeps telling me to have more children. So I told
her, there will be nothing left for us to eat if we keep giving birth ...
The elders need to understand things were different before and times have
changed now.*

6.6 Discussion and conclusion

The results of the analysis of social networks and the evidence from FGDs
reveal that the flow of information from the ASHAs to the target women is
not one-to-one. Rather the process is mediated by the senior female member
in the household, the mother-in-law. The latter plays the role of a gatekeeper,
mediating the interaction of the younger family members of reproductive age
with non-family members. This allows her to control the flow of information
to her daughter-in-law and enables her to sustain both social norms and her
position of authority.

Such a conceptualisation of the interaction between the target women and
the ASHA is a unique finding of this study. Existing studies of community
health workers in India and other developing countries have ignored the process of interaction, stressing on whether there is any behavioural change or
not (Andrews et al., 2004; Okuga et al., 2015; Panday et al., 2017; Wagner
et al., 2018; Agarwal et al., 2019; Bettampadi et al., 2019; Bonifácio et al.,
2019; Burnett-Zieman et al., 2021; Nadella et al., 2021). The finding that the
actual process of interaction is neither simple nor one-to-one has important
implications for research and policymaking.

With regard to research implications, this study argues that the traditional
approach to a male-centric patriarchal society may not be useful in analysing
the complex realities of the current society in Bihar. Existing studies have
argued that the patriarchal society existing in South Asian countries gener-
ates gendered norms that:

> associate men with authority and control over resources and women with
> submissive and reproductive roles. These norms ... constrain women's
> voice, freedom of physical mobility, and role in the economy, and repre-
> sent an important social mechanism by which gender inequality persists.
> (Petesch & Badstue, 2020, p. 291)

Given the limited interpersonal control of women over their lives and
dependence on husbands and older family members for health-related

decision-making researchers tend to focus on the role of male members, particularly husbands, in the utilisation of health care by women (Becker, 1996; Balaiah et al., 1999; Becker & Costenbader, 2001; Population Council, 2005; Walston, 2005; Chattopadhyay, 2012):

> Men play important and often dominant roles in making decisions that are crucial to women's reproductive health. Because of the low status of women in the Indian society, they still have to depend on their husbands in order to receive appropriate and adequate health care for their illnesses.
> (Singh & Arora, 2008, p. 219)

The findings of this chapter are more in line with those of recent studies have argued that an exclusive focus on the domination of women by male household members diverts attention from the fact that women's empowerment is also constrained by power relations between female members, leading to oppression of women by women (Cornwall, 2007; Vera-Sanso, 2012). The role of "inter-generational power struggles between daughters-in-law and mothers-in-law in shaping household dynamics in South Asia" (Gram et al., 2018, p. 194) has, in particular, been the focus of several studies (Bennet, 1983, 1992; Kandiyoti, 1988; Mandelbaum, 1993; Minturn & Kapoor, 1993; Vera-Sanso, 2012; Allendorf, 2017). It has been pointed out that, in the early years of marriage, the relations with her mother-in-law is more important than power relations with her husband in shaping her agency:

> Women ... have remarkably few social connections outside their homes, and co-residence with the mother-in-law is a significant barrier to a woman's mobility and ability to tap into her caste-based village networks, resulting in detrimental impacts on her access and utilisation of reproductive health services.
> (Anukriti et al., 2020, pp. 1–2)

This phenomenon may be attributed to the low mobility of South Asian women reported in various studies (Khan, 1999; Eswaran et al., 2013; Bankar et al., 2018; Kapur, 2019). Even though women above 30 years are more mobile now (Datta and Rustogi, 2012), movements of newly married women, or those with young children, are still severely restricted within the *tola* to ensure the paternity of children (Eswaran et al., 2013).

Given that "Relationships between mothers-in-law and daughters-in-law were notoriously fraught in the South Asian context as they competed for the affection and loyalty of the same man who is their primary source of support" (Kabeer, 2012), mother-in-law may exploit their gatekeepers' position to deprive their daughter-in-law of knowledge and maintain the traditional hierarchical order. This is also confirmed in the present study.

Our study also reveals the caste-based nature of information networks in Bihar. This is in line with the existing literature on the importance of caste as an important form of identity, or marker of community or cultural differ-ence in India (Fuller, 1996; Gupta, 2004), and strong caste-based networks reported in studies (Mobarak & Rosenzweig, 2012; Munshi & Rosenzweig, 2016; Munshi, 2019). In Bihar, given the importance of caste in economic, social, and political relations (Sahay, 1998, 2009), it is only to be expected that the social environment will favour an information diffusion mechanism that is restricted to the same caste members. Since caste is an immutable char-acteristic, the tendency of the actors to interact with other actors belonging to the same caste is an important form of self-selection (Easley & Kleinberg, 2010, p. 81) that has been documented in other studies (Mosse, 2018) as well.

To conclude, results from our analysis of networks indicate the need to consider the power relations within the society and family, and specifically the role of older female relatives. Such factors need to be incorporated into policymaking so that the outreach activities of ASHAs become more effective.

Notes

1 Self-ties are ignored. If ties are undirected (i.e. AB is the same as BA), potential ties will number n × (n - 1) /2.
2 Key players may be identified in four ways:

   (i) The concept of node centrality may be used to quantify the structural impor-tance of actors in a network (Bonacich, 1972; Freeman, 1978);
   (ii) It is also possible to identify key players by distinguishing between cores and peripheries (Seidman, 1983; Everett and Borgatti, 1999; Borgatti and Everett, 2000);
   (iii) Group-level centrality is another way to detect key players (Everett and Borgatti, 2000); and,
   (iv) Assess the contribution of a set of actors to the cohesion of the network (Borgatti, 2006).

   We have used the fourth method in our analysis.

References

Adams, A. M., Nababan, H. Y., & Hanifi, S. M. M. A. (2015). Building social networks for maternal and newborn health in poor urban settlements: A cross-sectional study in Bangladesh. *PLoS One*, 10(4), e0123817. http://doi.org/10.1371/journal.pone.0123817

Agarwal, S. et al. (2019). Are community health workers effective in retaining women in the maternity care continuum? Evidence from India. *BMJ Global Health*, 4(4), e001557. http://doi.org/10.1136/bmjgh-2019-001557

Allendorf, K. (2017). Like her own: Ideals and experiences of the mother-in-law/daughter-in-law relationship. *Journal of Family Issues*, 38(15), 2102–2127. http://doi.org/10.1177/0192513X15590685

Andrews, J. O. et al. (2004). Use of community health workers in research with ethnic minority women. *Journal of Nursing Scholarship*, 36(4), 358–365. http://doi.org/10.1111/j.1547-5069.2004.04064.x

Anukriti, S. et al. (2020). Curse of the Mummy-JI Irse oinfluence of mothers-in-law on women in India †. *American Journal of Agricultural Economics*, 102(5), 1328–1351. http://doi.org/10.1111/ajae.12114

Balaiah, D. et al. (1999). Contraceptive knowledge, attitude and practices of men in rural Maharashtra. *Advances in Contraception*, 15(3), 217–234. http://doi.org/10.1023/A:1006753617161

Bankar, S. et al. (2018). Contesting restrictive mobility norms among female mentors implementing a sport based programme for young girls in a Mumbai slum. *BMC Public Health*, 18(1), 471. http://doi.org/10.1186/s12889-018-5347-3

Barlett, C. P. et al. (2018). Social media use as a tool to facilitate or reduce cyberbullying perpetration: A review focusing on anonymous and nonanonymous social media platforms. *Violence and Gender*, 5(3), 147–152. http://doi.org/10.1089/vio.2017.0057

Barnett, G. A. (2001). A longitudinal analysis of the international telecommunication network, 1978–1996. *American Behavioral Scientist*, 44(10), 1638–1655. http://doi.org/10.1177/0002764201044010007

Bavelas, A. (1950). Communication patterns in task-oriented groups. *The Journal of the Acoustical Society of America*, 22(6), 725–730. http://doi.org/10.1121/1.1906679

Becker, S. (1996). Couples and reproductive health: A review of couple studies. *Studies in Family Planning*, 27(6), 291. http://doi.org/10.2307/2138025

Becker, S., & Costenbader, E. (2001). 'Husbands' and wives' reports of contraceptive use. *Studies in Family Planning*, 32(2), 111–129. http://doi.org/10.1111/j.1728-4465.2001.00111.x

Bennet, L. (1983). *Dangerous wives and sacred sisters*. Edited by C.U. Press.

Bennet, L. (1992). *Women, poverty and productivity in India (Report No. 10595)*. .

Bertin, J. (1983). *Semiology of graphics: Diagrams networks maps*. University of Wisconsin Press.

Bettampadi, D. et al. (2019). Are community health workers cost-effective for childhood vaccination in India? *Vaccine*, 37(22), 2942–2951. http://doi.org/10.1016/j.vaccine.2019.04.038

Blau, P. M. (1977). *Inequality and heterogeneity: A primitive theory of social structure*. Free Press.

Bonacich, P. (1972). Factoring and weighting approaches to status scores and clique identification. *The Journal of Mathematical Sociology*, 2(1), 113–120. http://doi.org/10.1080/0022250X.1972.9989806

Bonacich, P. (1987). Power and centrality: A family of measures. *American Journal of Sociology*, 92(5), 1170–1182. http://doi.org/10.1086/228631

Bonifácio, L. P., Marques, J. M. A., & Vieira, E. M. (2019). Assessment of the knowledge of Brazilian community health workers regarding prenatal care. *Primary Health Care Research & Development*, 20, e21. http://doi.org/10.1017/S1463423618000725

Borgatti, S. (1995). Centrality and AIDS. *Connections*, 18, 112–115.

Borgatti, S. P. (2006). Identifying sets of key players in a social network. *Computational and Mathematical Organization Theory*, *12*(1), 21–34. http://doi.org/10.1007/s10588-006-7084-x

Borgatti, S. P., & Everett, M. G. (2000). Models of core/periphery structures. *Social Networks*, *21*(4), 375–395. http://doi.org/10.1016/S0378-8733(99)00019-2

Burnett-Zieman, B. et al. (2021). Community-based postnatal care services for women and newborns in Kenya: An opportunity to improve quality and access? *Journal of Global Health*, *11*, 07006. http://doi.org/10.7189/jogh.11.07006

Burris, V. (2005). Interlocking directorates and political cohesion among corporate elites. *American Journal of Sociology*, *111*(1), 249–283. http://doi.org/10.1086/428817

Cook, K. S., Emerson, R. M., Gillmore, M. R., & Yamagishi, T. (1983). The distribution of power in exchange networks: Theory and experimental results. *American Journal of Sociology*, 89(2), 275–305. https://doi.org/10.1086/227866.

Chattopadhyay, A. (2012). Men in maternal care: Evidence from India. *Journal of Biosocial Science*, *44*(2), 129–153. doi:10.1017/S0021932011000502.

Coleman, J. S., Johnstone, J. W. C., & Jonassohn, K. (1981). *The adolescent society: The social life of the teenager and its impact on education*. Greenwood Press.

Coleman, J. S., Katz, E., & Menzel, E. (1966). *Medical innovations: A diffusion study*. Bobs-Merrill Company Inc.

Cornwall, A. (2007). Myths to live by? Female solidarity and female autonomy reconsidered. *Development and Change*, *38*(1), 149–168. http://doi.org/10.1111/j.1467-7660.2007.00407.x

Datta, A., & Rustogi, P. (2012). *Status of women in Bihar: Exploring transformation in work and gender relations*. Institute of Human Development.

Easley, D., & Kleinberg, J. (2010). *Networks, crowds, and markets: Reasoning about a highly connected world*. Cambridge University Press.

Eswaran, M., Ramaswami, B., & Wadhwa, W. (2013). Status, caste, and the time allocation of women in rural India. *Economic Development and Cultural Change*, *61*(2), 311–333. http://doi.org/10.1086/668282

Everett, M. G., & Borgatti, S. P. (1999). The centrality of groups and classes. *The Journal of Mathematical Sociology*, *23*(3), 181–201. http://doi.org/10.1080/0022250X.1999.9990219

Everett, M. G., & Borgatti, S. P. (2000). Peripheries of cohesive subsets. *Social Networks*, *21*(4), 397–407. http://doi.org/10.1016/S0378-8733(99)00020-9

Feld, S. L. (1981). The focused organization of social ties. *American Journal of Sociology*, *86*(5), 1015–1035. http://doi.org/10.1086/227352

Feld, S. L. (1982). Social structural determinants of similarity among associates. *American Sociological Review*, *47*(6), 797. http://doi.org/10.2307/2095216

Fowler, J. H., & Christakis, N. A. (2009). Dynamic spread of happiness in a large social network: Longitudinal analysis over 20 years in the Framingham Heart Study. *BMJ (Online)*, *338*(7685), 23–26. http://doi.org/10.1136/BMJ.A2338

Frank, K. A. (1996). Mapping interactions within and between cohesive subgroups. *Social Networks*, *18*(2), 93–119. http://doi.org/10.1016/0378-8733(95)00257-X

Freeman, L. C. (1978). Centrality in social networks conceptual clarification. *Social Networks*, *1*(3), 215–239. http://doi.org/10.1016/0378-8733(78)90021-7

Freeman, L. C. (1996). VIsualizing social networks. *Journal of Social Structure*, *1*. https://www.cmu.edu/joss/content/articles/volume1/Freeman.html

Freeman, L. C., Borgatti, S. P., & White, D. R. (1991). Centrality in valued graphs: A measure of betweenness based on network flow. *Social Networks*, 13(2), 141–154. http://doi.org/10.1016/0378-8733(91)90017-N

Fuller, C. (Ed.). (1996). *Caste today*. Oxford University Press.

Garip, F. (2008). Social capital and migration: How do similar resources lead to divergent outcomes? *Demography*, 45(3), 591–617. http://doi.org/10.1353/dem.0.0016

Gram, L. et al. (2018). Revisiting the patriarchal bargain: The intergenerational power dynamics of household money management in rural Nepal. *World Development*, 112, 193–204. http://doi.org/10.1016/j.worlddev.2018.08.002

Granoveter, M. (1994). *Getting a job: A study of contacts and careers*. Northwestern University Press.

Granovetter, M. (1983). The strength of weak ties: A network theory revisited. *Sociological Theory*, 1, 201. http://doi.org/10.2307/202051

Granovetter, M. S. (1982). Alienation reconsidered econsistrength of weak ties. *Connections*, 4–16.

Gupta, D. (Ed.). (2004). *Caste in question: Identity or hierarchy?* SAGE.

Hamberger, K, Houseman, M., & White, D. R. (2011). Kinship network analysis. In J. Scott & P. J. Carrington (Eds.), *The SAGE handbook of 2social network analysis* (pp. 533–549). Sage Publications.

Hanneman, R. A., & Riddle, M. (2011). Concepts and measures for basic network analysis. In J. Scott & P. J. Carrington (Eds.), *The SAGE handbook of social network analysis* (pp. 340–369). Sage Publications Inc.

Kabeer, N. (2012). The decline in 'missing women' in Bangladesh. *Blog posted on 9 November* [Preprint]. Retrieved January 18, 2021, from http://nailakabeer.net/2012/11/09/the-decline-in-missing-women-in-bangladesh/

Kandiyoti, D. (1988). Bargaining with patriarchy. *Gender & Society*, 2(3), 274–290. http://doi.org/10.1177/089124388002003004

Kapur, R. (2019). Status of women in rural areas. *Acta Scientific Agriculture*, 3(8), 17–24. http://doi.org/10.31080/ASAG.2019.03.0558

Khan, A. (1999). Mobility of women and access to health and family planning services in Pakistan. *Reproductive Health Matters*, 7(14), 39–48. http://doi.org/10.1016/S0968-8080(99)90005-8

Krackhardt, D. (1994). Graph theoretical dimensions of informal organizations. In K. Carley & M. Prietula (Eds.), *Computational organizational theory* (pp. 89–111). Lawrence Erlbaum Associates, Inc.

Krackhardt, D., & Stern, R. N. (1988). Informal networks and organizational crises: An experimental simulation. *Social Psychology Quarterly*, 51(2), 123. http://doi.org/10.2307/2786835

Krebs, V. E. (2002). Mapping networks of terrorist cells. *Connections*, 24(3), 43–52.

Lazarsfeld, P., & Merton, R. K. (1954). Friendship as a social process: A substantive and methodological analysis. In M. Berger, T. Abel, & C. H. Page (Eds.), *Freedom and control in modern society* (pp. 18–66). Van Nostrand Inc.

Leavitt, H. J. (1951). Some effects of certain communication patterns on group performance. *The Journal of Abnormal and Social Psychology*, 46(1), 38–50. http://doi.org/10.1037/h0057189

Lois, D. (2022). Social networks, family social capital, and child health. In *Social networks and health inequalities* (pp. 109–128). Springer International Publishing. http://doi.org/10.1007/978-3-030-97722-1_7

Mandelbaum, D. G. (1993). *Women's seclusion and men's honor: Sex roles in North India, Bangladesh, and Pakistan*. University of Arizona Press.

McPherson, M., Smith-Lovin, L., & Cook, J. M. (2001). Birds of a feather: Homophily in social networks. *Annual Review of Sociology, 27*(1), 415–444. http://doi.org/10.1146/annurev.soc.27.1.415

Minturn, L., & Kapoor, S. (1993). *Sita's daughters: Coming out of purdah: The Rajput women of Khalapur revisited*. Oxford University Press.

Mobarak, A. M., & Rosenzweig, M. R. (2012). *Selling formal insurance to the informally insured*. https://ssrn.com/abstract=2009528.

Mosse, D. (2018). Caste and development: Contemporary perspectives on a structure of discrimination and advantage. *World Development, 110*, 422–436. http://doi.org/10.1016/j.worlddev.2018.06.003

Mukong, A. K., & Burns, J. (2020). Social networks and antenatal care utilisation in Tanzania. *Scientific African, 9*, p. e00535. http://doi.org/10.1016/j.sciaf.2020.e00535

Munshi, K. (2011). Strength in numbers: Networks as a solution to occupational traps. *The Review of Economic Studies, 78*(3), 1069–1101. http://doi.org/10.1093/restud/rdq029

Munshi, K. (2019). Caste and the Indian economy. *Journal of Economic Literature, 57*(4), 781–834. http://doi.org/10.1257/jel.20171307

Munshi, K., & Rosenzweig, M. (2016). Networks and misallocation: Insurance, migration, and the rural-urban wage gap. *American Economic Review, 106*(1), 46–98. http://doi.org/10.1257/aer.20131365

Nadella, P., Subramanian, S. V., & Roman-Urrestarazu, A. (2021). The impact of community health workers on antenatal and infant health in India: A cross-sectional study. *SSM - Population Health, 15*, 100872. http://doi.org/10.1016/j.ssmph.2021.100872

Okuga, M. et al. (2015). Engaging community health workers in maternal and newborn care in eastern Uganda. *Global Health Action, 8*(1), 23968. http://doi.org/10.3402/gha.v8.23968

Panday, S. et al. (2017). The contribution of female community health volunteers (FCHVs) to maternity care in Nepal: A qualitative study. *BMC Health Services Research, 17*(1), 623. http://doi.org/10.1186/s12913-017-2567-7

Petesch, P., & Badstue, L. (2020). Gender norms and poverty dynamics in 32 Villages of South Asia. *International Journal of Community Well-Being, 3*(3), 289–310. http://doi.org/10.1007/s42413-019-00047-5

Population Council (2005). *Mixed success involving men in maternal care worldwide*. Available at: https://www.popcouncil.org/uploads/pdfs/factsheets/RH_MenInMaternalCare_A4.pdf.

Prell, C. (2012). *Social network analysis: History, theory and methodology*. Sage Publications.

Reyes, L. I. et al. (2022). Functions of social networks in maternal food choice for children in Mexico. *Maternal & Child Nutrition, 18*(1). http://doi.org/10.1111/mcn.13263

Rogers, E. (1962). *Diffusion of innovations* (5th ed.). The Free Press.

Sahay, G. R. (1998). Caste system in contemporary rural Bihar: A study of selected villages. *Sociological Bulletin*, *47*(2), 207–220. http://doi.org/10.1177/0038022919980205

Sahay, G. R. (2009). Major caste matters. *Contributions to Indian Sociology*, *43*(3), 411–441. http://doi.org/10.1177/006996670904300303

Scott, J. (2017). *Social network analysis* (4 ed.). Sage Publications Inc.

Seidman, S. B. (1983). Network structure and minimum degree. *Social Networks*, *5*(3), 269–287. http://doi.org/10.1016/0378-8733(83)90028-X

Singh, A., & Arora, A. (2008). How much do rural Indian husbands care for the health of their wives. *Indian Journal of Community Medicine*, *33*(1), 19. http://doi.org/10.4103/0970-0218.39238

Skvoretz, J. (1985). Random and biased networks: Simulations and approximations. *Social Networks*, *7*(3), 225–261. http://doi.org/10.1016/0378-8733(85)90016-4

Skvoretz, J. (1990). Biased net theory: Approximations, simulations and observations. *Social Networks*, *12*(3), 217–238. http://doi.org/10.1016/0378-8733(90)90006-U

Ssegujja, E., Ddumba, I., & Andipatin, M. (2022). Health workers' social networks and their influence in the adoption of strategies to address the stillbirth burden at a subnational level health system in Uganda. *PLOS Global Public Health*, *2*(7), p. e0000798. http://doi.org/10.1371/journal.pgph.0000798

Veblen, T. (1989). *The theory of the leisure class: An economic study of institutions*. Macmillan.

Vera-Sanso, P. (2012). Gender, poverty and old age, in urban south india in an era of globalisation. *Oxford Development Studies*, *40*(3), 324–340.

Wagner, A. L. et al. (2018). Have community health workers increased the delivery of maternal and child healthcare in India? *Journal of Public Health*, *40*(2), pp. e164–e170. http://doi.org/10.1093/pubmed/fdx087

Walston, N. (2005). *Challenges and opportunities for male involvement in reproductive health*. USAID.

Chapter 7

Signposts for the future

7.1 Recapitulation of objectives and methodology

7.1.1 Motivation of study

Health, nutrition, and population policies have a fundamental role in accelerating development and poverty alleviation. Improvements in the health status of individuals and populations – attained through health and nutrition policies – have contributed to economic growth. Acceleration of economic growth, in turn, leads to better health outcomes. This creates a virtuous cycle with good health boosting economic growth, thus facilitating economic growth and enabling improvements in health.

Despite the substantial investment in the health sector, and the associated improvement in health status, the progress in the domain of maternal and child health (MCH) has remained a major concern before policymakers and activists. In particular, the global performance in attaining Millenium Development Goals (MDGs) with respect to MCH targets demonstrates a dismal failure. India has been one of the underperformers; despite substantial improvement in the reduction of maternal and child mortality, India failed to attain the MDG targets (Shah, 2016). Moreover, there have been considerable regional variations related to improving MCH outcomes, with underperforming states being declared as the high focus states under the National Rural Health Mission (Balarajan et al., 2011; Bango & Ghosh, 2022; Baru & Bisth, 2010; Sanneving et al., 2013, 2013). Bihar is one such state.

In Bihar, at the onset of the National Health Mission, maternal health indicators like the proportion who received at least four antenatal care (ANC), full ANC, institutional delivery, and postnatal care (PNC) was significantly lower compared to the national average; this translated to higher than national average maternal mortality in Bihar (Ghosh & Husain, 2019). National Family Health Survey (NFHS) reports assert that infant and child mortality rates, too, substantially surpassed the all-India average, reflecting the poor nutritional status of children and failure to adopt recommended

DOI: 10.4324/9781003499251-7

dietary practices. Since 2005, however, there have been substantial efforts to improve the situation through a systematic and judicious implementation of health programmes by the Bihar government. Such efforts seem to have paid off as the level of utilisation of maternal health care services has improved in recent years (Ghosh & Husain, 2019). The last two rounds of NFHS also attest a steady improvement in MCH outcomes in Bihar.

While the progress in MCH outcomes was caused by both supply-side and demand-side factors, health communication – defined as "the art and technique of informing, influencing, and motivating individual, institutional, and public audiences about important health issues" (US Dept of Health and Human Services, 2000) – has also played a role in this process (Unnikrishnan et al., 2020) by dissemination of information and increasing awareness. However, the estimated impact of BCC reported in existing studies is often neither substantial in magnitude nor uniform across MCH practices and outcomes (Barnett et al., 2022). Given that BCC is undertaken in diverse socio-cultural contexts, it is not surprising that the effectiveness of such strategies is determined by constraints in the form of attitudes, norms, and practices embedded in the familial and community-level environment. Such community- and family-level features may pose bigger hindrances in a patriarchal society (Adhikari et al., 2020). Leveraging the different components of the BCC strategy to bypass or overcome such barriers to information dissemination and behavioural change requires a study of the diffusion of information and awareness within the community. Existing studies have focussed on the use of mass media (R. Ghosh et al., 2021), mobile phones (Rajkhowa & Qaim, 2022; Walia et al., 2020), microfinance institutions (Dehingia et al., 2019), and front-line health workers (Agarwal et al., 2019; Lyngdoh et al., 2018; Rammohan et al., 2021). Although the impact of peer effects on information dissemination (Katz & Lazarsfeld, 2005) and improving health outcomes (Bouckaert, 2014; Fletcher, 2014; Webel et al., 2010) has been widely reported, it has been largely neglected in the Indian context – with the exception of one study (Brooks et al., 2020).

7.1.2 Research questions

Based on this proposition, we framed our research questions as follows:

- What is the role of information networks and channels in improving MCH practices?
- What are the factors that determine the breadth of such networks?
- How effective are SHGs in improving MCH outcomes?
- Are there any peer effects from SHG members to non-members? What is their nature (viz. exogenous or endogenous)? Are they more effective than direct counselling by Accredited Social Health Activists (ASHAs)?
- What are the family and community-level obstacles to such information diffusion at the grass-roots level?

The broad areas in which behavioural change was examined are:

(i)   Controlling fertility,
(ii) Utilisation of ANC services,
(iii) Institutional delivery and availing of PNC services, and
(iv) Child health outcomes.

7.1.3 Data collection

Two sources of data were used in the study. The analysis undertaken in the chapter for the all-India level and for Bihar was based on the fifth round of the nationally representative National Family Health Survey (2019–20). In addition, data was collected through a primary survey conducted in six districts of Bihar. A multi-stage sampling design was adopted to select respondents. In the first stag-e, we selected 13 districts out of 38 districts of Bihar, where the JEEViKA Technical Support Programme (JTSP) and Health & Nutrition Strategy Programme (HNS) were in place during the last five years preceding the survey. In the second stage, these 13 districts were classified into three tercile groups based on a composite index of human development indicators, namely, percentages of non-scheduled castes (SC)/scheduled tribes (ST) population, female literacy, and male non-agricultural labourers. Data from the 2011 Census was used for this purpose. After selecting the study districts, i.e., at the fourth stage, four community development blocks were selected in each district based on the implementation of the JTSP and HNS programme. Two blocks were selected randomly where JTSP and HNS programmes had been implemented during the last five years, while another two blocks were also selected randomly from the rest of the blocks. In the fifth stage, five villages from each block were selected by employing the probability proportional to size sampling method. Thus, a total of 120 villages were selected. In the last stage, 20 women comprising ten JEEViKA members and ten non-members were selected from each village. Thus, the planned sample size of the study was 2400. The recruitment criterion was that the respondent had at least one living child aged below three years, and was a permanent resident of the village. Due to the lockdown and travel restrictions imposed following COVID-19, we could complete the survey for 2250 respondents.

The analysis of the sample profile reveals that JEEViKA members are older, less educated, poorer, and have a higher number of children. A higher proportion of JEEViKA members are engaged in income-earning activities, although the overall proportion of working women is low. Differences between districts with respect to the availability of health services are minimal; overall, the survey villages have access to healthcare facilities. Other backward castes (OBCs) comprise the majority of the population in the survey villages.

It should be noted that our analysis is based on self-reported data, which were not verified independently. The possibility of social desirability bias with respondents overstating uptake of MCH practices cannot be ruled out. This is a limitation of our study.

The quantitative data was supplemented by 12 focus group discussions (FGDs) and 12 network maps. The qualitative survey was undertaken in four districts because of travel restrictions.

7.2 Summing up of results

7.2.1 Networks and information dissemination: Evidence from NFHS

In the absence of direct indicators to measure network, the analysis from NFHS data used some proxy indicators to prepare indices of media/internet exposure, knowledge and participation in microfinance activities, women's mobility outside home, exposure to family planning messages in media, and contact with front-line health workers by employing advance statistical methods. The analyses found that these indices generally have a significant positive influence on the outcome variables representing maternal and child healthcare utilisation, and use of modern contraceptive methods, with some exceptions, even after controlling for a range of confounding covariates. Additionally, the study also identified that socially marginalised and economically deprived groups lack access to networks and sources of information. These groups may be targeted to improve their access to information and networks, thereby improving their MCH outcomes. By examining the results of the analyses it was concluded that the importance of networks in the form of sources of information and contacts with SHGs and health workers are important determinants of MCH outcomes.

The analysis of variations in access to sources of information and networks helps to identify regions and socio-economic groups that lack access to such forms of social capital. It may make certain population groups vulnerable and affect their MCH outcomes adversely. For instance, compared to all-India levels, the mechanism for information diffusion in Bihar appears relatively poor; the only exception is SHGs. At the same time, we should note that the same population group may lack access to some forms of access but may be better placed with respect to other channels of information diffusion. In other words, sources of information are complementary and lack of access to one channel may be compensated by greater to another source. In general, however, older women, those with low levels of education and from Muslim households, are disadvantaged with respect to their networks and ability to access information. Such groups need to be targeted in BCC strategies.

7.2.2 Health communication through SHGs

Results reveal that adoption rates of recommended MCH practices are higher than state-level rates as reported in the third round of the National Family Health Survey (NFHS-3). The high figures cannot be entirely attributed to over-reporting, because preliminary results from NFHS-5 also indicate that there has been an improvement in the adoption of recommended ANC, PNC, and feeding practices in recent times. Bivariate analysis shows that adoption rates of the MCH practices studied are, in general, higher among younger respondents (those aged 17–20 years), more educated women, those from affluent households, and among respondents belonging to deprived/under-privileged (i.e., SC and ST) households.

Adoption rates of modern contraception rates, availing post-partum contraception advice, exclusive breastfeeding of children below six months, and complementary feeding of children aged 6–23 months are significantly higher among JEEViKA members, relative to non-members. Given that the HNS introduced by JEEViKA in 2016 focuses on dietary practices, this is an expected result. Econometric analysis undertaken using a multi-level probit model confirms this. Although univariate tests indicate that institutional and assisted delivery is significantly higher among non-members, the difference disappears after controlling for socio-demographic characteristics in the multi-level probit model. However, it should be kept in mind that being a JEEViKA member does not necessarily mean that the respondent receives "treatment" in the form of counselling from Community Mobilisers in the JEEViKA meetings. We found that only 50% of members have attended meetings in the last six months, while about a third of JEEViKA members have not taken part in any meetings in the last six months. Nevertheless, even after controlling for attendance in JEEViKA meetings, a programme effect is observed for the two components of JEEViKA's HNS – exclusive breastfeeding and complementary feeding. There is also a spill over of this programme effect from JEEViKA members to non-members, representing a peer effect. It is also reported by non-members in focus group discussions (FGDs). Not surprisingly, the spill over effect is lower than the program effect.

Analysis of marginal effects of the multi-level probit model indicates that utilisation of ANC and PNC services, institutional and assisted delivery, is conspicuously low among Muslim and H-FC women. It is also found that the adoption rate of availing first ANC check-up within the first trimester, availing of the recommended four ANC check-ups, availing of full ANC services, delivering in institutions, availing the assistance of skilled health workers during delivery, availing post-partum services including contraception advice, and ensuring polio vaccine at birth for their children is likely to be higher among more educated women. On the other hand, an inverse U-shaped relationship is observed between education levels and the predicted likelihood of using modern contraception methods, availing protection against natal tetanus and supplementing breastfeeding of a child with semi-solid and solid food after six months. Variations in the predicted likelihood of adopting MCH practices across asset index scores show a positive trend for most practices, implying that women from affluent households are more likely to adopt such practices. However, exclusive breastfeeding till six months and complementary feeding after six months are less common among affluent households.

7.2.3 Peer effect and its nature

It is also found that village adoption rates had a significant and positive impact on the probability of respondents adopting the MCH practices studied. It indicates the possibility of a peer effect. Although there is evidence of a peer effect, this requires closer investigation before concluding that the adoption rate of MCH practices is influenced by the behaviour of peers. For instance, people may behave similarly without influencing each other if they are exposed to a common health shock (Manski, 1993). This would generate an exogenous peer effect. In Bihar, for instance, the activity of the Accredited Social Health Activists (ASHAs) workers and the HNS of JEEViKA are two important common factors that may influence the behaviour of respondents. After controlling for ASHA activity, however, we still find that respondents tend to influence each other. This is observed for all the MCH practices studied. So an endogenous peer effect cannot be ruled out.

7.2.4 Role of ASHA

Although an endogenous peer effect is observed, we find that ASHAs play a major role in motivating behaviour-related changes among respondents. Respondents report that ASHA workers exert the strongest influence on their behaviour, with family members as a distant second. Husbands play an important role in the choice of modern contraception methods. Other family members (mothers-in-law and sisters-in-law) play a significant role as well in encouraging respondents to adopt contraceptives, avail of ANC services, deliver in institutions, exclusively breastfeed children till six months, and supplement diet after six months. Although we had found a significant program effect for exclusive breastfeeding and supplementary feeding, only one out of seven respondents acknowledged the role of JEEViKA members and officers in the adoption of these two practices.

It is observed that the identity of the main motivator varies with the education of respondent, the wealth of family, and socio-religious identity. Less educated women or those from economically or socially disadvantaged households report that ASHAs are playing a fundamental role in spreading awareness about MCH practices. Strikingly the influence of ASHAs on women with more than ten years of education and affluent households is, however, limited. ASHAs report that such women do not trust public health facilities and rely on private facilities:

> *You know what happens to the upper caste? They think that they have money so they will not avail of any government facilities.*

ASHAs also complain that there is no use trying to motivate them (*"Un logon ko aab keya samjhaye")* as *"They have money! Now what we will explain to them, they know it all".* We also observe that the influence of family members, viz. husband and mother-in-law, is strongest among women belonging to SC, ST, and Muslim women.

Econometric analysis shows that the influence of ASHA and other health workers is greater on JEEViKA members in the case of MCH practices like availing of recommended four ANC check-ups, ensuring protection against tetanus, taking iron folic acid tablets or syrup, delivering in an institution, availing of assisted delivery, giving polio vaccine at birth to the child, and complementary feeding of children aged between 7 and 35 months. Regression results also confirm that ASHAs have less influence over women from affluent backgrounds and also the educated ones; however, the influence of ASHAs does not vary systematically across socio-religious groups.

7.2.5 Channels of information flow

The presence of an exogenous peer effect indicates the need to examine the channels through which information diffuses within the community. To undertake this analysis, we have studied the information networks existing between respondents and health workers, via other actors, existing in 12 villages.

Our analysis reveals that existing information networks are small, low-density, and they can operate with closely connected actors. The geodesic distance is low, on an average. It implies that the information will diffuse quickly within the networks. Networks are strongly hierarchical, with ASHAs playing the role of "boss" (Krackhardt, 1994), disseminating information throughout the community. Moreover, ASHAs can transmit information to respondents through alternative channels, increasing the credibility of the information. Values of β-centrality (Bonacich, 1972) indicate that respondents are well connected to the central players of the network. ASHAs, too, have strong connections to the family. The hierarchical nature of the networks, however, has one weakness. Such networks have high fragmentation values. It implies that such networks are unstable, and certain players can become key actors in the process of diffusion of information. In such a situation, a potential danger is that the key player may block or distort the flow of information to the respondent.

7.2.6 Saas *as gatekeepers*

Although ASHAs comprise the core from which information diffuses within the community, analysis of the networks reveals a potential problem. The networks are small, of low density, caste-based, and hierarchical. Despite the fact that ASHA is the source from whom information is disseminated throughout the community, such information generally proceeds through the mother-in-law (*saas*). Given that "married women ... live in households that are headed by an older woman, usually the mother-in-law" (Kabeer, 2010), the latter can become a key player in the network. If the mother-in-law becomes the gatekeeper through whom information flows from the ASHA to the respondent, the former is in a position to control the information flow – either withholding the information or distorting it – so that the "oppressive exercise of authority by mothers-in-law over their daughters-in-law" (Kabeer, 1999) persists. In line with a similar study undertaken in Mexico (Molyneux & Thomson, 2011), we have found that, if there is a conflict between the information being provided and existing practices, tension may be generated within the family; in such cases, the mother-in-law may even use her position as a gatekeeper to ensure that existing practices are adhered to.

7.3 Signposts for the future

The starting proposition of this study was that supply-side measures are not enough to improve MCH outcomes; investment to upgrade healthcare facilities must be supplemented by demand-side intervention to improve awareness, leading to behaviour change. Our analysis reveals that both the National Health Mission (NHM) and HNS of JEEViKA have implemented this principle, and focussed on creating awareness about recommended MCH practices through BCC strategies.

Now, the thrust of BCC policies before the NHM was on an aggregate level intervention through community-level campaigns, distribution of publicity material, advertisements over the mass media, etc. Such BCC strategies did not rely on individual-level counselling or face-to-face interactions with the target recipients. After the introduction of the NHM, front-line health workers like the ASHAs became an important component of the BCC strategy; given that such health workers were females, they were able to reach target groups at home and were largely successful in inducing behavioural change with respect to several MCH practices and outcomes (Agarwal et al., 2019; Nadella et al., 2021; Rammohan et al., 2021). Although a general increase in awareness and education was responsible for the improved rates of adoption of MCH practices as reported in the last two rounds of NFHS, and further confirmed in this study, in conformity to other studies (Bajpai et al., 2009; Panda et al., 2013; Paul & Pandey, 2020), the role of the ASHA workers is observed to be crucial in effecting such behavioural change.

The success of the ASHA workers may be attributed to the strategy adopted by them. While the literature has focussed on the role of husbands in decision-making on reproductive health (Blunch, 2008; Kaggwa et al., 2008; Myo-Myo-Mon & Liabsuetrakul, 2009; Samandari et al., 2010); in reality, it is the mother-in-law who is the main decision-maker and key actor in the household arena. By involving mother-in-laws in the discussions and motivating campaigns, ASHAs implicitly acknowledge and accept their dominance in the household arena; it avoids potential conflict but at the cost of allowing mothers-in-law to control the flow of information to the target recipients. This has both positive and negative consequences. In some cases, the mother-in-law has been very supportive and assisted their daughter-in-law to avail of ANC services; there are also many instances when the message of the ASHA has clashed with the traditional norms regarding notions of maintaining large families. Policy intervention must be directed to address the challenges posed by inter-generational power relations between women and aim to tackle the

> potential misalignment of fertility preferences and asymmetry of information and bargaining power between the MIL and DIL in a manner similar to the family planning interventions that have aimed to challenge the intra-household allocation issues between husbands and wives.
>
> (Anukriti et al., 2020)

Specific practices that stand in disagreement with traditional norms should be identified; in such cases, the resistance of the mother-in-law has to be eroded by creating an argument that is relevant to her.

Currently, the focus seems to be on using microcredit groups (like JEEViKA) to empower women and enhance their agency, especially in the MCH domain. The logic underlying this strategy is clear – the involvement of microcredit groups improves the economic value of women so that their welfare becomes an important factor contributing to household decision-making (Fikree & Pasha, 2004). In Bangladesh, for instance, a "rise of the daughter-in-law" has been reported in recent years (Kabeer, 2012). It has been attributed to the increasing entry of women into the labour market, associated with the spread of microfinance, the growth of the export-based garment industry, and the introduction of new agrarian technology (Kabeer, 2012). While microfinance has often been portrayed as a vehicle of social change and empowerment of women (Kabeer, 2011, 2017), there is growing evidence that it is essentially in the nature of a consumption loan – smoothening the consumption stream, and enabling more efficient household money management – but with limited capacity for stimulating production activities (Attanasio et al., 2013; Breza & Kinnan, 2018; Guérin et al., 2010; Johnston & Morduch, 2008). It implies that there are restrictions on the ability of microfinance to empower women.[1] This raises the question as to whether microfinance groups need to be substituted by new institutions that will be more effective in bringing about the desired social changes

Our study also highlights the role of caste. Networks were found to be strongly homophilic. Not surprisingly, women from backward castes are influenced by ASHAs, who are often members of backward social groups.[2] It implies that outreach activities of the ASHAs are restricted to SC, ST, and OBC households, as reported in other studies also:

> the rural health workers such as the auxiliary nurse midwives and accredited social health activists seem to have adequate access and acceptability among rural poor, uneducated or semi-educated and underprivileged households, thus enabling them to convince these women to accept family planning easily…it difficult to penetrate and persuade the educated and influential households for family planning acceptance in the rural areas because of social barriers.
>
> (Ghosh & Keshri, 2020)

In fact, FGDs revealed antagonism between ASHAs and upper-caste women. It implies that any intervention strategy must take into account caste-based relations. Appointment of ASHAs may be recruited from the numerically dominant caste in the locality. As ASHAs are able to reach women from socially and economically backward groups easily, but are ineffectual in reaching forward-caste women who are, in general, more educated and affluent, other catalytic agents must be used to target the latter. Similar arguments were put forth by Ghosh and Keshri (2020) while discussing the acceptance of ASHA in disseminating family planning methods in rural Bihar. Albeit, media may play a conducive role in assisting changes.

Poverty and low levels of education have often been considered to be functional barriers to improve MCH outcomes. Investing in education and increasing household income appear to be possible means to improve MCH:

> The levels of household income and women's education within the household were key drivers of maternal mortality reduction and the increased uptake of MRH (maternal health and reproductive) services. Outside the programmatic interventions, only these two factors stand out as they were strongly correlated with improved MRH outcomes. Related to women's education within the household, completion of secondary education of girls, an education sector intervention, was also strongly correlated with improved MRH outcomes.
>
> (El-Saharty et al., 2016)

This claim does not hold true in the case of Bihar. Analysis of Sample Registration System and NFHS data reveals that fertility is higher among affluent households and educated families, while contraception usage is lower (S. Ghosh & Keshri, 2020). The present study observes that the incidence of exclusive breastfeeding and complementary feeding is lower among such families. The reasons for this perverse relationship need to be examined, and taken into account when designing intervention strategies.

Finally, we should recognise that improvement of MCH outcomes is not merely a matter of health and awareness but is related to a range of issues like economic empowerment, agency in the household domain, access to social support systems, and capability to tap social networks. Addressing all these issues is a complex task. It calls for the introduction of a multi-pronged strategy, cooperation between governments, non-governmental organizations, and international aid agencies, and engagement of gatekeepers in the household domain. Such strategies need to incorporate the convoluted cultural realities of the caste-ridden patriarchal society of the state.

Notes

1 In our study we found, for instance, that only one out of two members attended the monthly meetings.
2 This observation also holds true for women belonging to less affluent households, and with low levels of education.

References

Adhikari, T., Gulati, B. K., Juneja, A., Nair, S., Rao, M. V. V., Sharma, R. K., Saha, K. B., & Singh, S. (2020). Development of behaviour change communication model for improving male participation in maternal and child health services among Saharia Tribes in Gwalior district of Madhya Pradesh: A mixed method approach. *International Journal Of Community Medicine And Public Health*, 7(12), 5134. https://doi.org/10.18203/2394-6040.ijcmph20205197

Agarwal, S., Curtis, S. L., Angeles, G., Speizer, I. S., Singh, K., & Thomas, J. C. (2019). The impact of India's accredited social health activist (ASHA) program on the utilization of maternity services: A nationally representative longitudinal modelling study. *Human Resources for Health*, 17(1), 68. https://doi.org/10.1186/s12960-019-0402-4

Anukriti, S., Herrera-Almanza, C., Pathak, P. K., & Karra, M. (2020). Curse of the Mummy-ji: the influence of mothers-in-law on women in India †. *American Journal of Agricultural Economics*, 102(5), 1328–1351. https://doi.org/10.1111/ajae.12114

Attanasio, O., Augsburg, B., De Haas, R., Fitzsimons, E., & Harmgart, H. (2013). Group lending or individual lending? Evidence from a randomized field experiment in rural Mongolia. *SSRN Electronic Journal*. https://doi.org/10.2139/ssrn.2365432

Bajpai, N., Sachs, J. D., & Dholakia, R. H. (2009). *Improving access, service delivery and efficiency of the public health system in rural India: Midterm evaluation of the national rural health mission*. Center on Globalisation and Sustainable Development.

Balarajan, Y., Selvaraj, S., & Subramanian, S. (2011). Health care and equity in India. *The Lancet, 377*(9764), 505–515. https://doi.org/10.1016/S0140 -6736(10)61894-6

Bango, M., & Ghosh, S. (2022). Social and regional disparities in utilization of maternal and child healthcare services in India: A study of the post-national health mission period. *Frontiers in Pediatrics, 10.* https://doi.org/10.3389/fped.2022 .895033

Barnett, I., Meeker, J., Roelen, K., & Nisbett, N. (2022). Behaviour change communication for child feeding in social assistance: A scoping review and expert consultation. *Maternal and Child Nutrition, 18*(3), 1–14. https://doi.org/10.1111 /mcn.13361

Baru, R. V., & Bisth, R. (2010). *Health service inequities as a challenge to health security.* http://hdl.handle.net/10546/346634

Blunch, N.-H. (2008). *Human capital, religion and contraceptive use in Ghana* (Working Paper). http://www.csae.ox.ac.uk/conferences/2008-EdiA/papers/184 -Blunch.pdf

Bonacich, P. (1972). Factoring and weighting approaches to status scores and clique identification. *The Journal of Mathematical Sociology, 2*(1), 113–120. https://doi .org/10.1080/0022250X.1972.9989806

Bouckaert, N. (2014). Neighborhood peer effects in the use of preventive health care. *SSRN Electronic Journal.* https://doi.org/10.2139/ssrn.2381880

Breza, E., & Kinnan, C. (2018). *Measuring the equilibrium impacts of credit: Evidence from the Indian microfinance crisis.* https://doi.org/10.3386/w24329

Brooks, S. K., Webster, R. K., Smith, L. E., Woodland, L., Wessely, S., Greenberg, N., & Rubin, G. J. (2020). The psychological impact of quarantine and how to reduce it: Rapid review of the evidence. *The Lancet, 395*(10227), 912–920. https://doi .org/10.1016/S0140-6736(20)30460-8

Dehingia, N., Singh, A., Raj, A., & McDougal, L. (2019). More than credit: Exploring associations between microcredit programs and maternal and reproductive health service utilization in India. *SSM - Population Health, 9*(August), 100467. https:// doi.org/10.1016/j.ssmph.2019.100467

El-Saharty, S., Chowdhury, S., Ohno, N., & Sarker, I. (2016). *Improving maternal and reproductive health in South Asia: Drivers and enablers.* Washington, DC: World Bank. https://doi.org/10.1596/978-1-4648-0963-7

Fikree, F. F., & Pasha, O. (2004). Role of gender in health disparity: The South Asian context. *BMJ, 328*(7443), 823–826. https://doi.org/10.1136/bmj.328.7443.823

Fletcher, J. M. (2014). Peer effects in health behaviors. In A. J. Culyer (Ed.), *Encyclopedia of health economics* (1 ed, pp. 467–472). Elsevier. https://doi.org/10 .1016/B978-0-12-375678-7.00311-4

Ghosh, R., Mozumdar, A., Chattopadhyay, A., & Acharya, R. (2021). Mass media exposure and use of reversible modern contraceptives among married women in India: An analysis of the NFHS 2015–16 data. *PLoS One, 16*(7 July), 1–23. https://doi.org/10.1371/journal.pone.0254400

Ghosh, S., & Husain, Z. (2019). Has the national health mission improved utilisation of maternal healthcare services in Bihar? *Economic & Political Weekly, 54*(31), 44–51.

Ghosh, S., & Keshri, V. (2020). Women's education and fertility in the Hindi heartland. *Economic and Political Weekly, LV*(12), 54–57.

Guérin, I., Kumar, S., & Agier, I. (2010). *Microfinance and women's empowerment: Do relationships between women matter? Lessons from rural Southern India* (Working Papers CEB, Issues 10–053). ULB -- Universite Libre de Bruxelles. https://econpapers.repec.org/RePEc:sol:wpaper:2013/68292

Johnston, D., & Morduch, J. (2008). The Unbanked: Evidence from Indonesia. *The World Bank Economic Review, 22*(3), 517–537. https://doi.org/10.1093/wber/lhn016

Kabeer, N. (1999). Resources, agency, achievements: Reflections on the measurement of women's empowerment. *Development and Change, 30*(3), 435–464. https://doi.org/10.1111/1467-7660.00125

Kabeer, N. (2010). Women's empowerment, development interventions and the management of information flows. *IDS Bulletin, 41*(6), 105–113. https://doi.org/10.1111/j.1759-5436.2010.00188.x

Kabeer, N. (2011). Between affiliation and autonomy: Navigating pathways of women's empowerment and gender justice in rural Bangladesh. *Development and Change, 42*(2), 499–528. https://doi.org/10.1111/j.1467-7660.2011.01703.x

Kabeer, N. (2012). The rise of the daughter in law: The decline of missing women in Bangladesh. In *Blog posted on 8 November*. http://nailakabeer.net/2012/11/08/the-rise-of-the-daughter-in-law-the-decline-of-missing-women-in-bangladesh/

Kabeer, N. (2017). Economic pathways to women's empowerment and active citizenship: What does the evidence from Bangladesh Tell Us? *The Journal of Development Studies, 53*(5), 649–663. https://doi.org/10.1080/00220388.2016.1205730

Kaggwa, E. B., Diop, N., & Storey, J. D. (2008). The role of individual and community normative factors: A multilevel analysis of contraceptive use among women in union in Mali. *International Family Planning Perspectives, 34*(2), 79–88. https://doi.org/10.1363/ifpp.34.079.08

Katz, E., & Lazarsfeld, P. F. (2005). *Personal influence the part played by people in the flow of mass communications*. Transaction.

Krackhardt, D. (1994). Graph theoretical dimensions of informal organizations. In K. Carley & M. Prietula (Eds.), *Computational Organizational Theory* (pp. 89–111). Lawrence Erlbaum Associates, Inc.

Lyngdoh, T., Neogi, S. B., Ahmad, D., Soundararajan, S., & Mavalankar, D. (2018). Intensity of contact with frontline workers and its influence on maternal and newborn health behaviors: Cross-sectional survey in rural Uttar Pradesh, India. *Journal of Health, Population and Nutrition, 37*(1), 1–11. https://doi.org/10.1186/s41043-017-0129-6

Manski, C. F. (1993). Identification of endogenous social effects: The reflection problem. *The Review of Economic Studies, 60*(3), 531. https://doi.org/10.2307/2298123

Molyneux, M., & Thomson, M. (2011). Cash transfers, gender equity and women's empowerment in Peru, Ecuador and Bolivia. *Gender & Development, 19*(2), 195–212. https://doi.org/10.1080/13552074.2011.592631

Myo-Myo-Mon, & Liabsuetrakul, T. (2009). Factors influencing married youths' decisions on contraceptive use in a rural area of Myanmar. *The Southeast Asian Journal of Tropical Medicine and Public Health, 40*(5), 1057–1064.

Nadella, P., Subramanian, S. V., & Roman-Urrestarazu, A. (2021). The impact of community health workers on antenatal and infant health in India: A cross-sectional study. *SSM - Population Health*, *15*, 100872. https://doi.org/10.1016/j.ssmph .2021.100872

Panda, P., Devgun, S., Gupta, V., Chaudhari, S., & Singh, G. (2013). Role of ASHA in improvement of maternal health status in northern India: An urban rural comparison. *Indian Journal of Community Health*, *25*, 465–471.

Paul, P. L., & Pandey, S. (2020). Factors influencing institutional delivery and the role of accredited social health activist (ASHA): A secondary analysis of India human development survey 2012. *BMC Pregnancy and Childbirth*, *20*(1), 445. https://doi .org/10.1186/s12884-020-03127-z

Rajkhowa, P., & Qaim, M. (2022). Mobile phones, women's physical mobility, and contraceptive use in India. *Social Science and Medicine*, *305*(January), 115074. https://doi.org/10.1016/j.socscimed.2022.115074

Rammohan, A., Goli, S., Saroj, S. K., & Jaleel, C. P. A. (2021). Does engagement with frontline health workers improve maternal and child healthcare utilisation and outcomes in India? *Human Resources for Health*, *19*(1), 1–21. https://doi.org /10.1186/s12960-021-00592-1

Samandari, G., Speizer, I. S., & O'Connell, K. (2010). The role of social support and parity in contraceptive use in Cambodia. *International Perspectives on Sexual and Reproductive Health*, *36*(3), 122–131. https://doi.org/10.1363/ipsrh.36.122.10

Sanneving, L., Trygg, N., Saxena, D., Mavalankar, D., & Thomsen, S. (2013). Inequity in India: The case of maternal and reproductive health. *Global Health Action*, *6*(1), 19145. https://doi.org/10.3402/gha.v6i0.19145

Shah, P. (2016). *MDGs to SDGs: Reproductive, maternal, newborn and child health in India*, *103* (December). https://orfonline.org/wp-content/uploads/2016/12/ORF _Occasional_Paper_103_RMNCH.pdf

Unnikrishnan, B., Rathi, P., Sequeira, R. M., Rao, K. K., Kamath, S., & K, M. A. K. (2020). Awareness and uptake of maternal and child health benefit schemes among the women attending a district hospital in coastal south India. *Journal of Health Management*, *22*(1), 14–24. https://doi.org/10.1177/0972063420908371

US Dept of Health and Human Services. (2000). *Healthy people 2010*. US Department of Health and Human Services: Washington D.C. Available from https://www.cdc. gov/nchs/healthy_people/hp2010/hp2010_final_review.htm.

Walia, M., Irani, L., Chaudhuri, I., Atmavilas, Y., & Saggurti, N. (2020). Effect of sharing health messages on antenatal care behavior among women involved in microfinance-based self-help groups in Bihar India. *Global Health Research and Policy*, *5*(1), 3. https://doi.org/10.1186/s41256-020-0132-0

Webel, A. R., Okonsky, J., Trompeta, J., & Holzemer, W. L. (2010). A systematic review of the effectiveness of peer-based interventions on health-related behaviors in adults. *American Journal of Public Health*, *100*(2), 247–253. https://doi.org/10 .2105/AJPH.2008.149419

Index

For Product Safety Concerns and Information please contact our EU
representative GPSR@taylorandfrancis.com
Taylor & Francis Verlag GmbH, Kaufingerstraße 24, 80331 München, Germany

www.ingramcontent.com/pod-product-compliance
Lightning Source LLC
Chambersburg PA
CBHW060241220326
41598CB00027B/4009

* 9 7 8 1 0 3 2 8 1 3 2 6 4 *